Current Advances in Neonatal Care

Editors

BEENA G. SOOD
DARA D. BRODSKY

PEDIATRIC CLINICS
OF NORTH AMERICA

www.pediatric.theclinics.com

Consulting Editor
BONITA F. STANTON

April 2019 • Volume 66 • Number 2

ELSEVIER

1600 John F. Kennedy Boulevard • Suite 1800 • Philadelphia, Pennsylvania, 19103-2899

http://www.theclinics.com

THE PEDIATRIC CLINICS OF NORTH AMERICA Volume 66, Number 2
April 2019 ISSN 0031-3955, ISBN-13: 978-0-323-67839-1

Editor: Kerry Holland
Developmental Editor: Casey Potter

© **2019 Elsevier Inc. All rights reserved.**

This periodical and the individual contributions contained in it are protected under copyright by Elsevier, and the following terms and conditions apply to their use:

Photocopying
Single photocopies of single articles may be made for personal use as allowed by national copyright laws. Permission of the Publisher and payment of a fee is required for all other photocopying, including multiple or systematic copying, copying for advertising or promotional purposes, resale, and all forms of document delivery. Special rates are available for educational institutions that wish to make photocopies for non-profit educational classroom use. For information on how to seek permission visit www.elsevier.com/permissions or call: (+44) 1865 843830 (UK)/(+1) 215 239 3804 (USA).

Derivative Works
Subscribers may reproduce tables of contents or prepare lists of articles including abstracts for internal circulation within their institutions. Permission of the Publisher is required for resale or distribution outside the institution. Permission of the Publisher is required for all other derivative works, including compilations and translations (please consult www.elsevier.com/permissions).

Electronic Storage or Usage
Permission of the Publisher is required to store or use electronically any material contained in this periodical, including any article or part of an article (please consult www.elsevier.com/permissions). Except as outlined above, no part of this publication may be reproduced, stored in a retrieval system or transmitted in any form or by any means, electronic, mechanical, photocopying, recording or otherwise, without prior written permission of the Publisher.

Notice
No responsibility is assumed by the Publisher for any injury and/or damage to persons or property as a matter of products liability, negligence or otherwise, or from any use or operation of any methods, products, instructions or ideas contained in the material herein. Because of rapid advances in the medical sciences, in particular, independent verification of diagnoses and drug dosages should be made.

Although all advertising material is expected to conform to ethical (medical) standards, inclusion in this publication does not constitute a guarantee or endorsement of the quality or value of such product or of the claims made of it by its manufacturer.

The Pediatric Clinics of North America (ISSN 0031-3955) is published bimonthly by Elsevier Inc., 360 Park Avenue South, New York, NY 10010-1710. Months of issue are February, April, June, August, October, and December. Periodicals postage paid at New York, NY and additional mailing offices. Subscription prices are $229.00 per year (US individuals), $653.00 per year (US institutions), $315.00 per year (Canadian individuals), $868.00 per year (Canadian institutions), $345.00 per year (international individuals), $868.00 per year (international institutions), $100.00 per year (US students and residents), and $165.00 per year (international and Canadian residents and students). To receive students/resident rare, orders must be accompanied by name of affiliated institution, date of term, and the signature of program/residency coordinator on institution letterhead. Orders will be billed at individual rate until proof of status is received. Foreign air speed delivery is included in all *Clinics* subscription prices. All prices are subject to change without notice. **POSTMASTER:** Send address changes to *The Pediatric Clinics of North America*, Elsevier Health Sciences Division, Subscription Customer Service, 3251 Riverport Lane, Maryland Heights, MO 63043. **Customer Service: 1-800-654-2452 (US and Canada). From outside of the US and Canada: 1-314-447-8871. Fax: 1-314-447-8029. For print support, E-mail: JournalsCustomerService-usa@elsevier.com. For online support, E-mail: JournalsOnlineSupport-usa@elsevier.com.**

Reprints. For copies of 100 or more, of articles in this publication, please contact the Commercial Reprints Department, Elsevier Inc., 360 Park Avenue South, New York, NY 10010-1710. Tel.: 212-633-3874; Fax: 212-633-3820; E-mail: reprints@elsevier.com.

The Pediatric Clinics of North America is also published in Spanish by McGraw-Hill Inter-americana Editores S.A., Mexico City, Mexico; in Portuguese by Riechmann and Affonso Editores, Rua Comandante Coelho 1085, CEP 21250, Rio de Janeiro, Brazil; and in Greek by Althayia SA, Athens, Greece.

The Pediatric Clinics of North America is covered in *MEDLINE/PubMed (Index Medicus), Excerpta Medica, Current Contents, Current Contents/Clinical Medicine, Science Citation Index, ASCA, ISI/BIOMED,* and *BIOSIS*.

Printed in the United States of America.

PROGRAM OBJECTIVE
The goal of the *Pediatric Clinics of North America* is to keep practicing physicians and residents up to date with current clinical practice in pediatrics by providing timely articles reviewing the state-of-the-art in patient care.

TARGET AUDIENCE
All practicing pediatricians, physicians and healthcare professionals who provide patient care to pediatric patients.

LEARNING OBJECTIVES
Upon completion of this activity, participants will be able to:
1. Review the post-discharge care of the NICU graduate
2. Discuss the current state of newborn screening, including special considerations and limitations of newborn screening in sick and premature infants
3. Recognize new advances in prenatal genetic testing options

ACCREDITATION
The Elsevier Office of Continuing Medical Education (EOCME) is accredited by the Accreditation Council for Continuing Medical Education (ACCME) to provide continuing medical education for physicians.

The EOCME designates this enduring material for a maximum of 15 *AMA PRA Category 1 Credit*(s)™. Physicians should claim only the credit commensurate with the extent of their participation in the activity.

All other healthcare professionals requesting continuing education credit for this enduring material will be issued a certificate of participation.

DISCLOSURE OF CONFLICTS OF INTEREST
The EOCME assesses conflict of interest with its instructors, faculty, planners, and other individuals who are in a position to control the content of CME activities. All relevant conflicts of interest that are identified are thoroughly vetted by EOCME for fair balance, scientific objectivity, and patient care recommendations. EOCME is committed to providing its learners with CME activities that promote improvements or quality in healthcare and not a specific proprietary business or a commercial interest.

The planning committee, staff, authors and editors listed below have identified no financial relationships or relationships to products or devices they or their spouse/life partner have with commercial interest related to the content of this CME activity:
Heron D. Baumgarten, MD, MPH; Jennifer E. Bentley, AuD; Andrew E. Bluher, MD; Dara D. Brodsky, MD; David H. Darrow, MD, DDS; Sherin U. Devaskar, MD; William A. Engle, MD; Marilyn B. Escobedo, MD; Noelle Andrea V. Fabie, MD; Gerald L. Feldman, MD, PhD; Alan W. Flake, MD; Ricki F. Goldstein, MD; Pamela I. Good, MD; Ish K. Gulati, MD; Nicole Harter, MD; Kerry Holland; Thomas A. Hooven, MD; Katie Huff, MD; Sudarshan R. Jadcherla, MD, FRCP (Irel), DCH, AGAF; Lauren M. Jansson, MD; Angie C. Jelin, MD; Paul B. Kaplowitz, MD, PhD; Alison Kemp; Kalpashri Kesavan, MD; Abhishek Makkar, MD; William F. Malcolm, MD; Elisabeth C. McGowan, MD; Kara B. Pappas, MD; Stephen W. Patrick, MD, MPH, MS; Rajkumar Mayakrishnan; Rebecca S. Rose, MD; Paul J. Rozance, MD; Katelynn G. Sagaser, MS; Birju A. Shah, MD, MPH, MBA; Clara Song, MD; Beena G Sood, MD, MS; Bonita F. Stanton, MD; Jane E. Stewart, MD; Edgardo Szyld, MD, MSc; Betty R. Vohr, MD; Louise Wilkins-Haug, MD, PhD; Joseph I. Wolfsdorf, MD, BCh.

The planning committee, staff, authors and editors listed below have identified financial relationships or relationships to products or devices they or their spouse/life partner have with commercial interest related to the content of this CME activity:
Anthony J. Mancini, MD: is a consultant/advisor for Pierre Fabre Pharmaceuticals Inc.

UNAPPROVED/OFF-LABEL USE DISCLOSURE
The EOCME requires CME faculty to disclose to the participants:
1. When products or procedures being discussed are off-label, unlabelled, experimental, and/or investigational (not US Food and Drug Administration [FDA] approved); and
2. Any limitations on the information presented, such as data that are preliminary or that represent ongoing research, interim analyses, and/or unsupported opinions. Faculty may discuss information about pharmaceutical agents that is outside of FDA-approved labelling. This information is intended solely for CME

and is not intended to promote off-label use of these medications. If you have any questions, contact the medical affairs department of the manufacturer for the most recent prescribing information.

TO ENROLL

To enroll in the *Pediatric Clinics of North America* Continuing Medical Education program, call customer service at 1-800-654-2452 or sign up online at http://www.theclinics.com/home/cme. The CME program is available to subscribers for an additional annual fee of USD 301.60.

METHOD OF PARTICIPATION

In order to claim credit, participants must complete the following:
1. Complete enrolment as indicated above.
2. Read the activity.
3. Complete the CME Test and Evaluation. Participants must achieve a score of 70% on the test. All CME Tests and Evaluations must be completed online.

CME INQUIRIES/SPECIAL NEEDS

For all CME inquiries or special needs, please contact elsevierCME@elsevier.com

Contributors

CONSULTING EDITOR

BONITA F. STANTON, MD
Founding Dean, Hackensack Meridian School of Medicine at Seton Hall University,
President, Academic Enterprise, Hackensack Meridian Health Robert C. and Laura C.
Garrett Endowed Chair for the School of Medicine, Dean Professor of Pediatrics, Nutley,
New Jersey

EDITORS

BEENA G. SOOD, MD, MS
Professor, Department of Pediatrics, Division of Neonatal Perinatal Medicine,
Wayne State University, Associate Neonatologist, Children's Hospital of Michigan
and Hutzel Women's Hospital, Detroit Medical Center, Detroit, Michigan

DARA D. BRODSKY, MD
Associate Professor of Pediatrics, Harvard Medical School, Director of Education,
Department of Neonatology, Beth Israel Deaconess Medical Center, Editor-in-Chief,
NeoReviews, Boston, Massachusetts

AUTHORS

HERON D. BAUMGARTEN, MD, MPH
Department of Surgery, Center for Fetal Diagnosis and Treatment, Children's
Hospital of Philadelphia, University of Pennsylvania School of Medicine, Philadelphia,
Pennsylvania

JENNIFER E. BENTLEY, AuD
Department of Neonatology, Beth Israel Deaconess Medical Center, Boston,
Massachusetts

ANDREW E. BLUHER, MD
Chief Resident, Department of Otolaryngology–Head and Neck Surgery, Eastern Virginia
Medical School, Norfolk, Virginia

DAVID H. DARROW, MD, DDS
Professor, Department of Otolaryngology–Head and Neck Surgery, Eastern Virginia
Medical School, Attending Otolaryngologist, Children's Hospital of The King's Daughters,
Norfolk, Virginia

SHERIN U. DEVASKAR, MD
Distinguished Professor of Pediatrics, Mattel Executive Endowed Chair, Department of
Pediatrics, David Geffen School of Medicine at UCLA, UCLA Mattel Children's Hospital,
Los Angeles, California

WILLIAM A. ENGLE, MD
Erik T. Ragan Emeritus Professor of Pediatrics, Department of Neonatology, Indiana University School of Medicine, Indianapolis, Indiana

MARILYN B. ESCOBEDO, MD
Professor Emeritus, Reba McEntire Chair, Neonatal-Perinatal Medicine, Department of Pediatrics, Children's Hospital, University of Oklahoma Health Sciences Center, Oklahoma City, Oklahoma

NOELLE ANDREA V. FABIE, MD
Division of Genetics, Genomics and Metabolic Disorders, Children's Hospital of Michigan, Detroit, Michigan; Department of Medical Genetics and Genomics, Children's Hospitals and Clinics of Minnesota, Minneapolis, Minnesota

GERALD L. FELDMAN, MD, PhD
Division of Genetics, Genomics and Metabolic Disorders, Children's Hospital of Michigan, Professor, Department of Pediatrics, Pathology and Center for Molecular Medicine and Genetics, Wayne State University School of Medicine, Detroit, Michigan

ALAN W. FLAKE, MD
Department of Surgery, Center for Fetal Diagnosis and Treatment, Children's Hospital of Philadelphia, University of Pennsylvania School of Medicine, Philadelphia, Pennsylvania

RICKI F. GOLDSTEIN, MD
Professor of Pediatrics, Director, Pediatric Complex Care Program for Infants and Children, Director, NICU Graduate Clinic, Department of Pediatrics/Neonatology, Kentucky Children's Hospital/University of Kentucky, Lexington, Kentucky

PAMELA I. GOOD, MD
Neonatal-Perinatal Medicine Fellow, Department of Pediatrics, Vagelos College of Physicians and Surgeons, Columbia University, New York, New York

ISH K. GULATI, MD
Assistant Professor of Pediatrics, Innovative Research Program in Neonatal Feeding Disorders, The Neonatal and Infant Feeding Disorders Program, Nationwide Children's Hospital, Columbus, Ohio

NICOLE HARTER, MD
Pediatric Dermatology Fellow, Division of Dermatology, Ann & Robert H. Lurie Children's Hospital of Chicago, Northwestern University Feinberg School of Medicine, Chicago, Illinois

THOMAS A. HOOVEN, MD
Assistant Professor, Department of Pediatrics, Vagelos College of Physicians and Surgeons, Columbia University, New York, New York

KATIE HUFF, MD
Fellow, Department of Neonatology, Indiana University School of Medicine, Indianapolis, Indiana

SUDARSHAN R. JADCHERLA, MD, FRCP (Irel), DCH, AGAF
Professor of Pediatrics, Associate Division Chief of Neonatology, Academics, Innovative Research Program in Neonatal Feeding Disorders, The Neonatal and Infant Feeding Disorders Program, Nationwide Children's Hospital, Divisions of Neonatology and Pediatric Gastroenterology and Nutrition, Department of Pediatrics, Principal Investigator, Center for Perinatal Research, The Research Institute at Nationwide Children's Hospital, The Ohio State University College of Medicine, Columbus, Ohio

LAUREN M. JANSSON, MD
Johns Hopkins School of Medicine, Baltimore, Maryland

ANGIE C. JELIN, MD
Assistant Professor, Division of Maternal Fetal Medicine, Department of Gynecology and Obstetrics, The Johns Hopkins Hospital, Baltimore, Maryland

PAUL B. KAPLOWITZ, MD, PhD
Division of Endocrinology, Children's National Health System, Professor Emeritus of Pediatrics, George Washington School of Medicine & Health Sciences, Washington, DC

KALPASHRI KESAVAN, MD
Assistant Professor, Division of Neonatology and Developmental Biology, Department of Pediatrics, David Geffen School of Medicine at UCLA, UCLA Mattel Children's Hospital, Los Angeles, California

ABHISHEK MAKKAR, MD
Assistant Professor, Medical Director of CCMH NICU, Neonatal-Perinatal Medicine, Department of Pediatrics, Children's Hospital, University of Oklahoma Health Sciences Center, Oklahoma City, Oklahoma

WILLIAM F. MALCOLM, MD
Professor of Pediatrics, Director, Special Infant Care Follow-up Program, Department of Pediatrics/Neonatology, Duke University Medical Center, Durham, North Carolina

ANTHONY J. MANCINI, MD
Head, Division of Dermatology, Ann & Robert H. Lurie Children's Hospital of Chicago, Professor of Pediatrics and Dermatology, Northwestern University Feinberg School of Medicine, Chicago, Illinois

ELISABETH C. McGOWAN, MD
Assistant Professor, Department of Pediatrics, The Warren Alpert Medical School of Brown University, Staff Neonatologist, Women & Infants Hospital, Providence, Rhode Island

KARA B. PAPPAS, MD
Division of Genetics, Genomics and Metabolic Disorders, Children's Hospital of Michigan, Assistant Professor, Department of Pediatrics, Wayne State University School of Medicine, Detroit, Michigan

STEPHEN W. PATRICK, MD, MPH, MS
Vanderbilt University School of Medicine, Nashville, Tennessee

REBECCA S. ROSE, MD
Assistant Professor of Clinical Pediatrics, Department of Neonatology, Indiana University School of Medicine, Indianapolis, Indiana

PAUL J. ROZANCE, MD
Frederick C. Battaglia Chair, Perinatal Research Center, Professor, Department of Pediatrics, Colorado Children's Hospital, University of Colorado School of Medicine, Aurora, Colorado

KATELYNN G. SAGASER, MS
Certified Genetic Counselor, Division of Maternal Fetal Medicine, Department of Gynecology and Obstetrics, The Johns Hopkins Hospital, Baltimore, Maryland

BIRJU A. SHAH, MD, MPH, MBA
Assistant Professor, Co-Director of Newborn Resuscitation, Neonatal-Perinatal Medicine, Department of Pediatrics, Children's Hospital, University of Oklahoma Health Sciences Center, Oklahoma City, Oklahoma

CLARA SONG, MD
Assistant Professor, Director of Education, Neonatal-Perinatal Medicine, Department of Pediatrics, Children's Hospital, University of Oklahoma Health Sciences Center, Oklahoma City, Oklahoma

JANE E. STEWART, MD
Department of Neonatology, Beth Israel Deaconess Medical Center, Harvard Medical University, Boston Children's Hospital, Boston, Massachusetts

EDGARDO SZYLD, MD, MSc
Professor of Research, Research Director, Neonatal-Perinatal Medicine, Department of Pediatrics, Children's Hospital, University of Oklahoma Health Sciences Center, Oklahoma City, Oklahoma

BETTY R. VOHR, MD
Professor, Department of Pediatrics, The Warren Alpert Medical School of Brown University, Director, Neonatal Follow-up Clinic, Women & Infants Hospital, Providence, Rhode Island

LOUISE WILKINS-HAUG, MD, PhD
Professor, Division of Maternal Fetal Medicine and Reproductive Genetics, Department of Obstetrics and Gynecology, Brigham and Women's Hospital, Boston, Massachusetts

JOSEPH I. WOLFSDORF, MB, BCh
Boston Children's Hospital Chair, Division of Endocrinology, Boston Children's Hospital, Professor of Pediatrics, Harvard Medical School, Boston, Massachusetts

Contents

> All patients should be offered prenatal screening and diagnosis. Testing options depend on many factors, including patient age, family history, and patient preference. Options are rapidly changing with emerging technology. Aneuploidy screening options include ultrasound, maternal analytes, and cell-free DNA. Prenatal chromosomal microarray is the recommended diagnostic test for patients with anomalies visualized on prenatal ultrasound. Prenatal whole exome sequencing is clinically available but is limited by challenges with counseling, interpretation, and turn-around time. Future technologies are emerging and may soon allow for translation of prenatal diagnosis to in utero therapy.

> Fetal surgery is an established but still rapidly evolving specialty, born from the rationale that destructive embryologic processes, recognized early in gestation, can be curtailed by prenatal correction. As more and more centers begin offering fetal interventions, quality of care must be verified through transparency about clinical capabilities and resources. Level designations should be assigned based on capability, as in trauma and neonatal ICU centers for excellence, and volume requirements must be set for fetal surgery certification. Regionalization of this specialty care may be required to optimize outcomes.

> The Neonatal Resuscitation Program, initially an expertise- and consensus-based approach, has evolved into an evidence-based algorithm. Ventilation remains the key component of successful resuscitation of neonates. Recent changes in recommendations include management of cord clamping, multiple methods to prevent hypothermia, rescinding of mandatory intubation and suction of the nonvigorous meconium-stained infant, electrocardiographic monitoring, and establishing an airway for ventilation before initiation of chest compressions. Emerging science,

including issues such as cord milking, oxygen targeting, and laryngeal mask use, may lead to future program modifications. Technology such as video laryngoscopy and telemedicine will affect the way training and care is delivered.

Early-onset sepsis (EOS) is an important cause of neonatal morbidity. Despite extensive study, identifying at-risk newborns remains challenging, especially if they are initially well appearing. Existing official EOS recommendations suggest a conservative approach that likely results in over-treatment of a low-risk population. Recent studies indicate that more precise risk assessment and alternative management strategies could decrease the number of infants exposed to blood draws and antibiotics during evaluations for EOS. This article reviews existing guidelines and provides an overview of the Bayesian sepsis calculator and serial observation as an alternative to laboratory studies and empirical antibiotics.

This article covers several aspects of the clinical management of neonatal hypoglycemia that have recently evolved, reviewing the evidence informing these recommended changes in practice. Topics covered include use of buccal dextrose gel, rationale for avoiding the traditional "mini dextrose bolus," and benefits of direct breastfeeding for the treatment of asymptomatic hypoglycemia in at-risk newborns. The reasons for increasing use of more accurate point-of-care devices for measuring neonatal glucose concentrations are discussed, as well as the implications of different published opinions regarding the determination of readiness for discharge and the most important considerations when making this determination.

Thyroid dysfunction that requires prompt diagnosis and treatment often becomes evident in the newborn period because of testing that is done as part of universal newborn screening. Primary congenital hypothyroidism is the most common treatable cause of mental retardation, requiring immediate treatment to prevent abnormal brain development. However, many of the abnormal thyroid test results are less abnormal and difficult to interpret, with a need for repeat testing and careful follow-up before initiation of treatment. Less often, neonatal hyperthyroidism is encountered. This article reviews and discusses management of thyroid dysfunction that may present in the first month after birth.

This review examines the continuum of care of opioid-exposed infants, including the assessment of the neonate, diagnosis of neonatal abstinence syndrome, management of the syndrome including nonpharmacologic and pharmacologic care, approach to breastfeeding, pediatric follow-up care, and integration of care of the mother-infant dyad.

Noelle Andrea V. Fabie, Kara B. Pappas, and Gerald L. Feldman

Newborn screening has evolved since its introduction in 1963. The disorders that are being screened for continue to evolve as new treatments and new technologies advance. In this review, the authors discuss the current state of newborn screening in the United States, including the disorders currently being screened for and how newborn screening is performed. They also discuss the special considerations and limitations of newborn screening in sick and premature infants and as well as some ethical issues related to newborn screening. Finally, new disorders being considered for testing and new technologies that may be used in the future of newborn screening are discussed.

Katie Huff, Rebecca S. Rose, and William A. Engle

Infants born between 34 weeks 0 days and 36 weeks 6 days of gestation are termed late preterm. This group accounts for the majority of premature births in the United States, with rates increasing in each of the last 3 years. This increase is significant given their large number: nearly 280,000 in 2016 alone. Late preterm infants place a significant burden on the health care and education systems because of their increased risk of morbidities and mortality compared with more mature infants. This increased risk persists past the newborn period, leading to the need for continued health monitoring throughout life.

Kalpashri Kesavan and Sherin U. Devaskar

Intrauterine growth restriction (IUGR) is an important cause of fetal, perinatal and neonatal morbidity and mortality. IUGR occurs because of multiple reasons. Neonates with IUGR experience acute problems in the perinatal and early neonatal period that can be life-threatening. The unfavorable uterine environment causing growth restriction results in programming that predisposes IUGR infants to long-term health issues such as poor physical growth, metabolic syndrome, cardiovascular disease, neurodevelopmental impairment and endocrine abnormalities, warranting careful monitoring. It is imperative to strike the balance between achieving optimal catch-up to promote normal development, while preventing the onset of cardiovascular and metabolic disorders in the long-term.

Jane E. Stewart and Jennifer E. Bentley

Screening infants for hearing loss at birth is a standard in most states in the United States, but follow-up continues to warrant improvement. Understanding the definition of hearing loss, its etiology, appropriate intervention options, and knowledge of methods to optimize an infant's outcomes through the medical home can help to maximize speech and language skills.

Infantile hemangiomas (IH) are a common benign tumor of infancy, most being uncomplicated and not requiring therapy. Some IH may, however, require treatment. The pediatric provider must be familiar with morphology, distribution, natural history, and associations of IH to determine when intervention is needed. Several treatment options are available for IH with the current standard of care being oral propranolol. Other therapies include wound care; topical beta-blocker therapy for small, superficial, and uncomplicated IH; and laser or surgical treatment of IH residua. In addition to functional compromise and other complications, the potential for permanent deformity and eventual psychosocial stigmatization are important when considering the need for treatment of IH in a neonate or young infant.

Gastroesophageal reflux (GER) and GER disease (GERD) pertaining to infants in the neonatal intensive care unit (NICU) are reviewed, based on research in this specific population. The developmental biology of the gastroesophageal junction, physiology of GER, and pathophysiology of GERD in this setting are summarized, and risk factors for GER and GERD identified. The epidemiology, economic burden, and controversies surrounding GERD in NICU infants are addressed, and an approach to GER and GERD in these patients formulated. Recent advancements in individual assessment of GER and GERD in the NICU infant are examined, and evidence-based guidelines for their adoption provided.

Stridor in the newborn period may result from numerous causes, both congenital and acquired. Its presentation is diverse, and understanding the subtleties of that diversity is the key to determining the likely cause of the stridor, as well as the urgency for specialist evaluation. This article presents a framework for evaluating the quality of stridor in the newborn, as well as a review of the characteristics of stridor associated with entities commonly encountered in the neonatal airway.

Premature and critically ill term infants are often discharged from the neonatal intensive care unit (NICU) with ongoing medical problems, including respiratory problems; growth, nutrition and feeding problems;

and neurologic injury. At discharge, they may also be dependent on technology such as supplemental oxygen, tracheostomy, mechanical ventilation, feeding tube, and monitors. Primary care physicians must have special knowledge and understanding of the medical complications of NICU graduates to coordinate post-discharge care. We examine the most common post-discharge medical problems in premature and critically ill term infants and inform the primary care provider about expected outcomes and possible new problems.

Neurodevelopmental Follow-up of Preterm Infants: What Is New?   509

Elisabeth C. McGowan and Betty R. Vohr

There is increasing evidence of ongoing changes occurring in short-term and long-term motor and language outcomes in former premature infants. As rates of moderate to severe cerebral palsy (CP) have decreased, there has been increased awareness of the impact of mild CP and of developmental coordination disorder on the preterm population. Language delays and disorders continue to be among the most common outcomes. In conjunction with medical morbidities, there is increased awareness of the negative impact of family psycho-socioeconomic adversities on preterm outcomes and of the importance of intervention for these adversities beginning in the neonatal ICU.

PEDIATRIC CLINICS OF NORTH AMERICA

SERIES OF RELATED INTEREST

Clinics in Perinatology
https://www.perinatology.theclinics.com/

THE CLINICS ARE AVAILABLE ONLINE!
Access your subscription at:
www.theclinics.com

Foreword

A Deep Dive into What Is New and Needed in the Care of Preterm Newborn Care

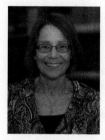

Bonita F. Stanton, MD
Consulting Editor

Universally, in most instances, the long-awaited arrival of a newborn is cause for joy and celebration. But not every birth goes as planned.

Huge advances have been made in the fields of obstetrics and neonatology over the last fifty years, but much remains to be done. Globally, an estimated 15 million babies are born prematurely annually, among whom approximately 1 million succumb to complications of premature birth. The neonatal period: the first month of life, holds the greatest risk of life (globally in 2017, an average rate of 18 deaths per 1000 live births). Overall, in the first month of life in 2017, an estimated 2.5 million children died, the majority of whom died in the first week.[1]

Morbidity and mortality related to the neonatal and infant period remains a significant problem in the United States. From 1970 to 2000, the rate of perinatal (defined as late fetal and the first week after birth) deaths had steadily decreased, although in the last decade of the twentieth century, the decrease was slight.[2] In the first decade of the new millennium, although perinatal deaths continued to show modest declines, the rate of infant and fetal mortality showed little decrease.[3,4] From 2014 to 2016, perinatal mortality was essentially flat (6.00 perinatal deaths per 1000 births and late fetal deaths).[5]

Closely correlated with perinatal mortality is the rate of premature births. While the opening years of the twenty-first century had witnessed close to a decade-long decline of this rate (from 2007 to 2015), most recently, for the third year in a row, the rate has shown a slight increase (9.85% in 2016 to 9.93% in 2017), according to the Centers for Disease Control and Prevention.[6]

In the sixteen articles constituting the current issue of *Pediatric Clinics of North America*, Beena Sood, Dara D. Brodsky, and their colleagues from across the nation

Pediatr Clin N Am 66 (2019) xv–xvi
https://doi.org/10.1016/j.pcl.2019.01.002
0031-3955/19/© 2019 Published by Elsevier Inc.

pediatric.theclinics.com

summarize many of the substantial advances that have been made over the last decade and discuss some of the remaining challenges confronting pediatricians, obstetricians, and other caregivers concerned with the perinatal period as they seek to further improve the health of this most vulnerable group of patients.

Bonita F. Stanton, MD
Hackensack Meridian School of Medicine at Seton Hall University
340 Kingsland Street, Building 123
Nutley, NJ 07110, USA

E-mail address:
bonita.stanton@shu.edu

REFERENCES

1. United Nations Children's Fund. Neonatal mortality. 2018. Available at: https://data.unicef.org/topic/child-survival/neonatal-mortality/. Accessed January 16, 2019.
2. Govande V, Ballard AR, Koneru M, et al. Trends in the neonatal mortality rate in the last decade with respect to demographic factors and health care resources. Proc (Bayl Univ Med Cent) 2015;28(3):304–6.
3. MacDorman MF. Race and ethnic disparities in fetal mortality, preterm birth, and infant mortality in the United States: an overview. Semin Perinatol 2011;35:200–8.
4. Gregory ECW, MacDorman MF, Martin JA. Trends in fetal and perinatal mortality in the United States, 2006-2012, #169. Center for Disease Control and Prevention, NCHS Data Brief; 2014.
5. Gregory ECW, Drake P, Martin JA. Lack of change in perinatal mortality in the United States, 2014-2016, #316. Center for Disease Control and Prevention, NCHS Data Brief; 2018.
6. Centers for disease control and prevention. Premature birth rates rise again, but a few states are turining things around. Available at: https://www.npr.org/sections/health-shots/2018/11/01/662683176/premature-birth-rates-rise-again-but-a-few-states-are-turning-things-around. Accessed January 16, 2019.

Preface
Current Advances in Neonatal Care

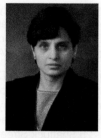 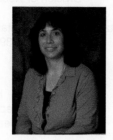

Beena G. Sood, MD, MS   Dara D. Brodsky, MD
Editors

The field of neonatology is constantly evolving. With the advent of new prenatal diagnostic options and fetal interventions, some newborns receive significant medical care even before delivery. After birth, advances in neonatal intensive care have led to improved survival in preterm infants born at progressively younger gestational ages. Advances in technology, surgical techniques, and therapeutics have dramatically changed the management, timing of treatment, and outcomes of common neonatal diseases. Frequently, former preterm infants require ongoing care long after hospital discharge. It is imperative that pediatric caregivers be aware of the changing spectrum of management of these infants during their initial hospital admission and become familiar with the ongoing care of complex medical problems after hospital discharge.

In this issue entitled, "Current Advances in Neonatal Care," we have recruited experts to summarize exciting new advances in prenatal genetic testing options, fetal surgery, neonatal resuscitation, and newborn screening that are relevant to the neonatal and pediatric care provider. We have also addressed recent progress in the understanding of pathogenesis and management of long-standing medical issues, such as intrauterine growth restriction, sepsis, gastroesophageal reflux disease, hypothyroidism, hypoglycemia, hemangiomas, and stridor, during initial hospital admission and following discharge. A review of the management of the mother-infant dyad following maternal substance abuse is opportune at a time when the opioid epidemic has taken center stage in health care. The reviews on the post-discharge care of the neonatal intensive care unit graduate and long-term neurodevelopmental outcomes address the complex needs of extremely preterm infants that are increasingly being observed in pediatric practice. We hope that readers will find that this issue enhances their knowledge and equips them with the skills to deliver evidence-based care to their patients.

We would like to thank the experts who, despite professional deadlines and personal commitments, have made the time to share their expertise. We would also like to thank

Pediatr Clin N Am 66 (2019) xvii–xviii
https://doi.org/10.1016/j.pcl.2019.01.001
0031-3955/19/© 2019 Published by Elsevier Inc.

Elsevier Inc for publishing this issue and would like to recognize Casey Potter for all of her editorial assistance. We dedicate this issue to our newborn patients and their families, who make us strive to improve our knowledge and expertise so that we can provide the best possible care.

Beena G. Sood, MD, MS
Department of Pediatrics
Division of Neonatal Perinatal Medicine
Wayne State University
Children's Hospital of Michigan & Hutzel Women's Hospital Detroit Medical Center
3901 Beaubien Boulevard
Detroit, MI 48201, USA

Dara D. Brodsky, MD
Harvard Medical School
Department of Neonatology
Beth Israel Deaconess Medical Center
25 Shattuck Street
Boston, MA 02115, USA

E-mail addresses:
bsood@med.wayne.edu (B.G. Sood)
dbrodsky@bidmc.harvard.edu (D.D. Brodsky)

Prenatal Genetic Testing Options

Angie C. Jelin, MD[a], Katelynn G. Sagaser, MS[a],
Louise Wilkins-Haug, MD, PhD[b],*

KEYWORDS

- Prenatal genetic testing • Cell-free DNA screening • Noninvasive prenatal testing
- Prenatal diagnosis

KEY POINTS

- Prenatal genetic testing options are evolving rapidly with emerging technology, including next generation sequencing and cell-free DNA.
- The number of diagnostic procedures has decreased in response to newer noninvasive screening options.
- Chromosomal microarray is recommended in the setting of fetal anomalies and can provide additional information over standard karyotype for all patients undergoing prenatal diagnosis.
- Whole exome sequencing is available for select prenatal cases but requires significant pre- and posttest counseling.

INTRODUCTION

The landscape of prenatal genetic testing and screening options has rapidly evolved in the past decade and shows no signs of slowing in the near future. Historically, the earliest available prenatal screening test was an elevated maternal serum alpha-fetoprotein (MS-AFP) level for detection of neural tube defects. Enhanced understanding of maternal serum biomarkers gradually paved the way for biochemical screening for common live-born aneuploidies, and such screening is now routinely available to all pregnant women, regardless of risk factors. Furthermore, completion of the Human Genome Project provided for rapid application of DNA sequencing technology to interpret circulating cell-free fetoplacental DNA (cfDNA) in the maternal circulation.

Funding sources: None.
Conflicts of Interest: None declared.
[a] Division of Maternal Fetal Medicine, Department of Gynecology and Obstetrics, Johns Hopkins Hospital, 600 N. Wolfe Street, Phipps 222, Baltimore, MD 21287, USA; [b] Division of Maternal Fetal Medicine and Reproductive Genetics, Department of Obstetrics and Gynecology, Brigham and Women's Hospital, 75 Francis Street, Boston, MA 02115, USA
* Corresponding author.
E-mail address: lwilkinshaug@bwh.harvard.edu

With the present-day ability to interpret the sequencing data of prenatal DNA specimens obtained from invasive diagnostic techniques, obstetricians, geneticists, genetic counselors, pediatric care providers, and patients alike look to the future with wonder and cautious awe as these technologies quickly become applied to noninvasively obtained samples.

Screening for Down syndrome, with a live birth incidence of approximately 1 in 700,[1] is readily available to women of all ages through a variety of methods.[2] Although Down syndrome is arguably the most well-known chromosomal trisomy to the general public, the option of screening for other rarer but viable forms of aneuploidy such as trisomy 18 (Edwards syndrome) and trisomy 13 (Patau syndrome) may also be desirable to many women, given the life-limiting nature of these conditions. The goal of prenatal screening is to identify as many pregnancies as possible at high risk for abnormal outcomes while simultaneously providing reassurance to women carrying typical pregnancies. Ideally, genetic screening achieves this high- and low-risk stratification as early as possible during pregnancy. Timely detection of genetic disease and/or fetal anomalies can allow for a potential pregnancy intervention (such as fetal surgery or pregnancy termination) as well as important pregnancy management considerations (including emotional, financial, and practical preparation of the parents, as well as delivery planning at tertiary care centers).

This review highlights the diverse offerings of prenatal genetic screening and testing options available now nearly a decade after the MELISSA study, which evaluated the sensitivity and specificity of cfDNA screening for trisomy 21[3]. For the purpose of this review, prenatal screening options refer to evaluations that provide assessment of fetal risk, whereas testing options refer to evaluations that provide diagnostic confirmation of fetal genetic status. Given the level of detail involved in determining a path through the maze of prenatal genetic screening and testing options, the authors recommend that obstetric providers refer their high-risk patients to prenatal genetic counseling services.

TIMELINE OF PRENATAL GENETIC SCREENING AND TESTING

An important factor in the decision of which prenatal genetic screen/test to choose is the matter of timing during pregnancy. Although early detection of fetal abnormalities is advantageous, confirmation of such at early gestational ages may be impeded by issues such as placental mosaicism in chorionic villus samples (CVS) and limited fetal views on sonographic imaging, among others. As demonstrated in **Fig. 1**, cfDNA screening is the earliest available aneuploidy risk assessment method and is clinically available at 9 weeks' gestational age (GA). Traditional aneuploidy screening methods, such as first trimester combined screening (FTS) and quad screening, are available from approximately 11 to 13 6/7 weeks' GA and 15 to 22 6/7 weeks' GA, respectively. The anatomy sonogram, which occurs between 18 and 22 weeks' GA, is the common focus of fetal sonographic imaging, because it provides detailed anatomic evaluation for congenital anomalies. Additional imaging recommendations may include the nuchal translucency (NT) sonogram (between ~11 and 13 6/7 weeks' GA, which is determined by crown rump length measurements between 45 mm–84 mm) as part of aneuploidy risk assessment and the fetal echocardiogram (between ~22–24 weeks' GA) for pregnancies at increased risk for congenital cardiac defects. In some centers, a fetal anatomy scan is attempted at 12 to 14 weeks' GA.

Prenatal confirmation of abnormal screening results is primarily achieved through either CVS beginning at 10 weeks' GA or amniocentesis after approximately 15 weeks'

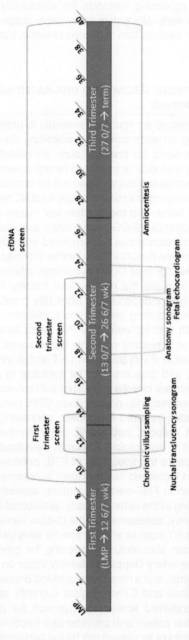

Fig. 1. Timeline of prenatal genetic screening and testing options.

GA, once amnion and chorion membrane fusion has occurred. Each of these procedures carries a less than 1% risk for pregnancy loss.

All pregnant women, regardless of gestational age and risk factors, should be offered the option to pursue prenatal genetic testing or screening.[2] The advent of serum- and DNA-based screening methods for aneuploidy risk assessment has provided women with an early alternative to invasive diagnostic testing, although such screening is limited in its detection of genetic disease, both in terms of sensitivity and specificity.

PRENATAL SCREENING OPTIONS: SERUM- AND DNA-BASED METHODS
Serum-Based Screening Methods

Serum-based screening options are routinely available to pregnant women across all risk categories. Depending on state screening practices, demographic factors, and GA at which a patient presents for prenatal care, an obstetric practice may offer one-step serum screening methods or multistep serum screening methods.

The FTS provides a personalized risk assessment for fetal Down syndrome and trisomy 18/trisomy 13 by combining the patient's age, fetal NT measurement, presence/absence of the fetal nasal bone, and the biochemical results of maternal serum free β-human chorionic gonadotropin (hCG), pregnancy-associated plasma protein A (PAPP-A), and AFP.[4] This screening can be performed in singleton and twin pregnancies only. Elevated levels of free β-hCG in conjunction with decreased levels of PAPP-A and AFP increase the risk for fetal Down syndrome, whereas decreased levels of free-β-hCG and PAPP-A increase the risk for fetal trisomy 18/trisomy 13. PAPP-A levels can also be examined independently from this combined screen, because poor pregnancy outcomes (including preeclampsia, stillbirth, and growth restriction) have been associated with first trimester PAPP-A levels less than or equal to fifth percentile.[5] This method of screening can only be achieved in centers certified by the Fetal Medicine Foundation (FMF) to perform NT scans, or those with internal review of their NT variation, and thus may not be available to patients in rural areas. Increased NT measurements are directly correlated with increased risks for fetal aneuploidy, and NT scan measurements greater than 99th percentile for crown-rump length should be immediately referred for genetic counseling to discuss additional risks for congenital heart defects, pathogenic copy number variants, and single gene disorders, in addition to aneuploidy. Accurate classification of fetal nasal bone presence/absence is critical to the specificity of FTS, because an absent fetal nasal bone is associated with an increased risk for Down syndrome, particularly in Caucasian populations. Yet, even in FMF-certified centers, assessment of the fetal nasal bone has proved challenging in the setting of early gestational ages and high maternal body mass indexes. Recently, assessment of the ductus venosus (a-wave or pulsatility index) was added to the NT scan as another tool for early detection of fetal congenital heart defects.[6] FTS can also include screening for preeclampsia through the incorporation of the uterine artery Doppler pulsatility index on the NT scan, maternal serum placental growth factor, and a mean arterial blood pressure, although the American College of Obstetricians and Gynecologists currently recommends a detailed medical history as the preferred screening approach for preeclampsia.[7] Results from FTS are provided to the patient and provider as a fractional risk that is also categorized as within normal limits or increased risk by the performing laboratory's cut-offs per condition screened. Results from this screening are generally available within several days of obtaining all elements of the screen and can therefore be used to determine the necessity of further screening or testing in a timely manner.

Second trimester serum screening options of the *quad screen* or *penta screen* are reasonable alternatives to the FTS for patients who do not present to prenatal care in time for first trimester aneuploidy risk assessment. The quad screen is composed of maternal serum AFP, unconjugated estriol (uE3), dimeric inhibin A (DIA), and hCG, whereas the penta screen uses these same analytes as well as hyperglycosylated hCG. The quad/penta screen provides risk information for fetal Down syndrome (associated with decreased AFP and uE3 levels and increased hCG and DIA levels), fetal trisomy 18 (associated with decreased levels of AFP, hCG, and uE3), and open neural tube defects (ONTDs, associated with an increased level of AFP). Detection rates for Down syndrome and trisomy 18 are decreased compared with FTS for singleton pregnancies (**Table 1**) and are thought to be quite significantly decreased for twin pregnancies. As both the quad and penta screens involve only a single blood draw, with no ultrasound information aside from accurate pregnancy dating, these screens are extremely useful in patient populations with limited access to prenatal care.

Some obstetricians may offer the option of standalone maternal serum AFP (MS-AFP) screening to patients with normal FTS results. In such cases, the full information provided by quad/penta screening would be redundant, but early detection of ONTDs through the identification of increased AFP levels may lead to earlier confirmatory imaging studies and, thus, fetal interventions. Yet, the sonographic imaging provided at the fetal anatomy scan has extremely high detection rates for ONTDs, and for this reason standalone MS-AFP may not be necessary.[2]

Multistep serum screening methods vary widely by provider preference, US state screening practices, and access to obstetric resources.[8] On the whole, these multistep screening methods use various combinations of the serum analyte and imaging metrics detailed earlier to provide aneuploidy risk assessment information throughout the first and second trimester of pregnancy, depending on results. The *integrated screen* combines the first trimester NT measurement and PAPP-A with the second trimester AFP, uE3, DIA, and hCG to provide increased detection rates and decreased false-positive rates for Down syndrome, although results are not provided to the patient until the completion of the screen in the second trimester. Patients who do not have access to an NT-certified sonographer can pursue the

Table 1
Detection rates for common aneuploidies provided by prenatal screening in singleton gestations

	Down Syndrome DR	Trisomy 18 DR	Trisomy 13 DR	SCA DR
Combined first trimester screen (NT, NB, and biochemistry)	96%–97% with fetal NB assessment	91%–96%	91%–96% (quoted by select laboratories)	N/A
Integrated screen (1st and 2nd trimester visits)	94%–96%	91%–96%	N/A	N/A
Serum integrated screen (1st and 2nd trimester visits)	87%–88%	82%	N/A	N/A
Stepwise sequential screen	91%–95%	91%–96%	N/A	N/A
Contingency screen	91%–92%	91%–96%	N/A	N/A
Quad screen/penta screen	75%–83%	60%–70%	N/A	N/A
Cell-free DNA screening	>99%	98%	99%	96%–100%

Abbreviations: DR, detection rate; NB, nasal bone; SCA, sex chromosome aneuploidy.
Data from Refs.[8,10,41,42–48]

serum integrated screen, with slightly lower detection rates, through obtaining the same information as the integrated screen save for the NT measurement. In contrast, the *sequential screen* uses first trimester PAPP-A, hCG, and NT measurement (if available), together with second trimester AFP, uE3, DIA, and hCG to determine Down syndrome and trisomy 18 risks. Patients determined to be at high risk for aneuploidy following the first trimester component of the screen are informed of their increased risk at that time, and the patient is referred for advanced screening/testing options in lieu of the second trimester portion of the sequential screen. Finally, the *contingency screen* is another option that may span both the first and second trimester, depending on patient risk. The first trimester evaluation of PAPP-A, hCG, and NT measurement categorizes patients into low-, moderate-, and high-risk groups. Patients in the high- and low-risk groups do not proceed to the second trimester analyte screening (AFP, uE3, DIA, and hCG), because the high-risk patients are referred for genetic counseling and diagnostic testing, whereas the low-risk groups are thought to have completed the screening sufficiently. Moderate-risk patients will receive the final results of their aneuploidy screening once the second trimester portion of the screen is complete.

DNA-Based Screening Methods

The clinical availability of cfDNA screening for aneuploidy in late 2011 revolutionized aneuploidy screening for many reasons.[3] cfDNA screening generally requires only a single blood draw at any time after 9 weeks' GA; this simplicity is attractive to the busy obstetric practice with both early- and late-to-care patient populations. cfDNA screening is not only the earliest method of fetal sex assessment (a feature popular with many patients) but also the earliest available aneuploidy screening method in pregnancy. The early aneuploidy risk assessment provided by cfDNA can aid prenatal genetic counselors in refining their diagnostic testing recommendations for patients with normal cfDNA results and fetal anomalies at the time of the NT ultrasound. Such refinement, however, currently applies only to the common aneuploidies leaving other chromosome and single gene disorders untested. Although this screening has quickly become a fixture in the American obstetric practice, many intricacies of cfDNA screening exist that are worth noting.

Today's cfDNA screening and its applications were made possible by the 1997 discovery that maternal plasma contained circulating cell-free fetal nucleic acids.[9] Although methodologies differ by performing laboratory, DNA sequencing technology allows for these circulating cfDNA fragments to be amplified, analyzed, and ultimately assigned to the chromosome of origin. The subsequent comparison of the quantities of the maternal and fetoplacental cfDNA in the sample to a normal reference allows for rather precise detection of aneuploidy. Presently, cfDNA screening is routinely available for analysis of trisomy 21 (99.7% detection rate and 0.04% false-positive rate), trisomy 18 (97.9% detection rate and 0.04% false-positive rate), trisomy 13 (99.0% detection rate and 0.04% false-positive rate), monosomy X (95.8% detection rate and 0.14% false-positive rate), and other sex chromosome aneuploidies.[10] cfDNA screening can also be offered to twin pregnancies, and currently available twin outcomes data suggest promising detection rates for trisomy 21 in particular.[10] However, additional limitations exist for cfDNA in twin gestations, such as the need for a higher overall fetal fraction rate for successful test performance, and disproportionate twin contribution to total fetal fraction, among others. For example, in the setting of a monochorionic/diamniotic twin pregnancy (presumed to be genetically identical) with abnormal cfDNA results, clinicians should take care to recall that cfDNA screening cannot account for the possibility (albeit rare) of postzygotic changes leading to discrepant twin karyotypes.

Within only a few years of becoming clinically available for aneuploidies of chromosomes 21, 18, 13, X, and Y, cfDNA screening technology was rapidly expanded to include optional assessment for certain chromosomal microdeletions, such as 22q11.2 deletion syndrome (DiGeorge syndrome). Various commercial laboratories may also offer additional evaluation for chromosomes 9, 16, or 22, because trisomies of these chromosomes are associated with early pregnancy loss. Genome-wide cfDNA screening for aneuploidy became clinically available in 2015 and is intended to screen for chromosomal aberrations greater than or equal to 7 Mb (similar to cytogenetically visible changes by karyotype analysis) across all 23 pairs of fetal chromosomes.[11] Although such offerings increase the yield of cfDNA screening for chromosomal abnormalities, it is crucial to understand that genome-wide and microdeletion screenings by cfDNA do not provide the same amount or depth of diagnostic information available through prenatal karyotype and single nucleotide polymorphism microarray analysis, respectively.

Although cfDNA screening boasts high detection rate for common live-born aneuploidies, detailed discussion of the concept of positive predictive value (PPV) is critical, both in the pretest counseling of patients seeking screening and in the posttesting counseling following abnormal results from such screening.[12] PPV, which refers to the likelihood that an abnormal screening result reflects a truly abnormal pregnancy, depends not only on the sensitivity and specificity of the screening test but also on the patient's *a priori* risk for the fetal condition. cfDNA screening for common live-born aneuploidies will have higher performance rates in the high-risk population (primarily women older than 35 years and women with abnormal serum screens), although obstetric providers may offer this screening to all women. Despite similar cfDNA sensitivities and specificities between these 2 patient populations, the prevalence of aneuploidy in average-risk women is decreased compared with their high-risk counterparts, and thus the PPV of cfDNA screening is reduced[2] (**Fig. 2**). Women with sonographically normal-appearing pregnancies and no prior risk factors

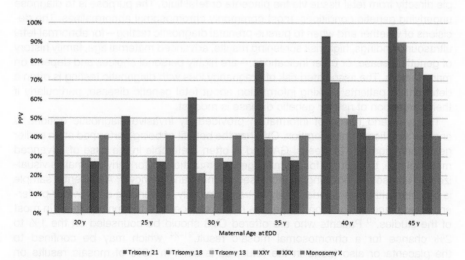

Fig. 2. Positive predictive value (PPV) of cfDNA screening for common aneuploidies. EDD, estimated date of delivery. (*Data from* NSGC & perinatal quality NIPT/cfDNA performance calculator. Available at: https://www.perinatalquality.org/vendors/nsgc/nipt. Accessed October 1, 2018.)

(eg, maternal age, abnormal serum screening results) for aneuploidy who have abnormal cfDNA results should especially receive a detailed discussion of the PPV of their cfDNA screening result. Furthermore, because of the low prevalence of certain chromosomal microdeletion syndromes (included on cfDNA screening expanded options) in the general population, limited outcomes data exist to support accurate sensitivity and specificity rates of commercially available products. As such, PPV calculation for patients with abnormal microdeletion syndrome screening results is challenging, which then creates difficulty in patient decision-making regarding confirmatory diagnostic testing.

Prompt and cautious follow-up is essential for all cfDNA screening results that do not convey a normal result. Patients with screen-positive cfDNA results should receive posttest counseling on the adjusted risk for an abnormal fetal diagnosis and be offered confirmatory prenatal diagnosis via CVS or amniocentesis.[2,12] As circulating cell-free fetal DNA is thought to be of trophoblastic (placental) origin, it is not possible to determine from cfDNA screening alone whether abnormal cfDNA results are reflective of a true fetal abnormality, confined placental mosaicism, or a vanished twin gestation. Patients with nonreportable cfDNA results, called "no call" results, that were failed due to a low fetal fraction of DNA should be counseled on the potential increased risk for fetal aneuploidy in this setting[13] and should also be offered a detailed discussion on the risks and benefits of repeat cfDNA screening or diagnostic testing.[2] In very rare circumstances, abnormal cfDNA results may be caused by underlying maternal cytogenetic abnormalities (such as a maternal sex chromosome abnormality or maternal deletion within a promised region of cfDNA evaluation) or even an underlying maternal malignancy.[14–16]

PRENATAL DIAGNOSTIC OPTIONS: ANEUPLOIDY AND BEYOND

All patients should be counseled in regard to the meaning and options of prenatal screening versus diagnosis regardless of maternal age.[17] Prenatal diagnosis differs from the previously presented prenatal screening by the acquisition of the DNA sample directly from fetal tissue via the placenta or fetal fluid. The purpose is to diagnose underlying genetic conditions, most commonly chromosomal abnormalities. The decisions of whether and when to pursue prenatal diagnostic testing—for abnormal fetal ultrasound findings, high-risk screening results, advanced maternal age, family history of genetic disease, or other indications —are highly personal choices and depend on many factors. The associated risk of pregnancy loss with diagnostic testing is often a deterrent to patients seeking information about fetal genetic disease, particularly if their perception of risk for genetic disease is modest.

The type and timing of information provided by invasive diagnostic options is another significant consideration. CVS has the benefit of being performed at an earlier gestational age (11–14 weeks' GA) and is often preferable in the case of advanced maternal age, to evaluate for a familial genetic mutation, or for early anomalies visualized on ultrasound including an increased nuchal translucency.[18] A placental sample is obtained either transabdominally or transcervically, depending on provider preference and placental location.[19] The loss rate is comparable to amniocentesis in most of the studies.[20] Patients who are offered CVS should be counseled on the 1% to 2% chance for a chromosomal mosaic result,[21–24] which may be confined to the placenta or also found in the fetus, as is seen in 10% of mosaic results on CVS.[25] Cell-free DNA is derived from the placenta, and therefore, the recommended follow-up procedure is an amniocentesis, rather than a CVS, to avoid the identification of placental mosaicism rather than true fetal aneuploidy.

Amniocentesis is performed for the same indications as CVS, for abnormal cell-free DNA results or for anomalies that are visualized on the anatomy ultrasound. It is performed after membranes are fused (>15 weeks' GA) due to the increased risks of miscarriage and limb anomalies associated with early amniocentesis. Amniocentesis in the second trimester affords the opportunity to measure amniotic fluid AFP for detection of ONTDs, whereas CVS does not. Yet, deferring prenatal diagnosis until the second trimester delays diagnostic results and also may be disagreeable to patients who might only consider pregnancy termination at earlier GAs.

Although amniocentesis specifically can be performed at any time greater than 15 weeks' GA, a complication in the early second trimester could result in miscarriage, whereas a complication later in pregnancy results in preterm delivery. The relative procedural risk for preterm labor from a third trimester procedure may be increased above the second trimester risk for miscarriage although this may be influenced by the indication for the third trimester amniocentesis. In addition, the utility of information derived from a third trimester amniocentesis may be limited to parental preparation, except in specific circumstances such as determining fetal ABO/Rh genotyping.[26] Some Maternal-Fetal Medicine Centers are able to facilitate fetal blood sampling in the third trimester, although this practice carries additional pregnancy risks and is performed less frequently than CVS and amniocentesis. In certain circumstances, genetic diagnosis can also be performed on fetal blood (percutaneous umbilical cord sampling), urine from the fetal bladder (shunt), fetal lung fluid (pleural shunt), ascites, or any other accumulation of fetal fluid that has substantial fetal cells.

The choice of testing that is performed on fetal cells depends on the indication for which the procedure was performed. Prenatal diagnosis was originally used to assess for chromosome abnormalities, which are present in 1/800 live births.[27] A karyotype is nearly 99% sensitive and specific for aneuploidy,[19] with the exception of confined placental mosaicism in the case of CVS. Although a karyotype is still a reasonable test if aneuploidy is suspected, in the case of fetal anomalies, a chromosomal microarray is recommended because of the approximately 6% increase in diagnostic yield.[28] Chromosomal microarrays are the recommended test of choice to detect smaller, micro, deletions or duplications that are too small for visualization cytogenetically by karyotype. These are referred to as copy number variants.[28]

Patients undergoing diagnostic testing require appropriate pre- and posttest counseling, including discussion of the risks and benefits, sensitivity, and specificity of each testing option. Any patient undergoing diagnostic evaluation not only should be offered a microarray but also should be counseled that there is an approximately 2% risk of obtaining a copy number variant of unknown significance.[29] A chromosomal microarray has several benefits when compared with a karyotype. Even in the absence of an ultrasound anomaly, there is a higher rate of detecting a syndromic diagnosis. In addition, as chromosomal microarray is performed on an uncultured (direct) amniotic fluid and does not require the cultured cells needed for a karyotype, divisional errors are avoided. The limitations of chromosomal microarray include limited detection of mosaicism (similar to karyotype) and inability to detect balanced translocations and inversions. Chromosomal microarray does not require cultured cells so a rapid turn-around time (3–5 days) is possible; however, the usual turn-around time (7–14 days) is comparable to the turn-around time for a karyotype. Fluorescence in situ hybridization analysis (FISH) can be performed on cells in interphase and is often used if rapid (2 days) results would assist with management; however, a FISH is a preliminary result and should be followed by either karyotype or microarray.[30]

Chromosomal microarray does not detect single nucleotide mutations that are responsible for many autosomal recessive and autosomal dominant conditions. If testing is being performed for a specific familial mutation (ie, cystic fibrosis, Marfan syndrome), then the genetic mutation should be established on the affected family member so that testing can be directed to this mutation on the fetal sample. Panel testing provides detection of known mutations of a disorder and can be performed on fetal DNA when anomalies visualized on prenatal ultrasound suggest a particular disorder. Panel testing typically is performed with genotyping, although sequencing or duplication/deletion analysis is becoming more readily available. Congenital anomalies that affect more than one organ system should be evaluated closely in conjunction with maternal exposure history and family history. Specific gene or panel testing should be individualized to assess for candidate syndromes. L1CAM testing is indicated in cases when aqueductal stenosis is suggested in a male fetus.[31] Examples of other panels include Noonan syndrome spectrum disorders[32] for a cystic hygroma with a normal microarray, a skeletal dysplasia panel when abnormalities of the long bones are visualized, or a heterotaxy panel for abnormal situs.

Whole exome sequencing (WES) is clinically available; however, prenatal utility is limited by turn-around time and interpretation.[33] WES detects changes that affect the protein coding regions of the genome. Changes in the exome that differ from the general population are referred to as variants. Each variant is characterized and reported as pathogenic, likely pathogenic, benign, likely benign, or a variant of unknown significance per the American College of Medical Genetics and Genomics.[34] Most of the prenatal WES is currently performed under the umbrella of research. Clinical WES is offered and recommended in specific cases for patients with a family history of a prior pregnancy with similar fetal anomalies (without a known genetic diagnosis), history of consanguinity, or for complex conditions where the yield of panel testing is low.[35] The diagnostic yield is case dependent, ranging from 10% to 50%[36,37] depending on the study.

When a genetic cause is not identified by genetic diagnosis, additional causes or testing options should be considered. Anomalies can also be attributed to mutations in the intronic area of the genome, a mitochondrial defect, or a defect in a trinucleotide repeat that was not detected by WES. Fetal abnormalities occur secondary to environmental exposures including medications (eg, thalidomide) and maternal conditions such as diabetes. In addition, many conditions are believed to be multifactorial, involving interplay between genes and environment. Patients should receive appropriate pre- and posttest genetic counseling specific to the recommended testing and understand that there is no test currently available that can completely exclude the possibility of a genetic condition that is undiagnosed.

SUMMARY AND FUTURE DIRECTIONS

In summary, prenatal screening and diagnosis requires a patient-centered approach. There are many prenatal aneuploidy screening options available. Prenatal nuchal translucency, in additional to first trimester analytes, remains an acceptable screening option for low-risk patients. Cell-free DNA has emerged as a favorable screening choice for patients at high risk for fetal chromosomal aneuploidy. Karyotype continues to be recommended when screening tests or ultrasound findings suggest aneuploidy; however, chromosomal microarray is now the preferred diagnostic test when fetal sonographic anomalies are visualized. Prenatal WES is now clinically available and should be considered for specific cases including those with complex findings, prior affected children, and consanguinity.

Future directions will likely allow for additional prenatal screening through cfDNA including screening for autosomal dominant conditions related to paternal age and foreseeably WES[38] through a maternal blood draw. Postnatal genetic therapy is being explored through clustered regularly interspaced short palindromic repeats technology[39] and will likely translate to in utero application. Indeed, in utero therapy is being explored for osteogenesis imperfecta by in utero mesenchymal stem cell transplantation via the fetal umbilical vein.[40] Applications of technology will promote prenatal testing and screening at earlier GAs, expanding the potential for in utero therapy.

REFERENCES

1. Parker SE, Mai CT, Canfield MA, et al. Updated national birth prevalence estimates for selected birth defects in the United States, 2004-2006. Birth Defects Res A Clin Mol Teratol 2010;88(12):1008-16.
2. Practice Bulletin No. 163: screening for fetal aneuploidy. Obstet Gynecol 2016; 127(5):e123-7.
3. Bianchi DW, Platt LD, Goldberg JH, et al. Genome-wide fetal aneuploidy detection by maternal plasma DNA sequencing. Obstet Gynecol 2012;119(5):890-901.
4. Bredaki FE, Wright D, Matos P, et al. First-trimester screening for trisomy 21 using alpha-fetoprotein. Fetal Diagn Ther 2011;30(3):215-8.
5. Dane B, Dane C, Kiray M, et al. Correlation between first-trimester maternal serum markers, second-trimester uterine artery Doppler indices and pregnancy outcome. Gynecol Obstet Invest 2010;70(2):126-31.
6. Wagner P, Sonek J, Kelin J, et al. First trimester ultrasound screening for trisomy 21 based on maternal age, fetal nuchal translucency, and different methods of ductus venosus assessment. Prenat Diagn 2017;37(7):680-5.
7. Committee on Obstetric Practice. ACOG committee opinion no. 638: First-trimester risk assessment for early-onset preeclampsia. Obstet Gynecol 2015; 126(3):e25-7.
8. Wilson KL, Czerwinksi JL, Hoskovec JM, et al. NSGC practice guideline: prenatal screening and diagnostic testing options for chromosome aneuploidy. J Genet Couns 2013;22:4-15.
9. Lo YM, Corbetta N, Chamberlain PF, et al. Presence of fetal DNA in maternal plasma and serum. Lancet 1997;350:485-7.
10. Gil MM, Accurti V, Santacruz B, et al. Analysis of cell-free DNA in maternal blood in screening for aneuploidies: updated meta-analysis. Ultrasound Obstet Gynecol 2017;50(3):302-14.
11. Ehrich M, Tynan J, Mazloom A, et al. Genome-wide cfDNA screening: clinical laboratory experience with the first 10,000 cases. Genet Med 2017;19(12):1332-7.
12. Committee on Genetics. ACOG committee opinion No. 693: counseling about genetic testing and communication of genetic test results. Obstet Gynecol 2017; 129(4):e96-101.
13. Pergament E, Cuckle H, Zimmerman B, et al. Single-nucleotide polymorphism-based noninvasive prenatal screening in a high-risk and low-risk cohort. Obstet Gynecol 2014;124(2Pt 1):210-8.
14. Amant F, Verheecke M, Wlodarska I, et al. Presymptomatic identification of cancers in pregnant women during noninvasive prenatal testing. JAMA Oncol 2015; 1(6):814-9.

15. Bianchi DW, Chudova D, Sehnert A, et al. Noninvasive prenatal testing and incidental detection of occult maternal malignancies. JAMA 2015;314(2):162–9.
16. Smith J, Kean V, Bianchi DW, et al. Cell-free DNA results lead to unexpected diagnosis. Clin Case Rep 2017;5(8):1323–6.
17. Practice bulletin no. 162 summary: prenatal diagnostic testing for genetic disorders. Obstet Gynecol 2016;127(5):976–8.
18. Benn PA. Prenatal diagnosis of chromosomal abnormalities through chorionic villus sampling and amniocentesis. In: Milunsky A, Milunsky JH, editors. Genetic disorders and the fetus: diagnosis, prevention and treatment. 7th edition. Hoboken (NJ): Wiley Blackwell; 2016. p. 178–266.
19. Jackson LG, Zachary JM, Fowler SE, et al. A randomized comparison of transcervical and transabdominal chorionic-villus sampling. The U.S. National Institute of Child Health and Human Development Chorionic-Villus Sampling and Amniocentesis Study Group. N Engl J Med 1992;327:594–8.
20. Akolekar R, Beta J, Picciarelli G, et al. Procedure-related risk of miscarriage following amniocentesis and chorionic villus sampling: a systematic review and meta-analysis. Ultrasound Obstet Gynecol 2015;45:16–26.
21. Ledbetter DH, Zachary JM, Simpson JL, et al. Cytogenetic results from the U.S. Collaborative Study on CVS. Prenat Diagn 1992;12(5):317–45.
22. Vejerselev LO, Mikkelsen M. The European collaborative study on mosaicism in chorionic villus sampling: data from 1986 to 1987. Prenat Diagn 1989;9(8):575–88.
23. Stetten G, Escallon CS, South ST, et al. Reevaluating confined placental mosaicism. Am J Med Genet A 2004;131(3):232–9.
24. Grati FR, Grimi B, Frascoli G, et al. Confirmation of mosaicism and uniparental disomy in amniocytes, after detection of mosaic chromosome abnormalities in chorionic villi. Eur J Hum Genet 2006;14(3):282–8.
25. Daniel A, Wu Z, Darmanian A, et al. Issues arising form the prenatal diagnosis of some rare trisomy mosaics – the importance of cryptic fetal mosaicism. Prenat Diagn 2004;24:524–36.
26. Bishop JC, Blakemore K, Vricella L, et al. Prenatal ABO/RHD genotyping: a new paradigm to allow for fresh whole blood for cardiopulmonary bypass in the immediate newborn period. Fetal Diagn Ther 2018;44(2):156–9.
27. Little BB, Ramin SM, Cambridge BS, et al. Risk of chromosomal abnormalities, with emphasis on live-born offspring of young mothers. Am J Hum Genet 1995;57(5):1178–85.
28. The use of chromosomal microarray analysis in prenatal diagnosis. Committee Opinion No. 581. American College of Obstetricians and Gynecologists. Obstet Gynecol 2013;122:1374–7.
29. Wapner RJ, Martin CL, Levy B, et al. Chromosomal microarray versus karyotyping for prenatal diagnosis. N Engl J Med 2012;367:2175–84.
30. Toutain J, Epiney M, Begorre M, et al. First-trimester prenatal diagnosis performed on pregnant women with fetal ultrasound abnormalities: the reliability of interphase fluorescence in situ hybridization (FISH) on mesenchymal core for the mail aneuploidies. Eur J Obstet Gynecol Reprod Biol 2010;21:293–301.
31. Fox NS, Monteagudo A, Kuller JA, et al. Mild fetal ventriculomegaly: diagnosis, evaluation, and management. Am J Obstet Gynecol 2018;219(1):B2–9.
32. Leach NL, Wilson Mathews DR, Rosenblum LS, et al. Comparative assessment of gene-specific variant distribution in prenatal and postnatal cohorts tested for Noonan syndrome and related conditions. Genet Med 2018. https://doi.org/10.1038/s41436-018-0062-0.

33. Harris S, Gilmore K, Hardisty E, et al. Ethical and counseling challenges in pre-natal exome sequencing. Prenat Diagn 2018. https://doi.org/10.1002/pd.5353.
34. Richards S, Aziz N, Bale S, et al. Standards and guidelines for the interpretation of sequence variants: a joint consensus recommendation of the American College of Medical Genetics and Genomics and the Association for Molecular Pathology. Genet Med 2015;17(5):405–24.
35. Jelin AC, Vora N. Whole exome sequencing: applications in prenatal genetics. Obstet Gynecol Clin North Am 2018;45(1):69–81.
36. Drury S, Williams H, Trump N, et al. Exome sequencing for prenatal diagnosis of fetuses with sonographic abnormalities. Prenat Diagn 2015;35:1010–7.
37. Alamillo CL, Powis Z, Farwell K, et al. Exome sequencing positively identified relevant alterations in more than half of cases with an indication of prenatal ultrasound anomalies. Prenat Diagn 2015;35:1073–8.
38. Ng SB, Turner EH, Robertson PD, et al. Targeted capture and massively parallel sequencing of 12 human exomes. Nature 2009;461(7261):272–6.
39. Finotti A, Breda L, Lederer CW, et al. Recent trends in the gene therapy of β-thalassemia. J Blood Med 2015;6:69–85.
40. Le Blanc K, Götherström C, Ringdén O, et al. Fetal mesenchymal stem-cell engraftment in bone after in utero transplantation in a patient with severe osteogenesis imperfecta. Transplantation 2005;79(11):1607–14.
41. Barkai G, Goldman B, Ries L, et al. Expanding multiple marker screening for Down's syndrome to include Edward's syndrome. Prenat Diagn 1993;13(9):843–50.
42. Cuckle HS, Malone FD, Wright D, et al. Contingent screening for Down syndrome – results from the FaSTER trial. Prenat Diagn 2008;28(2):89–94.
43. Malone FD, Canick JA, Ball RH, et al. First-trimester or second-trimester screening, or both, for Down's syndrome. N Engl J Med 2005;353(19):2001–11.
44. Palomaki G, Steinort K, Knight G, et al. Comparing three screening strategies for combining first- and second-trimester Down syndrome markers. Obstet Gynecol 2006;107(2 Pt 1):367–75. Erratum in: Obstet Gynecol 2006;107(4):955.
45. Spencer K, Nicolaides KH. A first trimester trisomy 13/trisomy 13 risk algorithm combining fetal nuchal translucency thickness, maternal serum free beta-hCG and PAPP-A. Prenat Diagn 2002;22(10):877–9.
46. Wald NJ, Rodeck J, Hackshaw AK, et al. First and second trimester antenatal screening for Down's syndrome: the results of the Serum Urine and Ultrasound Screening Study (SURUSS). J Med Screen 2003;10(2):56–104. Erratum in: J Med Screen 2006;13(1):51–2.
47. Wald NJ, Rodeck C, Hackshaw AK, et al. SURUSS in perspective. BJOG 2004;111(6):521–31.
48. Wapner RJ, Thorn E, Simpson JL, et al. First-trimester screening for trisomies 21 and 18. N Engl J Med 2003;349(15):1405–13.

Fetal Surgery

Heron D. Baumgarten, MD, MPH, Alan W. Flake, MD*

KEYWORDS

- Fetal surgery • Fetal myelomeningocele repair • Fetal tumor debulking
- Fetal hydrops • Fetal lobectomy for CPAM • Vesicoamniotic shunt
- Tracheal occlusion

KEY POINTS

- Fetal surgery is an established but still rapidly evolving specialty, born from the rationale that destructive embryologic processes, recognized early in gestation, can be curtailed by prenatal correction.
- As more and more centers begin offering fetal interventions, quality of care must be verified through transparency about clinical capabilities and resources.
- Level designations should be assigned based on capability, as in trauma and neonatal ICU centers for excellence, and volume requirements must be set for fetal surgery certification. Regionalization of this specialty care may be required to optimize outcomes.

INTRODUCTION

Fetal surgery is an established but still rapidly evolving specialty, born from the rationale that destructive embryologic processes, recognized early in gestation, can be curtailed by prenatal correction. As noninvasive, high-resolution fetal imaging has improved, the window of opportunity for intervention has widened; with expanding clinical experience and ongoing experimental work with animal models, there has been significant progress in the ability to safely implement fetal therapies.[1–3] Fetal surgery now offers validated and accepted treatments of several developmental defects and should be offered as an option for management of select anomalies.[4] There is now certainty that by intervening in utero, the outcome of selected fetal anomalies can be improved (**Table 1**).

BACKGROUND AND GENERAL PRINCIPLES OF FETAL SURGERY

Clinical application of fetal surgery was pioneered by Harrison and colleagues at the University of California, San Francisco (UCSF), in the late 1970s and early 1980s.[5] Using innovative laboratory research to design new tools and technical approaches, the group at UCSF set the standard for the field going forward. Their innovative effort took

Department of Surgery, Abramson Research Center, Room 1116B, 3615 Civic Center Boulevard, Philadelphia, PA 19104-4318, USA
* Corresponding author.
E-mail address: flake@email.chop.edu

Pediatr Clin N Am 66 (2019) 295–308
https://doi.org/10.1016/j.pcl.2018.12.001
0031-3955/19/© 2018 Elsevier Inc. All rights reserved.

Table 1
Defects currently treated prenatally

Anatomic Defect	Consequence(s)	Intervention(s)
Ultrasound-guided/fetoscopic		
Monochorionic twin pregnancies—twin-twin transfusion syndrome and twin reversed arterial perfusion	Perfusion imbalance with hydrops or renal failure/oligohydromnios	Laser coagulation Selective cord occlusion
Genitourinary obstruction	Renal dysplasia	Vesicoamniotic shunt Cystoscopic valve ablation
Diaphragmatic hernia	Pulmonary hypoplasia	Balloon tracheal occlusion
Hydrothorax/chylothorax	Hydrops	Thoracoamniotic shunt
Cardiac outflow tract obstruction	Single ventricle physiology	Balloon valvuloplasty
Macrocystic CPAM	Hydrops	Thoracoamniotic shunt
Open fetal surgery		
Microcystic CPAM[a]	Hydrops	Fetal lobectomy
SCT	High-output failure/hydrops	Tumor debulking
Pericardial teratoma	Cardiac compression/hydrops	Tumor debulking
MMC/myeloschisis[b]	Hydrocephalus/Arnold-Chiari malformation, bowel/bladder/lower extremity dysfunction	Closure of the MMC defect

[a] When associated hydrops is unresponsive to steroid treatment.
[b] Treated fetoscopically in some centers. Standard of care remains open fetal surgery.

hypotheses based on clinical need and tested these in animal models, allowing confirmation of the pathophysiology of the anomaly, the response to fetal surgical intervention, and the development of safe maternal anesthetic and surgical techniques.[6,7] The laboratory work was followed by clinical trials with presentations and critique of the clinical results.

The concept of a fetal treatment center was developed during that period and the importance of the multidisciplinary fetal treatment team was then appreciated. The disciplines required for fetal therapy include pediatric surgery, obstetrics, pediatric anesthesia, obstetric anesthesia, cardiology, radiology, otolaryngology, neonatology, neonatal nursing, operative room nursing, and other case-specific relevant pediatric surgical specialties.[8] The prerequisites for fetal surgery enumerated 4 decades ago still guide the field today:

1. The ability to establish an accurate prenatal diagnosis
2. A well-defined natural history of the disorder
3. The presence of a correctable lesion that, if untreated, will lead to fetal demise or irreversible organ dysfunction before birth
4. The absence of severe associated anomalies
5. An acceptable risk-to-benefit ratio for both the pregnant woman and the fetus[9]

Complex chromosomal or associated anatomic anomalies in the fetus; maternal risk factors, including maternal comorbidities, placentomegaly, a short cervix, and other predispositions to preterm delivery; and maternal mirror syndrome (a syndrome in which maternal status mirrors that of the fetus with onset of preeclampsia/edema) are all contraindications to selection for fetal surgery.[9]

Fetal surgery was first performed clinically for bilateral hydronephrosis in the human fetus in 1982 at UCSF.[5] Efforts to address congenital diaphragmatic hernia (CDH) followed, and, by 1998, myelomeningocele (MMC) repair, sacrococcygeal teratoma (SCT) debulking, and congenital cystic adenomatoid malformation resection had been successfully performed. Since the first fetal intervention for each of these devastating fetal defects, careful patient selection and analysis of accumulated experience have enabled ongoing progress and improved outcomes for fetus and mother. The impact of advances in fetal ultrasound and MRI techniques, as well as maternal serum screening, on patient selection cannot be understated. Accumulation of clinical experience in several centers has validated the efficacy of many of these procedures.[8] Still, the increased risk of preterm delivery and the impact of a large uterine incision on future reproductive risk remain. Recent advances in fetoscopic approaches seem promising in addressing both of these issues but require further study to prove fetal safety and technical equivalence to the open approach.

LOWER URINARY TRACT OBSTRUCTION

Fetal obstructive uropathy was the first anatomic anomaly treated with fetal surgery.[5] Lower urinary tract obstruction (LUTO) is a common congenital anomaly, occurring in up to 1% of all fetuses, which is caused by intermittent or incomplete blockages of the lower urinary tract. The associated morbidity is variable to the degree and duration of obstruction. Complete unrelenting obstruction is infrequent but results in neonatal death in 45% of cases, with worse prognoses associated with early onset and severity of the obstruction.[10] In female fetuses, LUTO is most often related to cloacal anomalies and, therefore, not amenable to intervention. In male fetuses, the most common cause of LUTO is posterior urethral valves, which obstruct urine outflow at the level of the prostate, resulting in bladder distension at gestational weeks 8 to 10, with subsequent renal pelviectasis and echogenicity of the renal cortex seen on fetal ultrasound at 18 to 20 weeks.[11–14]

Many fetuses with LUTO have irreversible kidney damage at the time of diagnosis, whereas others have preserved function despite persistent hydronephrosis through the duration of fetal development. Predicting which fetuses with LUTO will have poor outcomes is thus challenging. Oligohydramnios is required for consideration of fetal intervention, because those with preserved amniotic fluid indices are likely to have preserved renal function.[15] Once oligohydramnios is diagnosed, however, many affected fetuses already have evidence of fibrocystic dysplasia and renal cortical cysts, which are signs of a poor prognosis. Thus, analysis of fetal urine has been investigated as a method to screen for preserved renal function. This analysis began with Glick's Criteria, including urinary sodium, chloride, and hourly production. β-Microglobulin, calcium, total protein, and osmolality also have been analyzed, with calcium and sodium proving the best predictors of renal function and neonatal outcome.[11–13,16–18]

At Children's Hospital of Philadelphia (CHOP), 3 fetal urinary taps at 24-hour intervals are used to assess intrauterine renal function, allowing for collection of fresh urine for analysis.[19,20] Those fetuses with preserved function—decreasing electrolyte and protein profiles over the 3 collections—are believed to benefit from placement of a vesicoamniotic shunt.[8] Many patients, however, have bladder dysfunction and some level of renal failure on long-term follow-up despite vesicoamniotic shunting.

Fetal cystoscopy has been used for posterior valve ablation in select fetuses and has shown promise in the hands of some investigators.[21]

Furthermore, in fetuses with persistent oligohydramnios, despite placement of a vesicoamniotic shunt, amnioinfusion via placement of semipermanent uterine infusion ports is an option to prevent pulmonary hypoplasia. This approach has been used for patients with normal renal function on placement of the vesicoamniotic shunt but subsequent decline in urine production.[22] Controversially, amnioinfusion has also been proposed for use in fetuses with renal agenesis to prevent pulmonary hypoplasia.[23]

The treatment of LUTO in fetuses remains controversial due to a small number of candidates for fetal intervention in any single center and persistent debate over the embryologic pathophysiology of the disease and patient selection. The question of whether the renal dysplasia is a primary or secondary malformation is still definitively unanswered.[24] If it is a secondary malformation, the renal damage is caused by faulty urodynamics. It may be caused, however, by an abnormal lateral embryologic origin of the ureteric bud, resulting in both the presence of urethral valves and inherent renal dysplasia.[25]

The Percutaneous Shunting in Lower Urinary Tract Obstruction trial attempted to demonstrate efficacy of intervention for congenital LUTO but closed after enrolling only 31 patients.[26] Among those patients in the study, shunted patients had improved survival compared with nonshunted fetuses; however, no conclusions could be made about the effect on long-term renal function.[27] There is an ongoing need for improved understanding of this congenital process and the ability to affect long-term prognosis with fetal intervention.

SACROCOCCYGEAL TERATOMA

Teratomas are the most common congenital neoplasm, with an estimated incidence of 1 in 20,000 to 40,000 live births.[28–34] They occur with female predominance in a 3:1 ratio[35] and are most commonly found along the midline, with 60% sacrococcygeal.[30] Derived from the Greek word, *teratos*, meaning "monster,"[36] these tumors originate from the 3 germinal layers (ectodermal, mesodermal, or endodermal tissue) and are believed to originate from the totipotent cells of Hensen node, a remnant of the primitive streak in the coccyx.[36,37] As germ cell tumors, their natural history is characterized by rapid growth in utero.[29,30]

The natural history of prenatally diagnosed SCT is different from postnatally diagnosed SCT. A majority (83% to 90%) of SCTs presenting in the newborn are benign[36] and have excellent long-term outcomes, with malignancy the primary cause of death in postnatal SCT; 85% of patients with postnatally diagnosed SCTs survive.

This is in contrast to the perinatal mortality of prenatally diagnosed SCTs, which is reported in up to 50% of cases.[31,32,35,38] Mortality in fetal SCT is caused by a variety of mechanisms, including tumor dystocia, preterm delivery due to tumor mass and polyhydramnios, tumor rupture and hemorrhage, and, of greatest interest to fetal surgeons, high-output cardiac failure associated with arteriovenous shunting through a rapidly growing tumor.[39] This may be compounded by anemia caused by hemorrhage into the tumor,[31] which can lead to fetal hydrops.[28,32,36] A rapid phase of tumor growth frequently precedes the development of placentomegaly and hydrops, which are signs of impending fetal demise.[40] Actual reversal of diastolic flow in the umbilical arteries can be observed as the lower resistance in the tumor steals blood flow from the placenta. Abnormalities also occur in left and right ventricular end-diastolic diameters, placental thickness, diameter of the inferior vena cava, combined ventricular output, descending aortic flow, and umbilical venous flow. The ensuing placentomegaly and fetal hydrops can lead to maternal mirror syndrome, and fetal mortality approaches 100% once fetal hydrops develops.[28,31,32,35,40]

Ultrasonographic assessment of tumor size, growth rate, and fetal cardiac function allows for the identification of those fetuses with an SCT who at particular risk for decompensation. Ultrasound identifies a complex mass, located at the distal end of the spine, which has vascular solid components with increased echogenicity.[29] As a result of acoustic shadowing by the fetal pelvic bones, ultrasound cannot always define the most cephalad extent of SCT. Thus, ultrafast fetal MRI is used to delineate the intrapelvic extent of the tumor.[40,41] Close surveillance with serial ultrasounds and echocardiography is recommended so that fetal intervention or early delivery can be performed when necessary.[35] Staging of the SCT is based on the amount of external and internal pelvic component of the tumor. The classification system was established by the Section on Surgery of the American Academy of Pediatrics and divides SCTs into 4 types:

I. Entirely external with small tumor component at the coccyx (45.8%)
II. Predominantly external with smaller intrapelvic component (34%)
III. Predominantly intrapelvic with smaller external component (8.6%)
IV. Entirely intrapelvic or presacral (9.6%)

The value of this classification relates to the ease of surgical resection and prenatal detection as well as the likelihood of malignancy. Type I is easy to detect and relatively easy to resect with a very low incidence of malignancy. By contrast, type IV tumors are difficult to diagnose, not amenable to fetal resection, and frequently malignant when first diagnosed because of prolonged delay in recognition. Fortunately, a majority of tumors are type I or type II.[29,31,38] Among infants with SCTs, 5% to 25% have a spectrum of associated anomalies, including anal and vaginal stenosis, MMC, spina bifida, ventricular septal defect, Currarino triad (anorectal stenosis, anterior sacral defect, and presacral mass), and tracheoesophageal fistula.[36,42] Deletions on chromosomes 1 and 6 and increased N-Myc amplification in immature teratomas have been reported, but a clear genetic etiology for this tumor is not known.[30]

Timely fetal intervention is performed to remove the external tumor and effectively reverse the pathophysiology of the disease in selected fetuses affected by high-output cardiac failure and impending hydrops before the age of viability.[28,32] The first successful fetal surgery was reported in 1996 by Harrison's group at UCSF.[43] Since that time, additional open fetal surgeries for SCT have demonstrated that resection of a large tumor can reverse the pathophysiology of high-output cardiac failure and that early intervention offers the best hope for fetal survival once high-output cardiac failure is documented.[33] Fetuses with type I or type II SCT are eligible for fetal intervention. Patients should undergo serial ultrasound evaluation at least once a week and more frequently if there is any concern for evolving heart failure. Certainly, for intervention to be successful, the timing is critical, because once fetal hydrops is recognized, the potential for recovery is limited. At CHOP, survival after fetal debulking of SCT is approximately 60%.

Fetal intervention can be complicated by postoperative uterine irritability and preterm delivery with related fetal mortality (50%).[44] Beyond 28 weeks of gestation, the risks for these complications increase and begin to outweigh the potential survival benefit to the fetus. As a result, fetal intervention is typically offered for SCT fetuses younger than 28 weeks of gestation with impending or early hydrops.[30,44] If signs of high-output cardiac failure are absent, the fetus may be followed by serial sonography. Thus, if hydrops develops after 27 weeks' gestation, or in the setting of placentomegaly, preemptive early delivery should be pursued with immediate debulking or resection.[45] Review of the authors' patients managed with early delivery at CHOP shows that outcomes for infants who decompensate after 27 weeks are significantly improved as a result of early delivery and immediate debulking.[45]

There has been interest in the efficacy of minimally invasive approaches to fetal intervention for SCT. Several institutions have attempted fetoscopic laser ablation, radiofrequency ablation, coiling, and embolization for these tumors, with poor results.[32] As ablation technologies improve, however, and are able to more precisely target larger vessels, there may develop potential for a successful minimally invasive approach.

MYELOMENINGOCELE

Neural tube defects are the most common congenital structural anomalies worldwide. Folic acid supplementation has helped to reduce the incidence of these anomalies; however, in the Western world, 4 in 10,000 infants are affected.[9,10] MMC, or open spina bifida, is caused by incomplete closure of the neural tube and a defect in the vertebral arches, allowing herniation of the meninges and neural placode. The damage to the spinal cord is caused by abnormal neurulation beginning at the level of the defect and is exacerbated by exposure of the cord elements to the caustic amniotic fluid environment—this is the 2-hit hypothesis.[4,6,46] Furthermore, almost all patients with MMC have associated Arnold-Chiari type II malformation of the hindbrain, resulting in noncommunicating hydrocephalus requiring ventriculoperitoneal (VP) shunting.[47] This damage results in a range of morbidities, including paralysis, bladder and bowel dysfunction, and developmental delay. Although this defect is not fatal, the severe spectrum of morbidity attributed to the second hit and progressive loss of lower limb movement and ventriculomegaly seen on ultrasound imaging as gestation progresses prompted investigation into the feasibility of fetal intervention.[4,48,49] Furthermore, up to 30% of these patients do not survive to adulthood as a result of the long-term morbidity associated with the congenital anomaly.[6]

Human MMC repair in utero was first reported in 1997, and there were promising results, with a reduced requirement for VP shunting and improved motor function for those undergoing fetal repair. The risks of preterm labor, uterine dehiscence, and fetal or neonatal death, however, were not negligible. The Management of Myelomeningocele Study (MOMS) was started in 2003 and enrolled patients through 2010, with early termination for efficacy of prenatal repair after interim analysis. Patients after prenatal repair had half the incidence of VP shunting and were twice as likely to ambulate independently compared with postnatal repair. This was accomplished with acceptable levels of maternal morbidity and complications related to prematurity.[49] The findings of the MOMS have been sustained for the full cohort at the 30-month analysis[4] and the results of the MOMS II, which will provide follow-up at 5 years to 8 years of age, are pending.

Since the MOMS, the surgical technique for open repair at CHOP has evolved with further improvement in results. Critical aspects of the repair include the mobilization of myofascial flaps that provide a thick-tissue, watertight closure lined by dura. Initially, these defects were closed with skin only, and patients developed cord tethering related to scarring around the neural elements that did not stretch and grow as the child grew, thus requiring reoperation. The importance of closing a durally lined myofascial flap over the spinal cord and achieving a watertight closure cannot be overemphasized.[49–52]

Fetoscopic approaches to MMC repair have since been developed in an attempt to reduce the maternal morbidity related to open repair and to decrease preterm delivery.

Multiple techniques have been described by various centers. In general, fetoscopic repair has not resulted in reduced rates of prematurity or membrane disruption. In addition, most reports do not provide rigorous data on the patients' neurologic outcomes or significant lengths of follow-up. When reported, there have been high rates of cerebrospinal fluid leakage and postoperative wound revisions, suggesting that further development of the closure technique is needed.[53–55] Recent presentations from Belfort and colleagues[56] have shown promise using a technique that is similar to the open technique with average gestation at delivery of 38 weeks. If these results are sustained and reproducible, they may represent a significant advance in the prenatal treatment of MMC.[57,58] CO_2 insufflation is used to allow for visualization and does, unfortunately, interfere with continuous ultrasound monitoring of fetal cardiac function throughout the procedure. It has also been shown to cause significant fetal acidosis in the lamb model. In human fetuses, however, the same reactions to insufflation have not been documented. Furthermore, the anticipated decline in preterm labor has not yet been achieved, although the maternal morbidity certainly is significantly reduced.[59] Fetoscopic repair is promising and with continued refinement of the technique and surgical tools will likely become the preferred approach.[60,61]

Animal models for MMC have been essential for developing techniques for prenatal closure of MMC and will allow testing of new and promising strategies for fetal repair. The use of injectable scaffolds with or without stem cells or other tissue engineering strategies is particularly appealing as a noninvasive approach that could provide a watertight tissue closure earlier in gestation than open fetal surgery can be applied.[62,63] Although these tissue scaffolds and stem cell patches have yet to be used in humans, there have been promising results published in animal models, and they will likely soon contribute to success in human repair.[62–65]

CONGENITAL LUNG LESIONS

Lung lesions are identified by prenatal ultrasound in 1 of 10,000 to 35,000 pregnancies.[9] The differential for fetal lung lesion, identified on prenatal ultrasound, includes congenital cystic adenomatoid malformations (also referred to as congenital pulmonary airway malformations [CPAMs]), bronchopulmonary sequestrations (BPSs), bronchogenic cysts, congenital lobar emphysema, segmental bronchial stenosis, bronchial atresia, unilateral lung agenesis, CDH (in particular, right-sided), mediastinal tumors, and congenital high airway obstruction.[66] CPAMs are differentiated from BPSs based on arterial supply and pulmonary versus systemic, respectively, although there is some overlap in the classification of these lesions, such as CPAMs that have systemic arterial supply, which are referred to as hybrid lesions.

Many lung lesions do not require fetal intervention. The size, rate, and pattern of growth; macrocystic or microcystic appearance; and presence of pleural effusion are important prognosticators. Approximately 15% of CPAMs interfere with in utero development, causing mediastinal compression, cardiac failure, and fetal hydrops.[46] BPS lesions can cause lymphatic or venous congestion progressing to tension hydrothorax. CPAMs typically demonstrate growth until around the 26th week of gestation, followed by regression beginning the 28th week. This pattern of growth is described using the CPAM volume ratio (CVR), calculated by dividing the volume of the CPAM by the fetal head circumference. This ratio is the best predictor of impending hydrops. If the CVR is greater than 1.6, the risk of developing hydrops is 75%.[67] This measurement can help guide serial prenatal imaging schedules and maternal steroid therapy.

Although open fetal surgery for thoracotomy and resection of the lung lesion used to be the primary treatment of CPAMs with CVR greater than 1.6 and evolving hydrops prior to 32 weeks, maternal steroid therapy has proved effective in halting the growth of these tumors and/or inducing tumor regression.[66] The need for open fetal surgery has declined significantly since the introduction of maternal steroid therapy. Macrocystic tumors, however, do not respond to steroids and may require thoracoamniotic shunting. BPS lesions with a tension chylothorax should also undergo shunting. Furthermore, there are occasionally cases of unresponsive microcystic CPAMs that do require surgical excision. The success rate after fetal lobectomy at CHOP was reported at 54% without high rates of postnatal morbidity and compared with the nearly 100% mortality after hydrops occurs; thus, fetal surgery remains the recommendation for lesions unresponsive to steroid treatment.[38,40]

CONGENITAL DIAPHRAGMATIC HERNIA

CDH affects 1 of 2500 to 4000 live births.[68] The congenital anomaly is a result of persistence of the foramen of Bochdalek, which normally closes at 8 weeks' to 10 weeks' gestation.[46] The opening in the diaphragm results in herniation of abdominal viscera into the chest throughout gestation, which interferes with branching morphogenesis during lung development. The resulting pulmonary hypoplasia includes decreased surface area for gas exchange and hypermuscular pulmonary vasculature, which leads to increased vasoreactivity in the lung and clinical lability in these infants.[8] The pulmonary hypertension resulting from this hypervascularity results in persistence of fetal circulation, hypoxemia, acidosis, and further pulmonary vasospasm. This physiology can lead to rapid deterioration after birth. Neonatal management with extracorporeal membrane oxygenation, permissive hypercapnia, and delayed surgical repair have improved survival; however, the pulmonary insufficiency and need for prolonged ventilation can lead to chronic lung disease and significant lifelong morbidity.[69]

There is a range of severity for patients with CDH, and predicting the patients who will have severe pulmonary hypoplasia as a result of their defect is of paramount importance for selecting appropriate patients for fetal intervention. The best predictors of severity thus far have proved the presence of significant liver herniation combined with direct or indirect measurements of lung volume. The contralateral lung area–to–head circumference ratio (LHR), modified to the observed-to-expected LHR to standardize for gestational age, or observed-to-expected lung volume measurements obtained by MRI, have been validated and are currently used by most experienced fetal treatment centers in counseling CDH patients.[70,71] The ability to predict mortality in a specific fetus, however, is not reliable. This lack of confidence in understanding of the natural history of this disease results in considerable debate over patient selection for intervention.

In the late 1980s, the first attempts to treat CDH by open fetal surgery and diaphragmatic repair were performed. This was successful for fetuses without liver herniation, however, for the most severe fetuses with liver herniation, kinking of the umbilical vein on reduction of the liver resulted in fetal demise, and fetal CDH repair by open fetal surgery was abandoned.[9] Fetal endoscopic tracheal occlusion (FETO) has shown some promise in promoting lung growth by preventing the egress of pulmonary fluid, which results in increased intrabronchial pressure and stretch-induced growth of the airways. This approach has been shown to improve lung growth in animal models.[72–74] Analysis of pulmonary function in these lungs, however, did not show improved function as a result of the growth after tracheal occlusion.[75] Furthermore, a randomized controlled trial out of UCSF was unable to show improved outcomes for patients undergoing FETO.[76] Still, FETO has been performed for many fetuses with CDH, and there are several nonrandomized studies from Europe suggesting improved survival in patients with liver herniation and LHR of less than 1.0.[77] There is currently a multicenter randomized trial (TOTAL) started in Europe and now enrolling patients in the US, assessing the efficacy, if any, of FETO in the treatment of CDH. The results of these trials will be pivotal in determining the future of fetal therapy for CDH.

THE FUTURE

After 4 decades of work in the field of fetal surgery and medicine, several treatments of fetal disease have been validated as effective.[78,79] These therapies are now offered at an increasing number of institutions, with an increasing focus on the selection of patients for intervention and technologic advances that may further improve outcomes.[80,81] In the immediate future, there will be considerable effort directed toward perfecting the fetoscopic approach for prenatal repair of spina bifida that hopefully will lead to improved outcomes for mothers and their fetuses.[6] Success with fetoscopic repair of MMC may lead to further application of fetoscopy to other anatomic anomalies.

Cellular and genetic therapies continue to offer hope for a broad range of disorders, a majority of which do not manifest until after birth.[82–84] The first human clinical trials have begun, exploring the efficacy of these types of fetal interventions, which have been the focus of laboratory research at many centers.[85–88]

Artificial womb technology has shown promise in the lamb model, with the possibility of extending fetal development for the extremely premature neonate.[81] This technology would extend gestation in an extracorporeal environment and transform the neonatal ICU and the long-term outcomes for infants born at the lower limits of viability.[89,90]

As this field progresses and becomes part of the mainstream in prenatal medical care, the ethical integrity of all forms of fetal research will be equal in importance to the scientific integrity of the work.[91] There must exist a clear division between the personal drive of the researcher and innovator and the patient-centered guidance of the clinician.[7] This division must extend to the financial motivations of the hospital and preserve quality in the application of this specialty. This is a topic of particular relevance with the expansion of fetal care centers across the United States. As more and more centers begin offering fetal interventions—59 centers now in the United States—quality of care must be verified, through transparency about clinical capabilities and resources. Level designations should be assigned based on capability, as in trauma and neonatal ICU centers for excellence, and volume requirements must be set for fetal surgery certification. Regionalization of this specialty care may be required to optimize outcomes. Certainly, the leaders in the field should facilitate the organization of national consortiums and registries to improve outcomes for rare conditions requiring fetal intervention.[7]

REFERENCES

1. Harrison MR, Adzick NS. The fetus as a patient. Surgical considerations. Ann Surg 1991;213(4):279–91 [discussion: 277–278].

2. Danzer E, Victoria T, Bebbington MW, et al. Fetal MRI-calculated total lung volumes in the prediction of short-term outcome in giant omphalocele: preliminary findings. Fetal Diagn Ther 2012;31(4):248–53.

3. Hedrick HL. Management of prenatally diagnosed congenital diaphragmatic hernia. Semin Pediatr Surg 2013;22(1):37–43.

4. Farmer DL, Thom EA, Brock JW 3rd, et al. Management of Myelomeningocele Study. Full cohort 30-month pediatric outcomes. Am J Obstet Gynecol 2018; 218(2):256.e1-13.

5. Harrison MR, Golbus MS, Filly RA, et al. Management of the fetus with congenital hydronephrosis. J Pediatr Surg 1982;17(6):728–42.

6. Graves CE, Harrison MR, Padilla BE. Minimally invasive fetal surgery. Clin Perinatol 2017;44(4):729–51.

7. Antiel RM, Flake AW. Responsible surgical innovation and research in maternal-fetal surgery. Semin Fetal Neonatal Med 2017;22(6):423–7.

8. Watanabe M, Flake AW. Fetal surgery: progress and perspectives. Adv Pediatr 2010;57(1):353–72.

9. Partridge EA, Flake AW. Maternal-fetal surgery for structural malformations. Best Pract Res Clin Obstet Gynaecol 2012;26(5):669–82.

10. Wenstrom KD, Carr SR. Fetal surgery: principles, indications, and evidence. Obstet Gynecol 2014;124(4):817–35.

11. Glick PL, Harrison MR, Golbus MS, et al. Management of the fetus with congenital hydronephrosis II: prognostic criteria and selection for treatment. J Pediatr Surg 1985;20(4):376–87.

12. Glick PL, Harrison MR, Adzick NS, et al. Correction of congenital hydronephrosis in utero IV: in utero decompression prevents renal dysplasia. J Pediatr Surg 1984; 19(6):649–57.

13. Glick PL, Harrison MR, Noall RA, et al. Correction of congenital hydronephrosis in utero III. Early mid-trimester ureteral obstruction produces renal dysplasia. J Pediatr Surg 1983;18(6):681–7.

14. Estes JM, Harrison MR. Fetal obstructive uropathy. Semin Pediatr Surg 1993;2(2): 129–35.

15. Johnson MP, Danzer E, Koh J, et al, North American Fetal Therapy Network (NAFTNet). Natural history of fetal lower urinary tract obstruction with normal amniotic fluid volume at initial diagnosis. Fetal Diagn Ther 2018;44(1):10–7.

16. Crombleholme TM, Harrison MR, Longaker MT, et al. Prenatal diagnosis and management of bilateral hydronephrosis. Pediatr Nephrol 1988;2(3):334–42.

17. Enninga EA, Ruano R. Fetal surgery for lower urinary tract obstruction: the importance of staging prior to intervention. Minerva Pediatr 2018;70(3):263–9.

18. Morris RK, Quinlan-Jones E, Kilby MD, et al. Systematic review of accuracy of fetal urine analysis to predict poor postnatal renal function in cases of congenital urinary tract obstruction. Prenat Diagn 2007;27(10):900–11.

19. Johnson MP, Corsi P, Bradfield W, et al. Sequential urinalysis improves evaluation of fetal renal function in obstructive uropathy. Am J Obstet Gynecol 1995;173(1): 59–65.

20. Qureshi F, Jacques SM, Seifman B, et al. In utero fetal urine analysis and renal histology correlate with the outcome in fetal obstructive uropathies. Fetal Diagn Ther 1996;11(5):306–12.

21. Ruano R, Sananes N, Sangi-Haghpeykar H, et al. Fetal intervention for severe lower urinary tract obstruction: a multicenter case-control study comparing fetal cystoscopy with vesicoamniotic shunting. Ultrasound Obstet Gynecol 2015; 45(4):452–8.

22. Ruano R, Safdar A, Au J, et al. Defining and predicting 'intrauterine fetal renal failure' in congenital lower urinary tract obstruction. Pediatr Nephrol 2016;31(4): 605–12.

23. Sugarman J, Anderson J, Baschat AA, et al. Ethical considerations concerning amnioinfusions for treating fetal bilateral renal agenesis. Obstet Gynecol 2018; 131(1):130–4.
24. Vanderheyden T, Kumar S, Fisk NM. Fetal renal impairment. Semin Neonatol 2003;8(4):279–89.
25. Schwarz RD, Stephens FD, Cussen LJ. The pathogenesis of renal dysplasia. The significance of lateral and medial ectopy of the ureteric orifice. Invest Urol 1981; 19(2):97–100.
26. Morris RK, Malin GL, Quinlan-Jones E, et al. The Percutaneous Shunting in Lower Urinary Tract Obstruction (PLUTO) study and randomised controlled trial: evaluation of the effectiveness, cost-effectiveness and acceptability of percutaneous vesicoamniotic shunting for lower urinary tract obstruction. Health Technol Assess 2013;17(59):1–232.
27. Morris RK, Middleton LJ, Malin GL, et al, PLUTO Collaborative Group. Outcome in fetal lower urinary tract obstruction: a prospective registry study. Ultrasound Obstet Gynecol 2015;46(4):424–31.
28. Westerburg B, Feldstein VA, Sandberg PL, et al. Sonographic prognostic factors in fetuses with sacrococcygeal teratoma. J Pediatr Surg 2000;35(2):322–5 [discussion: 325–6].
29. Wilson RD, Hedrick H, Flake AW, et al. Sacrococcygeal teratomas: prenatal surveillance, growth and pregnancy outcome. Fetal Diagn Ther 2009;25(1):15–20.
30. Peiro JL, Sbragia L, Scorletti F, et al. Management of fetal teratomas. Pediatr Surg Int 2016;32(7):635–47.
31. Kitano Y, Flake AW, Crombleholme TM, et al. Open fetal surgery for life-threatening fetal malformations. Semin Perinatol 1999;23(6):448–61.
32. Van Mieghem T, Al-Ibrahim A, Deprest J, et al. Minimally invasive therapy for fetal sacrococcygeal teratoma: case series and systematic review of the literature. Ultrasound Obstet Gynecol 2014;43(6):611–9.
33. Adzick NS, Crombleholme TM, Morgan MA, et al. A rapidly growing fetal teratoma. Lancet 1997;349(9051):538.
34. Flake AW, Harrison MR, Adzick NS, et al. Fetal sacrococcygeal teratoma. J Pediatr Surg 1986;21(7):563–6.
35. Akinkuotu AC, Coleman A, Shue E, et al. Predictors of poor prognosis in prenatally diagnosed sacrococcygeal teratoma: a multiinstitutional review. J Pediatr Surg 2015;50(5):771–4.
36. Holcroft CJ, Blakemore KJ, Gurewitsch ED, et al. Large fetal sacrococcygeal teratomas: could early delivery improve outcome? Fetal Diagn Ther 2008;24(1): 55–60.
37. Gucciardo L, Uyttebroek A, De Wever I, et al. Prenatal assessment and management of sacrococcygeal teratoma. Prenat Diagn 2011;31(7):678–88.
38. Adzick NS, Kitano Y. Fetal surgery for lung lesions, congenital diaphragmatic hernia, and sacrococcygeal teratoma. Semin Pediatr Surg 2003;12(3):154–67.
39. Bond SJ, Harrison MR, Schmidt KG, et al. Death due to high-output cardiac failure in fetal sacrococcygeal teratoma. J Pediatr Surg 1990;25(12):1287–91.
40. Adzick NS. Open fetal surgery for life-threatening fetal anomalies. Semin Fetal Neonatal Med 2010;15(1):1–8.
41. Brace V, Grant SR, Brackley KJ, et al. Prenatal diagnosis and outcome in sacrococcygeal teratomas: A review of cases between 1992 and 1998. Prenat Diagn 2000;20(1):51–5.

42. Fadler KM, Askin DF. Sacrococcygeal teratoma in the newborn: a case study of prenatal management and clinical intervention. Neonatal Netw 2008;27(3): 185–91.

43. Graf JL, Albanese CT, Jennings RW, et al. Successful fetal sacrococcygeal teratoma resection in a hydropic fetus. J Pediatr Surg 2000;35(10):1489–91.

44. Ibele A, Flake A, Shaaban A. Survival of a profoundly hydropic fetus with a sacrococcygeal teratoma delivered at 27 weeks of gestation for maternal mirror syndrome. J Pediatr Surg 2008;43(8):e17–20.

45. Baumgarten HD, Gebb JS, Khalek N, et al. Preemptive delivery and immediate resection for fetuses with high-risk sacrococcygeal teratomas. Fetal Diagn Ther 2018;1–8 [Epub ahead of print].

46. Vrecenak JD, Flake AW. Fetal surgical intervention: progress and perspectives. Pediatr Surg Int 2013;29(5):407–17.

47. Danzer E, Johnson MP, Adzick NS. Fetal surgery for myelomeningocele: progress and perspectives. Dev Med Child Neurol 2012;54(1):8–14.

48. Adzick NS. Fetal Myelomeningocele: natural history, pathophysiology, and in-utero intervention. Semin Fetal Neonatal Med 2010;15(1):9–14.

49. Adzick NS, Thom EA, Spong CY, et al, MOMS Investigators. A randomized trial of prenatal versus postnatal repair of myelomeningocele. N Engl J Med 2011; 364(11):993–1004.

50. Adzick NS. Fetal surgery for spina bifida: past, present, future. Semin Pediatr Surg 2013;22(1):10–7.

51. Heuer GG, Adzick NS, Sutton LN. Fetal myelomeningocele closure: technical considerations. Fetal Diagn Ther 2015;37(3):166–71.

52. Kohl T, Hering R, Heep A, et al. Percutaneous fetoscopic patch coverage of spina bifida aperta in the human–early clinical experience and potential. Fetal Diagn Ther 2006;21(2):185–93.

53. Pedreira DA, Zanon N, Nishikuni K, et al. Endoscopic surgery for the antenatal treatment of myelomeningocele: The CECAM Trial. Am J Obstet Gynecol 2016; 214(1):e1–111.

54. Kohl T. Percutaneous minimally invasive fetoscopic surgery for spina bifida aperta. part I: surgical technique and perioperative outcome. Ultrasound Obstet Gynecol 2014;44(5):515–24.

55. Schoner K, Axt-Fliedner R, Bald R, et al. Fetal pathology of neural tube defects - an overview of 68 cases. Geburtshilfe Frauenheilkd 2017;77(5):495–507.

56. Belfort MA, Whitehead WE, Shamshirsaz AA, et al. Fetoscopic open neural tube defect repair: development and refinement of a two-port, carbon dioxide insufflation technique. Obstet Gynecol 2017;129(4):734–43.

57. Belfort MA, Whitehead WE, Bednov A, et al. Low-fidelity simulator for the standardized training of fetoscopic meningomyelocele repair. Obstet Gynecol 2018; 131(1):125–9.

58. Peiro JL, Fontecha CG, Ruano R, et al. Single-access fetal endoscopy (safe) for myelomeningocele in sheep model I: amniotic carbon dioxide gas approach. Surg Endosc 2013;27(10):3835–40.

59. Pedreira DA, Reece EA, Chmait RH, et al. Fetoscopic repair of spina bifida: safer and better? Ultrasound Obstet Gynecol 2016;48(2):141–7.

60. Kabagambe SK, Jensen GW, Chen YJ, et al. Fetal surgery for myelomeningocele: a systematic review and meta-analysis of outcomes in fetoscopic versus open repair. Fetal Diagn Ther 2018;43(3):161–74.

61. Joyeux L, Engels AC, Russo FM, et al. Fetoscopic versus open repair for spina bifida aperta: a systematic review of outcomes. Fetal Diagn Ther 2016;39(3):161–71.
62. Watanabe M, Li H, Kim AG, et al. Complete tissue coverage achieved by scaffold-based tissue engineering in the fetal sheep model of myelomeningocele. Biomaterials 2016;76:133–43.
63. Watanabe M, Kim AG, Flake AW. Tissue engineering strategies for fetal myelomeningocele repair in animal models. Fetal Diagn Ther 2015;37(3):197–205.
64. Brown EG, Saadai P, Pivetti CD, et al. In utero repair of myelomeningocele with autologous amniotic membrane in the fetal lamb model. J Pediatr Surg 2014;49(1):133–7 [discussion: 137–8].
65. Brown EG, Keller BA, Lankford L, et al. Age does matter: a pilot comparison of placenta-derived stromal cells for in utero repair of myelomeningocele using a lamb model. Fetal Diagn Ther 2016;39(3):179–85.
66. Adzick NS, Flake AW, Crombleholme TM. Management of congenital lung lesions. Semin Pediatr Surg 2003;12(1):10–6.
67. Crombleholme TM, Coleman B, Hedrick H, et al. Cystic adenomatoid malformation volume ratio predicts outcome in prenatally diagnosed cystic adenomatoid malformation of the lung. J Pediatr Surg 2002;37(3):331–8.
68. van der Veeken L, Russo FM, van der Merwe J, et al. Antenatal management of congenital diaphragmatic hernia today and tomorrow. Minerva Pediatr 2018;70(3):270–80.
69. Ruano R, Klinkner DB, Balakrishnan K, et al. Fetoscopic therapy for severe pulmonary hypoplasia in congenital diaphragmatic hernia: a first in prenatal regenerative medicine at Mayo Clinic. Mayo Clin Proc 2018;93(6):693–700.
70. Bebbington M, Victoria T, Danzer E, et al. Comparison of ultrasound and magnetic resonance imaging parameters in predicting survival in isolated left-sided congenital diaphragmatic hernia. Ultrasound Obstet Gynecol 2014;43(6):670–4.
71. Tsuda H, Kotani T, Miura M, et al. Observed-to-expected MRI fetal lung volume can predict long-term lung morbidity in infants with congenital diaphragmatic hernia. J Matern Fetal Neonatal Med 2017;30(13):1509–13.
72. Van der Veeken L, Russo FM, De Catte L, et al. Fetoscopic endoluminal tracheal occlusion and reestablishment of fetal airways for congenital diaphragmatic hernia. Gynecol Surg 2018;15(1):9.
73. Deprest J, Gratacos E, Nicolaides KH, et al. Fetoscopic Tracheal Occlusion (FETO) for severe congenital diaphragmatic hernia: evolution of a technique and preliminary results. Ultrasound Obstet Gynecol 2004;24(2):121–6.
74. Davey M, Shegu S, Danzer E, et al. Pulmonary arteriole muscularization in lambs with diaphragmatic hernia after combined tracheal occlusion/glucocorticoid therapy. Am J Obstet Gynecol 2007;197(4):381.e1-7.
75. Danzer E, Davey MG, Kreiger PA, et al. Fetal tracheal occlusion for severe congenital diaphragmatic hernia in humans: a morphometric study of lung parenchyma and muscularization of pulmonary arterioles. J Pediatr Surg 2008;43(10):1767–75.
76. Harrison MR, Keller RL, Hawgood SB, et al. A randomized trial of fetal endoscopic tracheal occlusion for severe fetal congenital diaphragmatic hernia. N Engl J Med 2003;349(20):1916–24.
77. Al-Maary J, Eastwood MP, Russo FM, et al. Fetal tracheal occlusion for severe pulmonary hypoplasia in isolated congenital diaphragmatic hernia: a systematic review and meta-analysis of survival. Ann Surg 2016;264(6):929–33.

78. Flake AW. Prenatal intervention: ethical considerations for life-threatening and non-life-threatening anomalies. Semin Pediatr Surg 2001;10(4):212–21.
79. Antiel RM, Curlin FA, Lantos JD, et al. Attitudes of paediatric and obstetric specialists towards prenatal surgery for lethal and non-lethal conditions. J Med Ethics 2018;44(4):234–8.
80. Flake AW. Surgery in the human fetus: the future. J Physiol 2003;547(Pt 1):45–51.
81. Flake AW. Fetal intervention: improving evidence and expanding applications. Semin Fetal Neonatal Med 2017;22(6):359.
82. Kumar P, Gao K, Wang C, et al. In utero transplantation of placenta-derived mesenchymal stromal cells for potential fetal treatment of hemophilia A. Cell Transplant 2018;27(1):130–9.
83. Riley JS, McClain LE, Stratigis JD, et al. Pre-existing maternal antibodies cause rapid prenatal rejection of allotransplants in the mouse model of in utero hematopoietic cell transplantation. J Immunol 2018;201(5):1549–57.
84. Witt R, MacKenzie TC, Peranteau WH. Fetal stem cell and gene therapy. Semin Fetal Neonatal Med 2017;22(6):410–4.
85. MacKenzie TC. Future AAVenues for in utero gene therapy. Cell Stem Cell 2018;23(3):320–32.
86. Kreger EM, Singer ST, Witt RG, et al. Favorable outcomes after in utero transfusion in fetuses with alpha thalassemia major: a case series and review of the literature. Prenat Diagn 2016;36(13):1242–9.
87. Ahn NJ, Stratigis JD, Coons BE, et al. Intravenous and intra-amniotic in utero transplantation in the murine model. J Vis Exp 2018;(140). https://doi.org/10.3791/58047.
88. Rossidis AC, Stratigis JD, Chadwick AC, et al. In utero CRISPR-mediated therapeutic editing of metabolic genes. Nat Med 2018;24(10):1513–8.
89. Partridge EA, Davey MG, Hornick MA, et al. An EXTrauterine environment for neonatal development: EXTENDING fetal physiology beyond the womb. Semin Fetal Neonatal Med 2017;22(6):404–9.
90. Partridge EA, Davey MG, Hornick MA, et al. An Extra-uterine system to physiologically support the extreme premature lamb. Nat Commun 2017;8:15112.
91. Chervenak FA, McCullough LB. The ethics of maternal-fetal surgery. Semin Fetal Neonatal Med 2018;23(1):64–7.

Recent Recommendations and Emerging Science in Neonatal Resuscitation

Marilyn B. Escobedo, MD*, Birju A. Shah, MD, MPH, MBA,
Clara Song, MD, Abhishek Makkar, MD, Edgardo Szyld, MD, MSc

KEYWORDS

• Resuscitation • Newborn • Delivery room • Training • Laryngeal mask • Simulation

KEY POINTS

• The Neonatal Resuscitation Program (NRP) has evolved in the last several decades from expert opinion to evidence-based practice.

• Effective positive pressure ventilation continues to be the most important intervention during neonatal resuscitation.

• Major recent changes in NRP recommendations include delayed cord clamping, use of electrocardiographic monitoring, and rescinding the mandate on endotracheal suctioning of nonvigorous infants born through meconium-stained amniotic fluid.

• Emerging science in the use of oxygen, cord management, and the use of laryngeal masks will contribute to future recommendations.

• New technologies such as video laryngoscopy and telemedicine hold promise for improving education, training, and delivery of practice.

BACKGROUND

The Neonatal Resuscitation Program (NRP) was launched by the American Academy of Pediatrics (AAP) in 1987 with the publication of the first textbook, an innovative algorithmic approach to newborn resuscitation.[1] The program was initiated as an expert and consensus-based guideline because resuscitation science was nascent at the time. This new paradigm had an ambitious goal of having a trained individual at the birth of every infant in the United States. To accomplish this aim, the committee embarked on training a pyramid of instructors: national instructors would train regional instructors who would train hospital instructors, and these instructors would teach the

Disclosure Statement: The authors have nothing to disclose.
Neonatal-Perinatal Medicine, Department of Pediatrics, Children's Hospital, University of Oklahoma Health Sciences Center, 1200 North Everett Drive, ETNP7504, Oklahoma City, OK 73104, USA
* Corresponding author. 118 Tower Drive, San Antonio, TX 78232.
E-mail address: Marilyn-Escobedo@ouhsc.edu

bedside providers. The tenet of equality of team members, which included doctors, nurses, and respiratory therapists, was established. The NRP Steering Committee (NRPSC), made up of volunteers with an interest and expertise in neonatal resuscitation, supported by staff from the AAP and joined by liaisons from other professional groups, has provided robust leadership for the program's development. The textbook has been periodically revised and is now in its seventh edition.[2] Major developments in the NRP over the past three decades include:

1. Fostering resuscitation research
2. Establishing scientific evidence-based guidelines
3. Integrating cognitive, technical, and behavioral skills into individual and team performance

The NRPSC has supported resuscitation research through an annual grant competition for both early and established investigators. Other funding sources for resuscitation have been actively encouraged, with positive results.

Establishing a neonatal work group within the International Liaison Committee on Resuscitation (ILCOR) has advanced the scientific evidence base for guidelines. The ILCOR Neonatal Work Group, composed of international volunteer neonatologists, reviews the scientific evidence of the world's literature and produces a consensus summary, which is the basis for guidelines created by neonatal resuscitation councils globally. This work is available as Consensus on Science and Recommendations at eccguidelines.heart.org. If there are scientific gaps with low level or absent scientific support, a pragmatic approach is taken.[3] The program continues to be faced with the challenge of training providers for low-frequency events that have significant consequences. Developing delivery room technologies, such as telemedicine and videolaryngoscopy, provide the opportunity for improvements in performance and practice.

CURRENT NRP GUIDELINES

The seventh edition of the Textbook of Neonatal Resuscitation includes changes in the NRP training program, mandated at the beginning of 2017.[2] The current guidelines, as well as a summary of the emerging science in that area, are summarized herein.

Predelivery Anticipatory Preparation

During the birth of every newborn, the potential need for resuscitation must be anticipated. Thus, at least one clinician who is skilled in basic neonatal resuscitation should be present at every delivery, and this person must be available exclusively to assess the infant and provide intervention (for example, positive pressure ventilation [PPV]) if needed. Risk factors that increase the likelihood for the need for resuscitation should be ascertained before delivery, if possible, and provision of additional personnel trained in advanced resuscitation should be arranged. Rapid neonatal response teams should be immediately available for the unanticipated infant who requires resuscitation.[2,4]

When neonatal resuscitation is anticipated based on maternal or fetal factors, neonatal providers should meet with family before delivery, when feasible. All perinatal team members (obstetric and neonatal care providers, and the parents) should discuss resuscitation options and agree on a plan.

Timing of Umbilical Cord Clamping

Previously the procedure of umbilical cord clamping had been considered the obstetric team's domain and was routinely performed soon after delivery of infants born in the United States and many other areas of the world.[5] More recently, with new data about the benefits of delayed cord clamping, the NRP has provided recommendations about this procedure. The 2017 NRP guidelines recommend a 30- to 60-second delay in clamping in all term and preterm infants not requiring resuscitation. If the placental circulation is disrupted (eg, placental abruption), the cord should be clamped immediately.[6] Major evidence gaps remain regarding the timing of cord clamping in newborns requiring resuscitation because these patients were generally excluded from many of the studies on the timing of cord clamping.[3]

Emerging science

Since the 2015 ILCOR review and publication of the seventh edition of the NRP textbook, the American College of Obstetricians and Gynecologists has recommended delayed (30–60 seconds) cord clamping for both term and preterm infants.[7,8] A recent systematic review and meta-analysis by Fogarty and colleagues[9] examined this new practice of delayed clamping (comparing a delay of 30 seconds or more with early clamping that was <30 seconds). The investigators analyzed data from 18 randomized controlled trials of 2834 preterm and term infants and found that delayed clamping reduced mortality before discharge.

Research is focused on determining the optimal timing of cord clamping in depressed infants. Many physiologic studies, both in animal models and in humans, of dynamic blood flow within and through the cord have deepened our understanding of the hemodynamic complexity of the placental transfusion at birth. In a preterm lamb model, Bhatt and coworkers[10] explored the hemodynamic differences between ventilation before and after cord clamping. They found that when the lung was not ventilated before cord clamping, the transitional circulation was characterized by bradycardia and cerebral blood pressure fluctuations. Katheria and colleagues[11] performed a clinical trial comparing delayed clamping with resuscitation performed on the delivery table versus early cord clamping with resuscitation performed on the warmer. They found no differences in outcomes such as hematocrit, need for phototherapy, or intraventricular hemorrhage. A large randomized controlled trial of resuscitation (VentFirst) of depressed preterm infants before cord clamping is under way.[12]

A possible alternative to delayed cord clamping for placental transfusion facilitation is the cord-milking technique. In this procedure the obstetric provider compresses the cord, moving the blood toward the newborn. This maneuver is accomplished by milking the intact unclamped cord 4 to 5 times. Another option is to clamp and cut a long segment of the cord immediately after birth and then milk the cord. The major advantage of either method of cord milking is that the newborn can be passed to the awaiting resuscitation team without delay while preserving the receipt of the placental transfusion. Katheria and colleagues[13] recently reviewed the evidence in term and preterm newborns supporting the practices of delayed cord clamping, intact umbilical cord milking, and cut-umbilical cord milking. However, Blank and colleagues[14] showed that umbilical cord–milking strategies compared with physiologically based cord clamping caused considerable hemodynamic disturbances in a preterm sheep model; thus, further study is warranted.

Initial Steps

Thermal defense of term and especially preterm infants remains a key factor in neonatal resuscitation. For small preterm infants, hypothermia is consistently associated with higher mortality and serious morbidities.[8] Delivery room temperatures should be at 23°C to 25°C (74°F–77°F).[15] A combination of techniques, including plastic wrapping, thermal mattresses, radiant warmers, caps, and warmed humidified gases for resuscitation are recommended for preterm infants born at <32 weeks' gestation. Nonasphyxiated newborns should have axillary temperatures of 36.5°C to 37.5°C (97.7°F–99.5° F). Hyperthermia should be avoided.[8]

Airway Management in the Event of Meconium-Stained Amniotic Fluid

Suctioning of newborns should be performed only if the airway is obstructed or if PPV is needed.[6,16] In nonvigorous infants born through meconium-stained amniotic fluid (MSAF), current recommendations include intubation and endotracheal suctioning only for those who need it for ventilation or airway obstruction.[3] Because MSAF remains an important risk factor for resuscitation need, a person skilled in intubation should still be immediately available for these births.[6]

Emerging science

The discontinuation of routine endotracheal suctioning in nonvigorous infants born through MSAF is supported by several small international studies. Singh and colleagues,[17] in a recent randomized controlled trial, found that although suctioned infants tend to have a lower incidence of meconium aspiration syndrome (MAS), the overall incidence of respiratory distress and mortality was similar in the suctioned and unsuctioned groups. Chettri and coworkers[18] and Nangia and colleagues[19] showed in two different randomized controlled trials, which included 297 infants, that there was no difference in the incidence of MAS severity or complications, mortality, or neurodevelopmental outcome measured by developmental assessment scales or incidence of hypoxic ischemic encephalopathy. A Cochrane review is in progress evaluating the efficacy of tracheal suctioning at birth in preventing MAS in this population.[20] Observational trials are beginning to provide evidence for the impact of this change in practice.[21]

Assessment of Heart Rate

Heart rate is the critical indicator for signaling the need for intervention in neonatal resuscitation and evaluating the patient's response to these interventions. Auscultation of the precordium has been the standard assessment method with the adjunctive use of pulse oximetry. However, studies comparing electrocardiogram (ECG) use with both auscultation and pulse oximetry show that ECG monitoring revealed the heart rate more rapidly and accurately.[3] Katheria and colleagues[22] found in a pilot trial that using ECG supported earlier and more accurate assessment, which in turn allowed earlier intervention. Current recommendations are to consider using a 3-lead ECG for rapid and accurate heart rate assessment when PPV is initiated. ECG is the preferred method of assessment once chest compressions begin.[6]

Oxygenation Assessment and Administration

It is recommended that room air (21% O_2 at sea level) be used at the initiation of resuscitation in infants born at ≥35 weeks' gestation. In healthy term infants, supplemental oxygen should be used as needed to achieve saturation targets using pulse oximetry.[6,8] For preterm infants less than 35 weeks' gestation, the current recommendation is to begin resuscitation with 21% to 30% supplemental O_2 and titrate to saturation targets similar to term infants.[6,8] An optimal approach is not yet determined.

Emerging science

Preterm infants may benefit from target oxygen saturations that are based on gestational age. Oei and colleagues[23] recently analyzed individual patient data for 768 patients with birth gestational ages less than 32 weeks from 8 randomized controlled trials of lower versus higher initial Fio_2 (fraction of inspired oxygen) strategies targeted to specific predetermined oxygen saturation (Spo_2) before 10 min of age. They found that failing to reach Spo_2 of 80% at 5 minutes was associated with adverse outcomes including intraventricular hemorrhage, and risk of death was significantly increased with time to reach Spo_2 80%.

Ventilation

PPV is indicated for apneic or gasping infants and when heart rate is <100 beats/min. PPV may also be initiated in spontaneously breathing infants with heart rates greater than 100 beats/min who do not maintain oxygen saturations within the target range despite continuous positive airway pressure or free-flowing oxygen. During PPV, the continued recommendation is to start with a positive inspiratory pressure of 20 to 25 cm H_2O. A positive end-expiratory pressure (PEEP) of 5 cm H_2O is recommended; to attain this goal with self-inflating bags, a PEEP valve is necessary.[6,8]

A rising heart rate remains the cardinal indicator of successful ventilation. If the infant's heart rate does not increase after 15 seconds, ventilation-corrective steps should be taken. If the heart rate continues to fail to increase, tracheal obstruction should be considered and suctioning of the airway performed.[6]

Endotracheal Intubation and Laryngeal Mask Airway

Endotracheal intubation is indicated for ineffective or prolonged PPV or for special circumstances such as an abnormal airway anatomy. Intubation is strongly recommended when chest compressions are needed. A laryngeal mask airway may serve as an alternative airway interface when endotracheal intubation is not successful in term or larger preterm neonates. Laryngeal mask usage remains limited, owing to the lack of appropriately sized devices for the smaller infant and limited data to support their use.[3,6,8]

Emerging science

Laryngeal mask airways, with technological advances, are now available in many forms and configurations (**Fig. 1**). Although the original laryngeal mask airway was a multiuse device, cleaning requirements and high cost have steered providers toward less costly, single-use devices. Newer-generation devices provide higher seal pressures resulting from improved seal material or design, and some feature a gastric access port to vent or aspirate gastric contents.[24] Evidence for the broader use of the laryngeal mask for airway management and medication administration is developing. In 3 studies evaluating 158 infants, there were no clinically significant differences in insertion time or failure to correctly insert a laryngeal mask when compared with endotracheal intubation.[25] The use of a laryngeal mask is particularly valuable with diminishing exposure of trainees in neonatal tracheal intubation. Interhospital transfers, including air transport, of infants with congenital airway malformations have been managed with a size 1 (infants weighing <5 kg) laryngeal mask without administering sedatives or anesthetic drugs before device insertion.[26] Laryngeal mask airways used to administer anesthesia were associated with significantly fewer respiratory adverse events compared with endotracheal tubes in a randomized controlled trial of 181 infants undergoing minor elective procedures.[27]

Although there is limited evidence of the safety and efficacy of epinephrine via laryngeal mask in human neonates, recent studies demonstrate the effectiveness of laryngeal mask devices as conduits for surfactant administration.[28] Three trials (conducted by Pinheiro, Barbosa, and Roberts) successfully used laryngeal masks for surfactant administration.[29–31]

The laryngeal mask airway could become the preferred primary interface in neonatal resuscitation. Providing effective PPV is considered the single most important

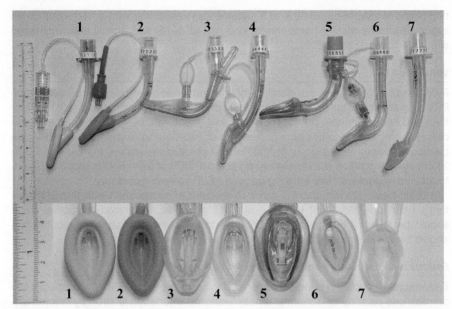

Fig. 1. Size 1 laryngeal masks. (1) Ultimate, (2) PRO-Breathe, (3) Supreme, (4) Unique, (5) air-Q, (6) AuroOnce, and (7) i-gel. (*From* Tracy MB, Priyadarshi A, Goel D, et al. How do different brands of size 1 laryngeal mask airway compare with face mask ventilation in a dedicated laryngeal mask airway teaching manikin? Arch Dis Child Fetal Neonatal Ed 2018;103(3):F273; with permission.)

component of successful neonatal resuscitation. Face mask ventilation may be difficult to perform successfully, resulting in prolonged resuscitation or neonatal asphyxia. A recent Cochrane review examining 5 trials with 661 infants showed superiority of laryngeal mask to face mask ventilation in achieving spontaneous breathing and decreasing the need for intubation.[25] This benefit is especially relevant for resources-limited environments including rural settings and/or developing countries. The pros and cons of using a laryngeal mask airway are summarized in **Table 1**.

Chest Compressions

Chest compressions are indicated when heart rate remains less than 60 beats/min after at least 30 seconds of PPV. When chest compressions begin, supplemental O_2

Table 1	
Pros and cons of use of laryngeal mask airway	
Pros	**Cons**
Quickly learnable by unskilled operators	Limited evidence for infants <34 wk gestation or birth weight <1500 g
Newer-generation devices with improved design and material	Potential for laryngospasm and soft-tissue injury (both are rare)
Faster placement as a result of easy insertion	
Better seal, negating the need for ventilation-corrective steps	Proper positioning needed for effectiveness
Better outcomes[25]	Potential for gastric distention (gastric vent available)

may be increased until the heart rate recovers and weaned rapidly afterward. In this scenario, ECG is preferred for assessing heart rate.[3,6,8]

Medications: Epinephrine

Epinephrine is indicated when the heart rate is <60 beats/min after 60 seconds of chest compressions coordinated with PPV using 100% O_2. Epinephrine can be administered by the intravenous (IV) or intraosseous (IO) route.[6,8] A higher dose may be given via the endotracheal route while IV or IO access is being obtained, although evidence for the efficacy of this practice remains lacking.[3,8]

Ethics and Care at End of Life

If the newborn is assessed to have no chance of survival by the responsible physician, initiating resuscitation is not an ethical option and should not be offered.[3,8] In conditions associated with a high risk of early death or significant burden of morbidity for the infant, decisions should be carefully discussed with parents.[3,6]

An Apgar score of 0 at 10 minutes of age remains highly correlated with mortality and serious morbidity. If a heartbeat remains undetectable after 10 minutes of resuscitative efforts, NRP states that it is reasonable to discontinue the efforts. This decision may be individualized depending on factors of the quality of the resuscitation efforts, the specific circumstances of the etiology of the event, and the availability/applicability of hypothermia treatment.[3,6,8]

EMERGING AREAS OF DEVELOPMENT IN RESUSCITATION TRAINING AND DELIVERY OF CARE
Education

The NRP instruction has progressively incorporated individual skills building and team function into the format of education since its inception. The most recent platform is Internet-based and uses both simulation and team performance.[32]

Emerging science

A growing body of evidence shows that simulation is a standardized technique for teaching neonatal resuscitation.[33] Simulation may be the preferred teaching model for resuscitation because of the need for quick critical analysis, communication skills, team-building behaviors, and procedural expertise, such as neonatal endotracheal intubation.[34]

Having a provider skilled at endotracheal intubation is key to preventing not only complications from birth asphyxia but also soft-tissue and airway damage, pneumothorax, esophageal perforation, and death that can arise as a result of deficient laryngoscope handling and tube positioning.[35] Proficiency in neonatal intubation is a procedural requirement for all pediatric trainees by the Pediatric Residency Review Committee of the Accreditation Council for Graduate Medical Education.[36] However, even after NRP training, numerous reports conclude that many providers remain feeling unprepared to resuscitate a newborn, much less being able to proficiently perform neonatal intubation.[37,38] Finer and Rich videotaped actual neonatal resuscitative efforts and identified gaps in acquired and maintained skills.[39] Simulation-based training was identified as a new teaching strategy to address these translational gaps and to foster mastery learning.[40–42]

Videolaryngoscopy (VL) is emerging as a helpful educational tool for endotracheal intubation. A randomized controlled trial by Volz and colleagues[43] revealed higher success rates for neonatal intubation among trainees after practice with VL, in comparison with traditional training, confirming previous studies.[44–46]

Real-time media-enhanced feedback may augment the simulation-based training experience. The authors demonstrated that the addition of Google Glass, wearable eyeglasses allowing real-time video feedback, when teaching neonatal endotracheal intubation to novice learners, shortens successful intubation time and increases confidence scores in a simulation environment.[47]

Ongoing simulation-based training is a step toward mastery learning. The most recent seventh edition of NRP stresses the importance of simulation debriefing, which encourages reflection on learning experiences for better retention of both knowledge and skills.[48]

Telemedicine

As the sophistication of the science and the demands of complex medical conditions advance, the difficulties of providing a high level of care in health care systems escalate. Telemedicine is a relatively new tool that can be used to extend the provision of low-frequency/high-consequence resuscitations for newborns and support resuscitation education.

Emerging science

Telemedicine is rapidly becoming an important tool for enhancing skilled provision of neonatal resuscitation. The AAP recommends that infants born at less than 32 weeks' gestation should be delivered at level III neonatal intensive care units (NICUs) because mortality rates are lower among very low birth weight infants delivered and treated at appropriate facilities.[49–52] Yet in many states less than 80% of women of reproductive age live within 50 miles of a level III NICU.[53] One promising solution to address the rural-urban disparity in access to subspecialty care is the use of telemedicine.[54–57] In simulated settings, telemedicine has been shown to decrease the time needed to establish effective ventilation. Fang and colleagues[58] compared the outcomes of infants who received a teleneonatology consult during resuscitation with controls who did not. Neonates who received a teleneonatology consult had a higher median quality rating evaluated by a blinded expert panel compared with the control group.

Recent work has demonstrated the feasibility and safety of a newborn resuscitation telemedicine program (NRTP) to remotely assist local providers with resuscitation.[59] Appropriate equipment for telemedicine application is essential for the audiovisual connection between the consultant at the remote site and the local provider. Both wired and wireless devices have been used in emergency telemedicine clinical settings. Beck and colleagues[60] recently conducted a study to compare the two technologies. A highly reliable connection is key for NRTP, owing to the critical nature of consults as assessments and interventions occur at 30-s to 1-min intervals during newborn resuscitation. Therefore, a wired connection device is probably the more reliable option to provide consultation in highly emergent settings.

Implementation of NRTP presents challenges because it differs substantially from the conventional way of providing neonatal resuscitation.[61] Key to the successful implementation of telemedicine is the inclusion of local stakeholders in the planning and design of clinical workflows. Although most providers in community settings are NRP trained, the lack of continued exposure to newborn resuscitation leads to decay in both knowledge and skills. Continuing education, including NRP and mock codes using telemedicine, are helpful to prepare the team for smooth application of NRTP when the need arises.

SUMMARY

Current recommendations in the seventh edition of the NRP textbook, effective in 2017 and reflected in the training program, were updated on the basis of the ILCOR review and consensus on science. Emerging science in many areas, including management of umbilical cord clamping, oxygen use, ventilation, rapid and accurate patient assessments, and laryngeal mask airway use will undoubtedly inform future recommendations. Exciting new technologies, such as telemedicine, may extend the benefits of our knowledge and improve our delivery of care. The developing science of human factors in neonatal resuscitation continues to improve the training and performance of skilled providers for these patients at the critical time of birth.

REFERENCES

1. Bloom R, Cropley C. Textbook of neonatal resuscitation/Ronald S, Vol 1. Elk Grove Village (IL): American Academy of Pediatrics; 1987.
2. Weiner G. Textbook of neonatal resuscitation. 7th edition. Elk Grove Village (IL): American Academy of Pediatrics; 2016.
3. Perlman JM, Wyllie J, Kattwinkel J, et al. Part 7: neonatal resuscitation: 2015 international consensus on cardiopulmonary resuscitation and emergency cardiovascular care science with treatment recommendations. Circulation 2015;132(16 Suppl 1):S204–41.
4. Foglia EE, Langeveld R, Heimall L, et al. Incidence, characteristics, and survival following cardiopulmonary resuscitation in the quaternary neonatal intensive care unit. Resuscitation 2017;110:32–6.
5. World Health Organization. Guideline: delayed umbilical cord clamping for improved maternal and infant health and nutrition outcomes. Geneva (Switzerland): World Health Organization; 2014.
6. Weiner GM, Zaichkin J, American Academy of Pediatrics, American Heart Association. Textbook of neonatal resuscitation (NRP). Elk Grove Village (IL): American Academy of Pediatrics; 2016.
7. Committee on Obstetric Practice. Delayed umbilical cord clamping after birth (Committee Opinion No 684). Obstet Gynecol 2017;129(1):e5–10.
8. Wyckoff MH, Aziz K, Escobedo MB, et al. Part 13: neonatal resuscitation: 2015 American Heart Association guidelines update for cardiopulmonary resuscitation and emergency cardiovascular care (reprint). Pediatrics 2015;136(2):14.
9. Fogarty M, Osborn DA, Askie L, et al. Delayed vs early umbilical cord clamping for preterm infants: a systematic review and meta-analysis. Am J Obstet Gynecol 2018;218(1):1–18.
10. Bhatt S, Alison BJ, Wallace EM, et al. Delaying cord clamping until ventilation onset improves cardiovascular function at birth in preterm lambs. J Physiol 2013;591(8):2113–26.
11. Katheria AC, Brown MK, Faksh A, et al. Delayed cord clamping in newborns born at term at risk for resuscitation: a feasibility randomized clinical trial. J Pediatr 2017;187:313–7.e1.
12. Winter J, Kattwinkel J, Chisholm C, et al. Ventilation of preterm infants during delayed cord clamping (VentFirst): a pilot study of feasibility and safety. Am J Perinatol 2017;34(2):111–6.
13. Katheria AC, Lakshminrusimha S, Rabe H, et al. Placental transfusion: a review. J Perinatol 2017;37(2):105–11.
14. Blank DA, Polglase GR, Kluckow M, et al. Haemodynamic effects of umbilical cord milking in premature sheep during the neonatal transition. Arch Dis Child Fetal Neonatal Ed 2018;103(6):F539–46.

15. Jia YS, Lin ZL, Lv H, et al. Effect of delivery room temperature on the admission temperature of premature infants: a randomized controlled trial. J Perinatol 2013; 33(4):264–7.

16. Perlman JM, Wyllie J, Kattwinkel J, et al. Part 11: neonatal resuscitation: 2010 international consensus on cardiopulmonary resuscitation and emergency cardiovascular care science with treatment recommendations. Circulation 2010;122(16 Suppl 2):S516–38.

17. Singh S, Saxena S, Bhriguvanshi A, et al. Effect of endotracheal suctioning just after birth in non-vigorous infants born through meconium stained amniotic fluid: a randomized controlled trial. Clin Epidemiol Glob Health 2018. https://doi.org/10.1016/j.cegh.2018.03.006.

18. Chettri S, Adhisivam B, Bhat BV. Endotracheal suction for nonvigorous neonates born through meconium stained amniotic fluid: a randomized controlled trial. J Pediatr 2015;166(5):1208–13.

19. Nangia S, Sunder S, Biswas R, et al. Endotracheal suction in term non vigorous meconium stained neonates-a pilot study. Resuscitation 2016;105:79–84.

20. Nangia S, Thukral A, Chawla D. Tracheal suction at birth in non-vigorous neonates born through meconium-stained amniotic fluid. Cochrane Library Syst Rev 2017. https://doi.org/10.1002/14651858.CD012671.

21. Viraraghavan VR, Nangia S, Prathik BH, et al. Yield of meconium in non-vigorous neonates undergoing endotracheal suctioning and profile of all neonates born through meconium-stained amniotic fluid: a prospective observational study. Paediatr Int Child Health 2018;38(4):266–70.

22. Katheria A, Arnell K, Brown M, et al. A pilot randomized controlled trial of EKG for neonatal resuscitation. PLoS One 2017;12(11):e0187730.

23. Oei JL, Finer NN, Saugstad OD, et al. Outcomes of oxygen saturation targeting during delivery room stabilisation of preterm infants. Arch Dis Child Fetal Neonatal Ed 2018;103(5):F446–54.

24. Tracy MB, Priyadarshi A, Goel D, et al. How do different brands of size 1 laryngeal mask airway compare with face mask ventilation in a dedicated laryngeal mask airway teaching manikin? Arch Dis Child Fetal Neonatal Ed 2018;103(3):F271–6.

25. Qureshi MJ, Kumar M. Laryngeal mask airway versus bag-mask ventilation or endotracheal intubation for neonatal resuscitation. Cochrane Database Syst Rev 2018;(3):CD003314.

26. Schmolzer GM, Agarwal M, Kamlin CO, et al. Supraglottic airway devices during neonatal resuscitation: an historical perspective, systematic review and meta-analysis of available clinical trials. Resuscitation 2013;84(6):722–30.

27. Drake-Brockman TF, Ramgolam A, Zhang G, et al. The effect of endotracheal tubes versus laryngeal mask airways on perioperative respiratory adverse events in infants: a randomised controlled trial. Lancet 2017;389(10070):701–8.

28. Wagner M, Olischar M, O'Reilly M, et al. Review of routes to administer medication during prolonged neonatal resuscitation. Pediatr Crit Care Med 2018;19(4): 332–8.

29. Pinheiro JM, Santana-Rivas Q, Pezzano C. Randomized trial of laryngeal mask airway versus endotracheal intubation for surfactant delivery. J Perinatol 2016; 36(3):196–201.

30. Barbosa RF, Simoes ESAC, Silva YP. A randomized controlled trial of the laryngeal mask airway for surfactant administration in neonates. J Pediatr (Rio J) 2017;93(4):343–50.

31. Roberts KD, Brown R, Lampland AL, et al. Laryngeal mask airway for surfactant administration in neonates: a randomized, controlled trial. J Pediatr 2018;193: 40–6.e41.
32. Zaichkin J, McCarney L, Weiner G. NRP 7th edition: are you prepared? Neonatal Netw 2016;35(4):184–91.
33. Ades A, Lee HC. Update on simulation for the neonatal resuscitation program. Semin Perinatol 2016;40(7):447–54.
34. Rubio-Gurung S, Putet G, Touzet S, et al. In situ simulation training for neonatal resuscitation: an RCT. Pediatrics 2014;134(3):e790–7.
35. Haubner LY, Barry JS, Johnston LC, et al. Neonatal intubation performance: room for improvement in tertiary neonatal intensive care units. Resuscitation 2013; 84(10):1359–64.
36. Accreditation Council for Graduate Medical Education. ACGME program require- ments for graduate medical education in pediatrics. 2017. Available at: https:// www.acgme.org/Portals/0/PFAssets/ProgramRequirements/320_pediatrics_2017- 07-01.pdf. Accessed August 29, 2018.
37. Cordero L, Hart BJ, Hardin R, et al. Pediatrics residents' preparedness for neonatal resuscitation assessed using high-fidelity simulation. J Grad Med Educ 2013;5(3):399–404.
38. Robinson ME, Diaz I, Barrowman NJ, et al. Trainees success rates with intubation to suction meconium at birth. Arch Dis Child Fetal Neonatal Ed 2018;103(5): F413–6.
39. Finer NN, Rich W. Neonatal resuscitation: toward improved performance. Resus- citation 2002;53(1):47–51.
40. Halamek LP, Kaegi DM, Gaba DM, et al. Time for a new paradigm in pediatric medical education: teaching neonatal resuscitation in a simulated delivery room environment. Pediatrics 2000;106(4):E45.
41. Wood FE, Morley CJ, Dawson JA, et al. Improved techniques reduce face mask leak during simulated neonatal resuscitation: study 2. Arch Dis Child Fetal Neonatal Ed 2008;93(3):F230–4.
42. Sawyer T, Sierocka-Castaneda A, Chan D, et al. Deliberate practice using simu- lation improves neonatal resuscitation performance. Simul Healthc 2011;6(6): 327–36.
43. Volz S, Stevens TP, Dadiz R. A randomized controlled trial: does coaching using video during direct laryngoscopy improve residents' success in neonatal intuba- tions? J Perinatol 2018;38(8):1074–80.
44. Moussa A, Luangxay Y, Tremblay S, et al. Videolaryngoscope for teaching neonatal endotracheal intubation: a randomized controlled trial. Pediatrics 2016;137(3):e20152156.
45. O'Shea JE, Thio M, Kamlin CO, et al. Videolaryngoscopy to teach neonatal intu- bation: a randomized trial. Pediatrics 2015;136(5):912–9.
46. Pouppirt NR, Foglia EE, Ades A. A video is worth a thousand words: innovative uses of videolaryngoscopy. Arch Dis Child Fetal Neonatal Ed 2018;103(5): F401–2.
47. Song CH, Choi A, Roebuck B, et al. Real-time, media-enhanced feedback im- proves neonatal intubation skills. Am Acad Pediatr 2018.
48. Sawyer T, Ades A, Ernst K, et al. Simulation and the neonatal resuscitation pro- gram 7th edition curriculum. Neoreviews 2016;17(8):e447–53.
49. Dooley SL, Freels SA, Turnock BJ. Quality assessment of perinatal regionalization by multivariate analysis: Illinois, 1991-1993. Obstet Gynecol 1997;89(2):193–8.

50. Gortmaker S, Sobol A, Clark C, et al. The survival of very low-birth weight infants by level of hospital of birth: a population study of perinatal systems in four states. Am J Obstet Gynecol 1985;152(5):517–24.

51. American Academy of Pediatrics Committee on Fetus and Newborn. Levels of neonatal care. Pediatrics 2012;130(3):587–97.

52. Lorch SA, Baiocchi M, Ahlberg CE, et al. The differential impact of delivery hospital on the outcomes of premature infants. Pediatrics 2012;130(2):270–8.

53. Brantley MD, Davis NL, Goodman DA, et al. Perinatal regionalization: a geospatial view of perinatal critical care, United States, 2010-2013. Am J Obstet Gynecol 2017;216(2):185.e1–10.

54. Wang SK, Callaway NF, Wallenstein MB, et al. SUNDROP: six years of screening for retinopathy of prematurity with telemedicine. Can J Ophthalmol 2015;50(2): 101–6.

55. Makkar A, McCoy M, Hallford G, et al. A hybrid form of telemedicine: a unique way to extend intensive care service to neonates in medically underserved areas. Telemed J E Health 2018;24(9):717–21.

56. Jain A, Agarwal R, Chawla D, et al. Tele-education vs classroom training of neonatal resuscitation: a randomized trial. J Perinatol 2010;30(12):773–9.

57. Wenger TL, Gerdes J, Taub K, et al. Telemedicine for genetic and neurologic evaluation in the neonatal intensive care unit. J Perinatol 2014;34(3):234–40.

58. Fang JL, Carey WA, Lang TR, et al. Real-time video communication improves provider performance in a simulated neonatal resuscitation. Resuscitation 2014; 85(11):1518–22.

59. Fang JL, Campbell MS, Weaver AL, et al. The impact of telemedicine on the quality of newborn resuscitation: a retrospective study. Resuscitation 2018;125:48–55.

60. Beck JA, Jensen JA, Putzier RF, et al. Developing a newborn resuscitation telemedicine program: a comparison of two technologies. Telemed J E Health 2018;24(7):481–8.

61. Fang JL, Asiedu GB, Harris AM, et al. A mixed-methods study on the barriers and facilitators of telemedicine for newborn resuscitation. Telemed J E Health 2018; 24(10):811–7.

Evaluating Newborns at Risk for Early-Onset Sepsis

Pamela I. Good, MD, Thomas A. Hooven, MD*

KEYWORDS

- Early-onset sepsis • Sepsis calculator • Serial physical examination
- Rule-out sepsis

KEY POINTS

- The incidence of early-onset sepsis (EOS) is low; however, it is associated with significant morbidity and mortality. Identifying well-appearing newborns at risk for EOS is essential.
- Several guidelines for evaluating and managing infants at risk for EOS have been published; however, these recommendations likely result in extensive laboratory screening and treatment of low-risk newborns.
- Cautious use of risk assessment tools such as the Bayesian sepsis calculator can decrease the number of infants exposed to blood draws and antibiotics.
- Serial physical examinations can be used to manage well-appearing at-risk newborns; however, this approach requires significant resources.
- Protocols and escalation plans must be clearly established before instituting new risk prediction and management tools.

INTRODUCTION

The concern for early-onset sepsis (EOS) often causes treatment dilemmas for clinicians. One of the major challenges is identifying well-appearing infants at highest risk of infection. Between 20% and 50% of late preterm or term infants with EOS seem well on initial examination,[1,2] yet those who develop EOS have significantly increased morbidity and mortality,[3] making identification of the highest risk individuals and early antibiotic therapy essential.[4,5]

The pathophysiology and treatment of EOS have been extensively reviewed in the literature.[6-8] In brief, the neonate is infected through ascending spread of organisms from the maternal genital tract into the sterile intraamniotic compartment—often triggering early labor and preterm birth—or through exposure during delivery.[9] The most common cause of EOS is group B *Streptococcus* (GBS), with recent data showing an

Disclosures: The authors have no commercial or financial conflicts of interest to disclose.
Department of Pediatrics, Vagelos College of Physicians and Surgeons, Columbia University, 630 West 168th Street, PH-17, New York, NY 10032, USA
* Corresponding author.
E-mail address: tah2120@cumc.columbia.edu

0031-3955/19/© 2018 Elsevier Inc. All rights reserved.

incidence of 0.25/1000 live births.[10] The second leading cause of EOS is *Escherichia coli*, with an incidence of 0.18/1000 live births, although *E coli* is the leading cause of EOS in preterm infants.[1,10]

Several risk factors for EOS have been recognized, including preterm birth, maternal colonization with GBS, rupture of membranes for longer than 18 hours, maternal signs or symptoms of intraamniotic infection, and various demographic factors.[11,12] However, associations between each individual risk factor and EOS are weak, and some risk factors are inconsistently diagnosed.[13] Intraamniotic infection, or chorioamnionitis, is particularly problematic. It is a clinical diagnosis based on a combination of maternal fever with maternal leukocytosis, maternal or fetal tachycardia, uterine tenderness, and/or purulent or foul-smelling amniotic fluid,[14] yet multiple combinations of diagnostic criteria are used in clinical practice and research studies.[15,16] In 2017, the American College of Obstetricians and Gynecologists published updated guidelines for diagnosis and treatment of intraamniotic infection, which may help standardize practices.[17]

Current management of infants at risk of EOS is heterogeneous. Although several sets of practice guidelines exist to help manage at-risk newborns, different centers use different combinations of risk factors, clinical assessment tools, and protocols for evaluation and clinical monitoring.[15] For equivocal and well-appearing at-risk infants, management varies. Options include close clinical monitoring, screening laboratory assessments (complete blood count and C-reactive protein or procalcitonin), blood culture, and empirical antibiotics.[13,15,18,19] For ill-appearing infants, there is much less variability: blood culture with or without lumbar puncture and empirical antibiotics are prescribed.

This article summarizes the recent evolution in how neonatal providers assess sepsis risk factors and new trends in the management of at-risk neonates. It is divided into a review of published official guidelines, an overview of the Bayesian sepsis calculator, and a discussion of new trends in using serial observation as an alternative to laboratory studies. This paper concludes with a suggested approach based on this information.

CURRENT GUIDELINES

Several sets of clinical guidelines for evaluation and management of EOS have been issued by government agencies and professional societies during the past decade. Many of the recommendations for specific clinical scenarios overlap, but there have been enough differences among the various guidelines to cause confusion among practitioners seeking consensus.[20] The most important and current sets of guidelines are briefly summarized in the next section.

Centers for Disease Control and Prevention

In 2010, the United States Centers for Disease Control and Prevention (CDC) issued revised guidelines for prevention of perinatal GBS disease.[21] This publication was the second major revision of CDC GBS prevention recommendations since the adoption of consensus guidelines for universal antepartum GBS screening and intrapartum antibiotic prophylaxis in 1996.[22]

The CDC 2010 guidelines included an updated algorithm for management of newborns with risk factors and/or clinical symptoms concerning for EOS. The algorithm, whose structure and key features are summarized and compared with contemporaneous recommendations (**Table 1**), was based on binary decision points. For example, was there maternal chorioamnionitis or not? Is the infant healthy appearing

Table 1
Summary and comparison of major governmental and professional society recommendations for evaluation and treatment of suspected early-onset sepsis

Guideline	Year	Evaluation and Treatment Algorithm Structure	Subsequent Revision	Recommendation for Asymptomatic Infants Born Following Suspected Chorioamnionitis
Centers for Disease Control and Prevention[21]	2010	Single flow chart with binary branch points, encompassing symptomatic and asymptomatic presentations	None	Laboratory evaluation and empirical antibiotics
American Academy of Pediatrics Committee on Fetus and Newborn[13]	2012	Three branching flow charts (each assumes asymptomatic): 1. Term following chorioamnionitis 2. Term following PROM or inadequate IAP 3. Preterm following chorioamnionitis, PROM, or inadequate IAP	Clarification publication (2013)[23]	Laboratory evaluation and empirical antibiotics
National Institute for Health and Clinical Excellence[24]	2012	Single branching flow chart combining clinical observations with tallied risk factors and "red flag" risk factors	In progress (update expected 2020)	Laboratory evaluation and empirical antibiotics

Abbreviations: IAP, intrapartum antibiotic prophylaxis; PROM, prelabor rupture of membranes.

or clinically ill? Answers to those questions led to 1 of 6 recommended courses of action.

American Academy of Pediatrics

Two years later, the American Academy of Pediatrics (AAP) Committee on Fetus and Newborn issued its own set of guidelines for management of proved or suspected EOS.[13] As with the CDC guidelines, the AAP recommendations were summarized in a series of branching decision point algorithms (see **Table 1**).

The major evaluation and treatment recommendations from the CDC and the AAP were mostly concordant. In contrast to the CDC, the AAP initially recommended administering empirical antibiotic therapy to asymptomatic preterm infants with sepsis risk factors other than chorioamnionitis (such as prolonged rupture of membranes or inadequate intrapartum antibiotic therapy administration). Under the CDC guidelines, these patients would undergo screening laboratory evaluation without receiving empirical antibiotics. In a subsequent clarification publication from the AAP, the Committee on Fetus and Newborn agreed with the CDC approach to these circumstances.[23]

National Institute for Health and Clinical Excellence

A third set of guidelines, issued in the United Kingdom by the National Institute for Health and Clinical Excellence (NICE) in 2012, provided yet another algorithm for evaluation and management of newborns with risk factors for sepsis (see **Table 1**).[24] The NICE guidelines separate risk factors into 2 tiers: plain risk factors and "red flags;" the latter includes confirmed infection of a sibling in a multiple gestation pregnancy and maternal antibiotic therapy for chorioamnionitis or intrapartum sepsis. The algorithm is structured around the number of risk factors and red flags present at initial evaluation, combined with clinical signs of EOS. Of note, the NICE guidelines are undergoing revision in order to assess several concerns raised among experts about the 2012 recommendations. Among the issues being considered are the possible importance of maternal obesity as an EOS risk factor and the possibility that the current guidelines result in unnecessary overtreatment of patients with very low likelihood of developing EOS (discussed further later).

It is significant that all 3 groups agreed that all infants born to mothers diagnosed with chorioamnionitis should undergo a screening laboratory evaluation and receive empirical antibiotic therapy until EOS could be ruled out based on a negative blood culture. This recommendation for universal empirical treatment of all newborns born in the setting of chorioamnionitis eventually drew criticism (summarized later) which in recent years has prompted ongoing reevaluation of how best to manage well-appearing newborns with sepsis risk factors.

RECENT GUIDELINES IN PRACTICE

Although the independent impact of any single set of guidelines is difficult to ascertain, epidemiologic reports after 2010, when the last set of CDC guidelines was published, suggest a trend toward gradually decreasing EOS rates. Population-based surveillance by the CDC from 2005 through 2014 demonstrated a drop in overall EOS rates from approximately 0.8 cases per 1000 live births to a nadir of just over 0.6 cases per 1000 live births.[10] The drop is largely attributable to an ongoing decrease in rates of EOS due to GBS, which probably reflects the continuing impact of universal intrapartum antibiotic prophylaxis for GBS colonized deliveries.

One theoretic concern that decreased incidence of GBS EOS would be offset by an increase in gram-negative infections has fortunately not occurred.[1,10] However, several studies and commentaries have highlighted unintended consequences of the 3 major EOS guidelines. Of greatest concern is the burden posed on patients and hospitals by "rule-out sepsis" admissions (to the Special Care Nursery or Neonatal Intensive Care Unit) for asymptomatic, term or near-term newborns born after a maternal diagnosis of chorioamnionitis who require intravenous antibiotics.[16,25,26] Even these low-acuity admissions subject families and patients to emotional stress and can have additional costs as a result of missed opportunities for early breast feeding and bonding.[27] They also subject infants to rare but potentially consequential medical errors.[25]

From a hospital standpoint, rule-out sepsis admissions can pose infrastructure and staffing challenges. Epidemiologic studies performed in the years following publication of the major guidelines have raised questions about the medical value of treating all asymptomatic newborns delivered after a diagnosis of chorioamnionitis. This practice has been shown to result in hundreds of admissions for every treated case of culture-confirmed sepsis,[28] and several studies have used different approaches to demonstrate that close serial observation of infants at risk of sepsis may be as effective as the traditional screen-and-treat protocol.[29,30] Serial observation of at risk infants is an emerging trend discussed in more detail later in this article.

RISK PREDICTION MODELS

Because of the challenges outlined earlier, neonatal clinicians have been motivated to develop flexible, quantitative models to estimate the probability of EOS in at-risk newborns. The first risk prediction tool was developed using the results of a nested, case control study performed at 12 Kaiser Permanente Medical Centers in Northern California and Brigham and Women's Hospital and Beth Israel Deaconess Medical Center in Boston.[31] This was a large study that included more than 600,000 births. Cases were defined as culture-proven sepsis within 72 hours of birth in infants born at 34 weeks gestation or greater.[31] Three controls per case were selected from the birth cohort; controls were matched with cases using birth hospital and year. Preterm birth, postterm birth, maternal fever, and prolonged rupture of membranes were associated with increased risk of infection in a bivariate analysis and the associations held true on multivariate analysis.[31] On multivariate analysis, GBS colonization was also associated with increased odds of EOS; maternal antibiotics more than 4 hours before delivery was associated with decreased odds of EOS. The strongest predictors of infection were low gestational age and highest intrapartum temperature, which accounted for 17% and 58% of the model's predictive ability, respectively.[31] The risk of EOS decreased with increasing gestational age from 34 to 40 weeks and then increased again after 40 weeks. EOS risk increased linearly with maternal temperature greater than 99.5°F (37.5°C), with the highest correlation greater than 100.4°F (38°C).[31]

Using pretest probability based on the incidence of EOS in the population, and incorporating risk factor data, the group was able to create a risk prediction tool for infants at risk of EOS. This tool was turned into a sepsis calculator and published online (https://neonatalsepsiscalculator.kaiserpermanente.org).[31] The sepsis calculator was modified in 2014 to incorporate physical examination findings during the first 12 hours of age in the risk stratification algorithm.[32] Clinical illness was defined as a 5-minute Apgar score less than 5 as well as continuous positive airway pressure requirement, continuous vasoactive medication infusion, mechanical ventilation, or clinical seizure in the first 12 hours of age. Respiratory distress with an oxygen requirement during the first 6 hours of age was also included in the category of clinical illness. An equivocal presentation was defined as 2 or more of the following: tachycardia, tachypnea, fever, hypothermia, or respiratory distress. Well-appearing infants were those without clinical illness or equivocal presentations.

Likelihood ratios were identified for each illness category and, when combined with the sepsis risk at birth based on risk factors alone, a posttest probability of EOS was generated. The updated version of the sepsis calculator provides 3 management recommendations: treat empirically, observe and evaluate, or observe. These recommendations are derived from a combination of clinical status and posttest probability based on maternal risk factors.[32]

Several subsequent studies have sought to validate the sepsis calculator as a useful clinical tool. One study by Kuzniewicz and colleagues[2] compared infants evaluated for EOS before and after the introduction of the sepsis calculator at Kaiser Permanente Oakland.[1] The investigators assessed infants greater than 35 weeks gestation born between 2010 and 2015 and included 204,485 births.[1,2] When comparing the era before the sepsis calculator with the era after the sepsis calculator, the researchers found decreased antibiotic use (5%–2.6%), a lower number of antibiotic days (16/100 births–8.5/100 births), and a decreased number of sepsis evaluations with blood culture (14.5%–4.9%).[1,2] They also found no increase in adverse events (readmission of infants within 7 days of discharge, late initiation of antibiotics for EOS, inotrope use, mechanical ventilation, meningitis, or death).[1,2]

Kuzniewics and colleagues[2] also found that of the 12 infants with culture-confirmed EOS during the postcalculator era, 6 were well-appearing at birth and had calculated EOS risks below the threshold for initial evaluation or empirical treatment for EOS.[1] These infants were identified when they became symptomatic after their initial evaluation.[2] This highlights the fact that the sepsis calculator will inevitably miss some cases of EOS, especially in those infants who are asymptomatic during the first several hours after birth, a finding that recurs in other studies and underscores the importance of close clinical follow-up in the first week after birth. The mechanism of delayed presentation is likely intrapartum colonization of the mucous membranes, with subsequent bacterial growth and eventual systemic invasion during the intervening, asymptomatic hours.[33] Because the Kuzniewics and colleagues' study population was the same as the population used to formulate the sepsis calculator, it was an ideal study for post hoc validation of the tool. However, the design prevented conclusions about how well the calculator might be generalized to broader populations.

When the sepsis calculator is applied to different patient populations, it leads to more mixed results. One recent study in Utah examined retrospective data on 698 well-appearing infants admitted for maternal chorioamnionitis and compared their management with the management prescribed by the sepsis calculator.[34] Adhering to sepsis calculator treatment recommendations would have allowed a significant decrease in the number of blood draws; while complete blood counts and blood cultures were obtained in 64% and 65% of cases respectively, this testing would only have been recommended by the sepsis calculator in 12% of cases.

The same Utah study showed a likely drop in antibiotic usage with use of the sepsis calculator.[34] Although 62% of infants in this cohort were treated with antibiotics, only 6% to 12% of infants would have received antibiotics if the sepsis calculator had been used. Importantly, all infants who received a 7-day course (or longer) of antibiotics for suspected or "culture-negative" EOS would have been identified by the sepsis calculator as infants who needed to be observed or treated, suggesting that this approach would be safe in this population.

Although the Utah study shows the generalizability of the sepsis calculator to a broader American population, care must be taken when interpreting the results. The incidence of EOS in this cohort was low, with only a single case of EOS due to a known pathogen occurring during the study period.[34] The sepsis calculator may not be a safe alternative to current practice in populations with a higher incidence of EOS. For example, a Netherlands study by Kerste and colleagues[35] also retrospectively applied the sepsis calculator to 2094 newborns with a birth gestational age of 34 weeks or greater who were evaluated for EOS, with 111 (5.3%) who were treated with antibiotics. Similar to the Utah study, the investigators found that application of the sepsis calculator would have led to a significant decrease in antibiotic exposure by more than 50%.[35] However, approximately half of the infants who received antibiotics in this study started treatment beyond 12 hours of age due to clinical deterioration—mostly from well appearing to equivocal. This contrasted with earlier investigations in American cohorts, where most of the patients with clinical illness presented within 12 hours of birth. This study, conducted in a country where universal maternal GBS colonization screening is not performed—among other differences in health care delivery—suggests the possibility that the sepsis calculator might not generalize to all populations.

Carola and colleagues[36] also retrospectively compared actual management with sepsis calculator recommendations for a cohort of 896 late preterm and term newborns born in Philadelphia to mothers with clinically diagnosed chorioamnionitis. In this group, 5 patients developed culture-confirmed sepsis, all of whom received empirical antibiotics based on precalculator management strategies. Three of these five newborns would have had empirical antibiotics recommended using the sepsis calculator. For the remaining 2, one would have received a recommendation for laboratory screening and close observation, and the other would have received a recommendation for close observation without laboratory assessment. Similar to the Dutch study by Kerste and colleagues, this work raises important questions about the generalizability of the sepsis calculator to diverse populations. It also highlights the importance of clinical monitoring in infants with EOS risk factors, which is discussed in detail below.

SERIAL OBSERVATION OF INFANTS AT RISK OF SEPSIS

Recent data indicate that 80% to 100% of infants with culture-proven sepsis develop symptoms in the first 48 hours of age, suggesting that careful clinical monitoring during the postpartum hospitalization may be a safe alternative to the management strategies described earlier.[1,16,37]

Several studies have examined the feasibility of monitoring infants at risk for EOS with serial physical examinations alone.

In Emilia Romagna, Italy, before June 2005, at-risk infants were screened and managed for EOS using the 2002 CDC guidelines. After June 2005, a subset of newborns was evaluated with serial physical examinations alone. Outcomes in almost 12,000 term infants were compared before and after this practice change. Assessments involved examination of skin perfusion and respiratory symptoms at prespecified time points after birth (1, 2, 4, 8, 12, 16, 20, 24, 30, 36, 42, and 48 hours). The group of infants managed with serial physical examinations had fewer blood draws and less antibiotic exposure (1.2% of infants during the CDC guideline period vs 0.5% of infants during the observation period). There was no difference in time from symptom onset to antibiotics, level of respiratory support required, or length of stay. None of the infants became ill after discharge during the first week of age. This study was limited by a low incidence of EOS, an absence of GBS EOS, and the exclusion of preterm infants.[38]

Several subsequent studies have assessed the safety of serial physical examinations for late preterm and term infants at risk for EOS. One was performed at The Modena University Hospital in Italy.[29] During the first phase of the study (2005–2007), at-risk neonates were assessed with blood cultures at birth and screening laboratories (complete blood count and C-reactive protein levels at 6–12 hours after birth). Antibiotics were administered to infants born to mothers with intrapartum fever and to infants with abnormal screening laboratories. From 2007 to 2011, most of the infants were assessed with serial physical examinations that documented the infant's overall appearance, perfusion, and respiratory status at 3 to 6, 12 to 18, and 36 to 48 hours of age. After performing a random sampling of 1000 charts, the investigators found that the observation-only group had less antibiotic exposure (0.6% in the observation period compared with 2.8% in the preobservation period) and shorter length of stay (medians of 3 days in the observation period compared with 4 days in the preobservation period). There was no delay in antibiotic administration, and none of the infants became ill within the first week of age.[29] Compared with the previously described study in Emilia Romagna, Italy, this study captured more cases of EOS, including 2 cases of GBS EOS.

A second retrospective cohort study in Emilia Romagna, Italy further validated the safety of serial physical examinations in well-appearing late-preterm and term neonates at risk for EOS.[30] During a 4-month period in 2015, well-appearing newborns born to mothers with untreated or partially treated GBS colonization were exclusively managed with a serial physical examination strategy (n = 216). Laboratory evaluations and antibiotics were initiated only if patients had symptoms of illness. The investigators compared hospital course and outcome data among this cohort with those of a larger control population: term or late-preterm newborns without risk factors and those whose mothers received appropriate intrapartum antibiotic prophylaxis. These control patients received routine care in the well-baby nursery, without formal serial observations, unless they developed symptoms of sepsis. In total, 1.6% of 2092 of infants born during the study period received empirical antibiotics. Among the cohort managed with serial physical examination, 1.9% received antibiotics. No cases of EOS were missed among any cohort. Most of the symptomatic infants during the study interval had no appreciable risk factors at birth and therefore were not followed with a formal serial physical examination protocol. This study was small and did not capture any cases of GBS EOS. In addition, more than half (58.6%) of the patients who developed symptoms presented later than 6 hours after birth, signifying the importance of continued clinical monitoring.[30]

In the United States, Joshi and colleagues[39] recently described a quality improvement effort at Lucile Packard Children's Hospital that assessed 277 well-appearing newborns with a birth gestational age greater than or equal to 34 weeks born following maternal chorioamnionitis. This cohort received serial clinical observations (assessed every 30 minutes for the first 2 hours of life, then continuous cardiorespiratory monitoring with vital signs checked every 4 hours for 2–24 hours of life) unless they became symptomatic. If infants were symptomatic, care was escalated to include laboratory evaluation with or without antibiotic administration (the decision of whether to treat was at the clinician's discretion, without formal guidelines).[39] This approach resulted in a 55% reduction in antibiotic exposure, with no missed cases of EOS (although there were no positive cultures among the cohort) or other significant complications. As a result of this outcome, the investigators report plans to make serial clinical observation the default protocol for well-appearing newborns with maternal chorioamnionitis at their institution.

SUMMARY AND RECOMMENDATIONS

The most recent guidelines from the CDC, AAP, and NICE—if rigorously followed—result in laboratory screening and treatment of many neonates at risk for EOS. Recent studies suggest that newer risk assessment and management tools could be used to decrease the number of infants exposed to antibiotics and minimize separation of infants from their parents. Although the use of risk prediction models can reduce the number of infants evaluated and treated for EOS, caution is needed when applying the sepsis calculator to patient populations that differ dramatically from those used to generate the tool.[31,32]

Serial physical examinations are also an effective alternative to laboratory evaluations of at-risk neonates; however, serial examinations require considerable resources. Serial physical examination strategies have been successfully implemented by groups that incorporated clear and rigorous protocols about how often the examinations are performed, who performs them, and what clinical findings require escalation of care. Institutions seeking to use a serial examination approach are advised to clearly define and carefully monitor their protocols.

With the development of risk stratification tools and validated standardized assessments, the authors anticipate updated official guidelines for the assessment and management of EOS in the near future. For now, it is recommended that all infants with persistent symptoms beyond the physiologic postnatal transition be evaluated and treated for EOS. Equivocal appearing late-preterm and term infants can be closely monitored for disease progression, as local resources allow. If the observed infants fail to improve (or if close monitoring is not feasible), these patients should be evaluated and treated for EOS. Infants who improve should, at a minimum, be monitored with serial physical examinations for 48 hours before discharge. Well-appearing late-preterm and term infants with risk factors for EOS can be assessed using a combination of the sepsis calculator and serial physical examinations. Both approaches are evidence-based and are likely to be part of future official recommendations. Those with multiple risk factors for EOS can be risk stratified using tools such as the sepsis calculator. Highest risk individuals require evaluation and treatment, whereas moderate and lower-risk newborns can be assessed with serial examinations or routine care with discharge at least 48 hours after birth, respectively.

The past decade has witnessed significant changes in how the neonatology community views EOS evaluations. It is thought that the field is moving toward a new consensus that is rational, cost-effective, and safe for the patients.

ACKNOWLEDGMENTS

We are grateful to Dr Richard Polin for his editing assistance and advice on this topic.

REFERENCES

1. Stoll BJ, Hansen NI, Sánchez PJ, et al. Early onset neonatal sepsis: the burden of group B Streptococcal and E. coli disease continues. Pediatrics 2011;127(5): 817–26.
2. Kuzniewicz MW, Puopolo KM, Fischer A, et al. A quantitative, risk-based approach to the management of neonatal early-onset sepsis. JAMA Pediatr 2017;171(4):365–71.
3. Pugni L, Pietrasanta C, Acaia B, et al. Chorioamnionitis and neonatal outcome in preterm infants: a clinical overview. J Matern Fetal Neonatal Med 2016;29(9): 1525–9.
4. Weston EJ, Pondo T, Lewis MM, et al. The burden of invasive early-onset neonatal sepsis in the United States, 2005-2008. Pediatr Infect Dis J 2011;30(11):937–41.
5. Shane AL, Stoll BJ. Neonatal sepsis: progress towards improved outcomes. J Infect 2014;68:S24–32.
6. Thomas W, Speer CP. Chorioamnionitis: important risk factor or innocent bystander for neonatal outcome? Neonatology 2011;99(3):177–87.
7. Newton ER. Chorioamnionitis and intraamniotic infection. Clin Obstet Gynecol 1993;36(4):795–808.
8. Simonsen KA, Anderson-Berry AL, Delair SF, et al. Early-onset neonatal sepsis. Clin Microbiol Rev 2014;27(1):21–47.
9. Seong HS, Lee SE, Kang JH, et al. The frequency of microbial invasion of the amniotic cavity and histologic chorioamnionitis in women at term with intact membranes in the presence or absence of labor. Am J Obstet Gynecol 2008;199(4): 375.e1-5.
10. Schrag SJ, Farley MM, Petit S, et al. Epidemiology of invasive early-onset neonatal sepsis, 2005 to 2014. Pediatrics 2016;138(6) [pii:e20162013].
11. Benitz WE, Gould JB, Druzin ML. Risk factors for early-onset group B streptococcal sepsis: estimation of odds ratios by critical literature review. Pediatrics 1999;103(6):e77.

12. Parente V, Clark RH, Ku L, et al. Risk factors for group B streptococcal disease in neonates of mothers with negative antenatal testing. J Perinatol 2017;37(2): 157–61.

13. Polin RA, Committee on Fetus and Newborn. Management of neonates with suspected or proven early-onset bacterial sepsis. Pediatrics 2012;129(5):1006–15.

14. Higgins RD, Saade G, Polin RA, et al. Evaluation and management of women and newborns with a maternal diagnosis of chorioamnionitis: summary of a workshop. Obstet Gynecol 2016;127(3):426–36.

15. Mukhopadhyay S, Taylor JA, Kohorn Von I, et al. Variation in sepsis evaluation across a national network of nurseries. Pediatrics 2017;139(3) [pii:e20162845].

16. Benitz WE, Wynn JL, Polin RA. Reappraisal of guidelines for management of neonates with suspected early-onset sepsis. J Pediatr 2015;166(4):1070–4.

17. Committee on Obstetric Practice. Committee Opinion No. 712: intrapartum management of intraamniotic infection. Obstet Gynecol 2017;130(2):e95–101.

18. Benitz WE, Han MY, Madan A, et al. Serial serum C-reactive protein levels in the diagnosis of neonatal infection. Pediatrics 1998;102(4):E41.

19. Guibourdenche J, Bedu A, Petzold L, et al. Biochemical markers of neonatal sepsis: value of procalcitonin in the emergency setting. Ann Clin Biochem 2002;39(2):130–5.

20. Which is the optimal algorithm for the prevention of neonatal early-onset group B streptococcus sepsis? Early Hum Dev 2014;90(Suppl 1):S35–8.

21. Verani JR, McGee L, Schrag SJ, Division of bacterial diseases, National Center for Immunization and Respiratory Diseases, Centers for Disease Control and Prevention (CDC). Prevention of perinatal group B streptococcal disease–revised guidelines from CDC, 2010. MMWR Recomm Rep 2010;59(RR-10):1–36.

22. Centers for Disease Control and Prevention (CDC). Prevention of perinatal group B streptococcal disease: a public health perspective. Centers for Disease Control and Prevention. MMWR Recomm Rep 1996;45(RR-7):1–24.

23. Brady MT, Polin RA. Prevention and management of infants with suspected or proven neonatal sepsis. Pediatrics 2013;132(1):166–8.

24. National Collaborating Centre for Women's and Children's Health (UK). Antibiotics for early-onset neonatal infection: antibiotics for the prevention and treatment of early-onset neonatal infection. London: RCOG Press; 2012.

25. Hooven TA, Randis TM, Polin RA. What's the harm? Risks and benefits of evolving rule-out sepsis practices. J Perinatol 2018;59(Suppl 1):1.

26. Polin RA, Watterberg K, Benitz W, et al. The conundrum of early-onset sepsis. Pediatrics 2014;133(6):1122–3.

27. Mukhopadhyay S, Lieberman ES, Puopolo KM, et al. Effect of early-onset sepsis evaluations on in-hospital breastfeeding practices among asymptomatic term neonates. Hosp Pediatr 2015;5(4):203–10.

28. Wortham JM, Hansen NI, Schrag SJ, et al. Chorioamnionitis and culture-confirmed, early-onset neonatal infections. Pediatrics 2016;137(1):e20152323.

29. Berardi A, Fornaciari S, Rossi C, et al. Safety of physical examination alone for managing well-appearing neonates ≥ 35 weeks' gestation at risk for early-onset sepsis. J Matern Fetal Neonatal Med 2015;28(10):1123–7.

30. Berardi A, Buffagni AM, Rossi C, et al. Serial physical examinations, a simple and reliable tool for managing neonates at risk for early-onset sepsis. World J Clin Pediatr 2016;5(4):358–64.

31. Puopolo KM, Draper D, Wi S, et al. Estimating the probability of neonatal early-onset infection on the basis of maternal risk factors. Pediatrics 2011;128(5): e1155–63.

32. Escobar GJ, Puopolo KM, Wi S, et al. Stratification of risk of early-onset sepsis in newborns ≥ 34 weeks' gestation. Pediatrics 2014;133(1):30–6.
33. Baker CJ. The spectrum of perinatal group B streptococcal disease. Vaccine 2013;31(Suppl 4):D3–6.
34. Shakib J, Buchi K, Smith E, et al. Management of newborns born to mothers with chorioamnionitis: is it time for a kinder, gentler approach? Acad Pediatr 2015; 15(3):340–4.
35. Kerste M, Corver J, Sonnevelt MC, et al. Application of sepsis calculator in newborns with suspected infection. J Matern Fetal Neonatal Med 2016;29(23): 3860–5.
36. Carola D, Vasconcellos M, Sloane A, et al. Utility of early-onset sepsis risk calculator for neonates born to mothers with chorioamnionitis. J Pediatr 2018;195: 48–52.e1.
37. Bromberger P, Lawrence JM, Braun D, et al. The influence of intrapartum antibiotics on the clinical spectrum of early-onset group B streptococcal infection in term infants. Pediatrics 2000;106(2 Pt 1):244–50.
38. Cantoni L, Ronfani L, Da Riol R, et al. Perinatal Study Group of the region friulivenezia giulia. Physical examination instead of laboratory tests for most infants born to mothers colonized with group B Streptococcus: support for the Centers for Disease Control and Prevention's 2010 recommendations. J Pediatr 2013; 163(2):568–73.
39. Joshi NS, Gupta A, Allan JM, et al. Clinical monitoring of well-appearing infants born to mothers with chorioamnionitis. Pediatrics 2018;141(4):e20172056.

Hypoglycemia in the Newborn

Paul J. Rozance, MD[a], Joseph I. Wolfsdorf, MB, BCh[b],*

KEYWORDS

- Neonatal hypoglycemia • Glucose • Dextrose • Dextrose gel • Glucose meter
- Discharge readiness

KEY POINTS

- Buccal dextrose gel should be considered in the management of asymptomatic hypoglycemia in at-risk newborns based on effectiveness in preventing neonatal intensive care unit admissions for neonatal hypoglycemia and safety (assessed at 2 years of age).
- The traditional 200 mg/kg dextrose "mini-bolus" given before instituting a continuous dextrose infusion for the treatment of neonatal hypoglycemia may not be necessary in asymptomatic hypoglycemic newborns.
- Direct breastfeeding should be encouraged for the treatment of asymptomatic hypoglycemia in at-risk newborns.
- The use of more accurate point-of-care devices for measuring neonatal glucose concentrations is becoming more prevalent.
- When discharge of a previously hypoglycemic newborn is being planned, several patient-specific factors should be considered, including the history, physical examination, glucose concentration trends, and feeding pattern.

INTRODUCTION

During the transition from intrauterine to extrauterine life, normal neonates typically have plasma glucose concentrations that are lower than those later in life.[1–5] In term appropriate for age healthy newborns, normal blood glucose concentrations can range between 25 and 110 mg/dL within the first few hours after birth; however, by about 72 hours of age, glucose values typically reach at least 60 to 100 mg/dL.[6] It may be difficult to recognize the uncommon or rare newborn with a persistent hypoglycemia disorder among the common infants with transitional low glucose levels in the initial 48 hours after birth. Nonetheless, it is crucial to distinguish between

Disclosures: Dr P.J. Rozance has received a Nova Statstrip for use in his animal laboratory.
[a] Perinatal Research Center, Department of Pediatrics, Colorado Children's Hospital, University of Colorado School of Medicine, 13243 E 23rd Avenue, Aurora, CO 80045, USA; [b] Division of Endocrinology, Boston Children's Hospital, Harvard Medical School, 300 Longwood Avenue, Boston, MA 02115, USA
* Corresponding author.
E-mail address: joseph.wolfsdorf@childrens.harvard.edu

transitional neonatal glucose regulation and hypoglycemia that persists beyond 72 hours of age to ensure a prompt diagnosis and effective treatment, which may prevent permanent brain injury leading to neurodevelopmental delay, learning difficulties, and seizures.

Hypoglycemia cannot be defined by a particular plasma glucose value, especially in the newborn period. Several different methods have been used to define hypoglycemia but none are entirely satisfactory.[6,7] Furthermore, there is controversy concerning when and how to manage symptomatic and asymptomatic hypoglycemia in the newborn period. This article reviews several aspects of the clinical management of neonatal hypoglycemia in which new research has informed changes in practice. Specifically, the following are addressed: the implications of a large associative study in asymptomatic hypoglycemic newborns and their 2-year and 4.5-year outcomes; the risks and benefits of using dextrose gel, breast milk, and formula to treat neonatal hypoglycemia; controversies around the determination of safety for discharge of previously hypoglycemic newborns; and how the diagnostic accuracy of certain types of point-of-care (POC) devices for measuring glucose concentrations in the newborn may change clinical practice. Not addressed herein are the pathophysiology of neonatal hypoglycemia, the mechanisms and clinical data related to hypoglycemic brain injury, or a specific algorithm for the screening, diagnosis, and management of neonatal hypoglycemia; nor are potential future additions to the diagnostic and management tools available for this problem discussed, such as continuous interstitial glucose monitoring, as these have been well covered in several other review articles and commentaries.[5,7–17]

MANAGEMENT OF ASYMPTOMATIC AT-RISK NEWBORNS

Two-year and 4.5-year outcome data from a cohort of newborns with and without asymptomatic hypoglycemia were recently reported in 2 separate publications.[18,19] This cohort comprised subjects who had the most common risk factors for asymptomatic hypoglycemia: late preterm birth, large for gestational age (LGA), infant of a diabetic mother (IDM), or small for gestational age/intrauterine growth restriction (SGA/IUGR). In this study, hypoglycemia was defined as any glucose concentration less than 47 mg/dL. Not only was 47 mg/dL the threshold for diagnosing hypoglycemia, it also was the target glucose concentration for treatment with oral feedings, buccal dextrose gel, and/or intravenous dextrose. The control group consisted of contemporaneously identified and studied newborns with the same risk factors for hypoglycemia, but who never had a clinically documented glucose concentration less than 47 mg/dL. Initial neurodevelopmental outcomes were prospectively assessed by neurologic examination, tests of executive function, the Bayley Scales of Infant Development III, vision screening, and global motion perception testing. Caregivers also completed an assessment of the child's health and executive function. At 2 years of age, these outcomes were not different between the hypoglycemic and nonhypoglycemic groups. However, overall impairments were frequent, indicating the high-risk nature of this patient population; for example, developmental delay was identified in 33% of hypoglycemic newborns and 36% of nonhypoglycemic newborns.[18]

Of interest, other associations between abnormal outcomes and glycemic patterns were noted at 2 years of age.[18] First, it seemed that newborns who did not have a recorded glucose concentration less than 54 mg/dL actually had worse neurosensory impairment, suggesting that higher glucose concentrations were detrimental. Indeed, although there were few cases of true neonatal hyperglycemia (eg, only 3 newborns had a glucose concentration >144 mg/dL), newborns with neurosensory impairment had an average glucose concentration (measured by continuous interstitial glucose monitoring) 2.9 mg/dL greater than those infants who did not have neurosensory impairment. Another important association observed in these studies was that the more time glucose concentrations were outside the range of 54 to 72 mg/dL, the more likely the newborn was to have neurosensory impairment and cognitive delay at 2 years of age. An additional important association was found among children who had neonatal hypoglycemia: compared with subjects without neurosensory impairment, children with neurosensory impairment at 2 years of age had a steeper initial increase in interstitial glucose concentration and higher glucose concentrations for 12 hours after receiving treatment for hypoglycemia. This study did not establish a cause-and-effect relationship between these neonatal glycemic patterns and worse outcomes at 2 years of age. The relationships may well be causative; however, an alternative explanation may be that within this high-risk group are subjects with increased metabolic instability as fetuses, which independently leads to increased glucose concentrations, increased glycemic variability, or a steeper rise in glucose concentrations after treatment and impaired outcomes at 2 years of age. Regardless, in an effort to reduce the rapidity with which low glucose concentrations are corrected and to avoid increased glucose variability, some experts have suggested that when an asymptomatic hypoglycemic newborn is treated with intravenous dextrose, a constant infusion of dextrose should be administered without a preceding "mini-bolus" of 200 mg/kg.[20]

More recently, outcomes of this cohort at 4.5 years of age also have been reported.[19] The outcomes assessed at this age focused on cognitive, executive, visual, and motor function. Parental questionnaires also were used to assess emotional and behavioral problems, executive dysfunction, and autistic traits. At 4.5 years of age, the children who experienced neonatal hypoglycemia had worse executive and visual motor integration compared with those who did not. Impairments appeared to be worse in those children who had more severe and frequent low glucose concentrations. Furthermore, children who had the lowest mean and lowest maximum interstitial glucose concentrations in the first 12 hours after birth had an increased risk of neurosensory impairment. Parental report of outcomes revealed no differences between the 2 groups, indicating that the impairments in executive and visual motor function were not apparent to caregivers. However, the investigators caution that the impairments may not become clinically apparent until school age, when these subtle defects may affect school performance. Other associations detected at 2 years of age were not apparent at 4.5 years of age.

When determining whether and how this study and its reported outcomes should affect clinical practice, there are several features to consider.[18,19] Most importantly, this association study did not compare different neonatal hypoglycemia management strategies. Although the management strategy used, treating at-risk newborns to keep their glucose concentrations higher than 47 mg/dL, is common, it is by no means universal.[17,21–23] There are no outcomes data from randomized controlled trials comparing this strategy with any other strategy. Therefore, the clinician is left to consider various strategies based on expert and consensus analysis of associative, statistical, and physiologic data. The current study (including the 4.5-year outcomes) does not provide evidence indicating that one strategy is superior to another. It is plausible that a management strategy targeting higher or lower glucose concentrations could produce the same, better, or worse outcomes. This gap in knowledge combined with the high rates of abnormal outcomes in this recent study only reinforces the previously recognized need for further studies to determine optimal approaches to the management of neonatal hypoglycemia.[23,24] The 2-year and 4.5-year outcomes data from the current study are apparently contradictory.[18,19] One interpretation is that 2 years of age may be too soon to assess outcomes related to asymptomatic neonatal hypoglycemia. This reasoning is particularly relevant for the design of future studies aimed at demonstrating the efficacy of a particular intervention for hypoglycemia in high-risk neonates.

BUCCAL DEXTROSE GEL FOR NEONATAL HYPOGLYCEMIA

As previously noted, there are also concerns with both overtreatment and undertreatment of neonatal hypoglycemia. Concerns with overtreatment include a greater number of blood draws, use of formula to provide an enteral source of carbohydrate, admission of the newborn to an intensive care nursery, separation from the mother, decreased breastfeeding success, use of intravenous catheters and medications, and iatrogenically increasing glucose concentration variability or a rapid rate of elevation in the glucose concentration after treatment. Risks of undertreatment include potential harm caused by asymptomatic hypoglycemia, progression to symptomatic hypoglycemia, and a delay in the diagnosis and treatment of a serious endocrinologic disorder such as congenital hyperinsulinism, hypopituitarism, or adrenal insufficiency or an inborn error of carbohydrate, fat, or amino acid metabolism.

To balance these risks, a single-center, double blind, placebo-controlled trial in New Zealand has recently evaluated dextrose gel.[25,26] In this study, at-risk infants (defined as late preterm [35–36 weeks gestational age], LGA [>90th percentile or >4500 grams], SGA/IUGR [<10th percentile or <2500 grams], and IDM), were randomized to receive dextrose buccal gel (200 mg/kg) or placebo, followed by feedings, if they had a glucose concentration less than 47 mg/dL. Newborns in the dextrose gel group had less treatment failure, defined as a blood glucose concentration less than 47 mg/dL, after the second of 2 doses of dextrose buccal gel. In addition, newborns in the dextrose gel group had lower rates of admission to the neonatal intensive care unit (NICU) for hypoglycemia and increased rates of exclusive breastfeeding at 2 weeks of age. In this study, the number needed to treat to prevent one NICU admission was 8. A subsequent cost analysis of the initial trial demonstrated reduced hospital costs associated with the use of buccal dextrose gel to treat asymptomatic hypoglycemia in this population.[27] Continuous interstitial glucose monitoring was used in a subset of the subjects with the data blinded to caregivers. Analysis of these data showed no evidence of recurrent or rebound hypoglycemia and no delay of definitive treatment of serious hypoglycemia with intravenous dextrose.[25]

However, despite these short-term data supporting the safety of dextrose gel, it should be noted that continuous interstitial glucose measurement was only used in a subset of patients. Therefore, it was encouraging that when 2-year outcomes were published there were no differences between the dextrose gel and placebo groups.[26] These outcomes data have led some to recommend adoption of dextrose gel in clinical practice.[20] When one is considering this option, several factors should be evaluated. First, it should be noted that this study only included the most common at-risk groups for asymptomatic neonatal hypoglycemia. Second, the definition of hypoglycemia was less than 47 mg/dL, the treatment goal was greater than 47 mg/dL, and the screening frequency and duration were different from what has been recommended by some investigators.[8,17] Third, in this study the clinicians used a very reliable POC device (a bedside blood gas analyzer) for measuring glucose concentrations. Fourth, by study design, the maximum number of doses of study gel an infant could receive was 6, and the average number of study doses actually administered was 2 to 3. Finally, practitioners should continue close follow-up of glucose concentrations, observation for clinical signs of hypoglycemia, and documentation of resolution of the hypoglycemia when using dextrose gel. Although the dextrose gel itself does not cause impaired feeding immediately after gel administration,[28] there is potential for the dextrose gel to mask serious problems related to poor feeding or a more persistent hypoglycemia disorder. Based on the 2-year data and with these caveats, dextrose gel therapy seems to be safe and effective at preventing NICU admissions for hypoglycemia based on the single-center study from New Zealand.[29] Following publication of the results from this trial, several smaller historically controlled trials have demonstrated benefits from the implementation of dextrose gel similar to those described in the New Zealand trial.[30–33]

There are several arguments against use of dextrose gel for the management of neonatal hypoglycemia. First, longer-term outcomes, which might be more informative than 2-year outcomes, have not been published. Second, the original trial was only powered to detect a difference in short-term treatment failure (a blood glucose concentration <47 mg/dL after the second of 2 doses of dextrose or placebo buccal gel) and was not specifically powered to detect longer-term differences between the groups or rare outcomes. Third, one must consider that most forms of dextrose gel readily available contain preservatives, artificial flavoring, and sometimes artificial coloring. All of these must be weighed against the likelihood that dextrose gel will decrease the number of newborns admitted to an NICU for management of hypoglycemia and increase rates of breastfeeding.

ENTERAL FEEDING FOR NEONATAL HYPOGLYCEMIA

Another controversial issue has been the use of breastfeeding, expressed breast milk, or formula for the treatment of neonatal hypoglycemia. A recent secondary analysis of the dextrose gel study offers some of the first evidence of short-term benefits of breastfeeding over formula feeding for the treatment of neonatal hypoglycemia.[34] This study analyzed glucose concentrations before and approximately 30 minutes after treatment of 295 episodes of hypoglycemia (glucose concentrations <47 mg/dL) with breastfeeding, expressed breast milk, formula, dextrose gel, and/or placebo gel. Feeding type was based on maternal preference and placebo versus dextrose gel was determined by randomization in the original study.[25] When formula was used with or without breastfeeding and breast milk, there was a higher initial increase in glucose concentrations. The initial increase in the formula fed infants was approximately 3.8 mg/dL higher than the increase observed in infants who did not receive formula. These data are not surprising given that the median volume of breast milk expressed, and likely transferred to the infant in the case of direct breastfeeding, was significantly lower than the volume of formula fed to the infant (0.5 versus 4.5 mL/kg per feeding). In older infants, glucose concentrations increase similarly if comparable volumes of breast milk and formula are used.[35]

Regardless, although these data seem to favor formula feeding over use of breast milk if the goal is immediately to increase glucose concentrations as high as possible, there are other considerations. First, the observation was also made in this study that breastfed infants had significantly less recurrent low glucose concentrations.[34] Importantly, this benefit was only found in infants who were breastfed and did not occur in those who received expressed breast milk. Second, early formula feeding can have a negative impact on overall breastfeeding success.[36] Finally, no study in this patient population has demonstrated that quickly increasing glucose concentrations improves outcomes. In fact, one should consider the data from this same group demonstrating an association between a faster increase in glucose concentrations following treatment of hypoglycemia and worse 2-year outcomes.[18] Therefore, when considering the long-term benefits of breastfeeding,[37] any strategy that might decrease breastfeeding rates and lead to more recurrent hypoglycemia may not be advisable.

Another observation made in this study was that use of dextrose gel led to a 3 mg/dL higher increase in glucose concentration compared with placebo gel.[34] Therefore, one might consider the application of 40% buccal dextrose gel followed by encouragement of breastfeeding as an appropriate strategy to treat low glucose concentrations in these patients. The dextrose gel achieves a similar immediate postprandial increase in glucose concentrations compared with formula feeding. The use of breastfeeding after dextrose gel might also lead to less recurrent or rebound hypoglycemia. Although limited to short-term outcomes, these data are among the first to show short-term benefits of breastfeeding over formula feeding in asymptomatic hypoglycemic newborns.[34]

OTHER HIGH-RISK NEWBORNS AND CONSIDERATIONS FOR DISCHARGE

The observations in the studies by McKinlay and colleagues[18,19] and findings in the dextrose gel studies cannot necessarily be extrapolated to groups of newborns with clinical characteristics that were not included in these studies. This population includes newborns with symptomatic hypoglycemia, newborns without a risk factor for hypoglycemia in whom persistently low glucose concentrations are not improving, and those with a family history of a hypoglycemia disorder or sudden unexplained neonatal death. Therefore, dextrose gel may not be appropriate in these situations. In the case of symptomatic newborns, especially those with neurologic symptoms, administration of intravenous dextrose with the 200 mg/kg (or 2 mL 10% dextrose/kg) "mini-bolus" should be considered, followed by a thorough evaluation for neonatal hypoglycemia disorders, especially if no prenatal risk factors for hypoglycemia are identified. In the case of a family history of a hypoglycemia disorder, or specific physical signs consistent with a hypoglycemia disorder (eg, midline facial defect, micropenis, hepatomegaly), appropriate diagnostic tests for the disorder being considered should be undertaken in consultation with an endocrinologist or metabolic specialist. Another clinical situation that must be carefully evaluated is the infant who was feeding well and then develops poor feeding and hypoglycemia. These patients should not be discharged until appropriate feedings have been re-established and glucose concentrations have normalized. It also is important to appreciate that although low glucose concentrations are common in the first several hours of age, newborn glucose concentrations typically increase steadily over time.[2,4,5] By contrast, a newborn in whom the initial low glucose concentration remains persistently low or decreases further must be monitored more closely before discharge to ensure that glucose homeostasis has normalized.

Opinions differ regarding the glucose concentration at which previously hypoglycemic patients may be safely discharged. These opinions are not founded on studies demonstrating that one discharge strategy is safer and more effective than another. The 2011 American Academy of Pediatrics (AAP) guideline states that in newborns with documented low glucose concentrations, the clinician must be certain that the infant can maintain normal glucose concentrations on a routine diet through at least 3 feed-fast periods before discharge.[8] However, no guidance was provided for what constituted an acceptable glucose concentration *after* 24 to 48 hours of age.[8] The 2015 Pediatric Endocrine Society (PES) recommendations state that for most newborns, preprandial glucose concentrations consistently greater than 60 mg/dL represent a safe range for discharge. The PES recommendations also state that for some at-risk infants without a suspected persistent hypoglycemia disorder and in whom hypoglycemia is considered likely to resolve within a short time, a "safety fast" of 6 to

8 hours (essentially omitting one feeding) with measurement of glucose concentrations during the fast should be considered. If these infants are unable to maintain a plasma glucose concentration higher than 60 mg/dL, additional management or investigations will be required. For infants with a known risk of a genetic or other persistent form of hypoglycemia (eg, congenital hyperinsulinism, glucose-6-phosphatase deficiency, fatty acid oxidation disorder), the safety fast should ensure that they can maintain their plasma glucose higher than 70 mg/dL.[17] After publication of the PES recommendations, the lead author of the 2011 AAP guidelines suggested that in older infants previously treated with intravenous glucose for symptomatic or asymptomatic hypoglycemia or in those with borderline glucose concentrations, prandial glucose concentrations should consistently be greater than 70 mg/dL before discharge.[10] Most experts agree that there are infants with certain clinical characteristics in whom persistent hypoglycemia should be excluded before discharge (Box 1). However, given the variability in the strategies describing how to exclude persistent hypoglycemia and determine that a patient is ready for discharge, it is important to consider carefully the history, physical examination, and feeding pattern of each formerly hypoglycemic infant at the time discharge is being contemplated. These considerations will inform whether specific glucose concentrations are sufficient to indicate probable resolution of hypoglycemia, or whether a safety fast is necessary to exclude a persistent hypoglycemia disorder and which plasma glucose concentrations should be used when evaluating the response to a fast.

METHODS FOR MEASURING GLUCOSE CONCENTRATIONS

The accuracy of different devices used to measure glucose concentrations can vary substantially.[38] Recommendations for the screening and treatment of neonatal hypoglycemia have involved the use of POC glucose meters for initial screening.[15] These devices tend to be somewhat inaccurate, especially at the low glucose concentrations characteristic of newborns. However, because of the inconvenience of obtaining blood samples (eg, larger blood volume) and the delay in obtaining values from accurate analytical instruments in clinical laboratories, the recommendations have been to send a confirmatory sample to the clinical laboratory after identification of a low glucose concentration with a POC glucose meter, and to treat the low glucose concentration without waiting for the confirmatory result.[15]

An alternative strategy that combines the rapidity of a POC glucose meter with the accuracy of the clinical laboratory methodology is use of POC blood gas analyzers with specific glucose cartridges. The drawbacks of using these devices are that they are not universally available in all hospitals and nurseries, they require more blood

---

Box 1
Neonates in whom to exclude persistent hypoglycemia before discharge

- Severe hypoglycemia (symptomatic or required treatment with intravenous dextrose)
- Inability consistently to maintain preprandial glucose >50 mg/dL for up to 48 hours of age and >60 mg/dL after 48 hours of age
- Family history of a genetic form of hypoglycemia
- Congenital syndromes (eg, Beckwith-Wiedemann), abnormal physical features (eg, midline facial malformation, microphallus)

Adapted from Thornton PS, Stanley CA, De Leon DD. Recommendations from the Pediatric Endocrine Society for evaluation and management of persistent hypoglycemia in neonates, infants, and children. J Pediatr 2015;167:238–45.

than POC glucose meters, and testing is more expensive compared with POC glucose meters. Despite these drawbacks, some organizations are advocating for the use POC blood gas analyzers with specific glucose cartridges for screening and management of neonatal hypoglycemia. In 2017, the British Association of Perinatal Medicine (BAPM; www.bapm.org/resources) published its recommendation that all hospitals caring for newborns should use these accurate POC devices for the initial screening and management of neonatal hypoglycemia. The rationale for this recommendation is that more accurate glucose measurements would decrease admission of some newborns to the NICU for treatment of neonatal hypoglycemia. Because of decreased NICU admission rates, using these more accurate POC devices may actually lower the costs associated with managing neonatal hypoglycemia.[39] This argument makes sense when one considers that bedside POC glucose meters are known to be less accurate at low concentrations and may underreport low glucose concentrations.[40]

Highly accurate hand-held glucose meters have been recently approved by the Food and Drug Administration for use in all hospital settings, including nurseries.[41–43] The accuracy of these devices is similar to that of gold-standard laboratory analytical methods, and they also have the advantage of using small blood volumes and quickly providing results. These devices have been successfully used in intensive care unit studies of insulin infusions to keep glucose concentrations within a narrow range.[44] As evidenced by the BAPM recommendations, we anticipate that with the advent of accurate POC glucose meters they will become the standard devices used to screen for and manage neonatal hypoglycemia. Other anticipated advances in biochemical monitoring will likely include the use of continuous interstitial glucose monitors and POC devices that measure alternative fuels such as ketones and lactate.

SUMMARY

This article reviews recent evidence underlying potential changes in clinical practice related to the management of neonatal hypoglycemia. With the exception of the buccal dextrose gel study, none of the data are from randomized trials comparing one management strategy with another, thus highlighting the need for ongoing research in this area. Even though the buccal dextrose gel study was only a single-center study it was randomized, blinded, and placebo controlled. Based on the apparent safety at 2 years of age and effectiveness with respect to preventing NICU admissions for neonatal hypoglycemia, many practitioners have adopted buccal dextrose gel into their management strategy for this condition. Other topics addressed in this review include the rationale for not administering a 200 mg/kg dextrose "mini-bolus" before starting a continuous dextrose infusion, and for using direct breastfeeding in the treatment of asymptomatic hypoglycemia in at-risk newborns. Also briefly described is the increasing use of more accurate POC devices for measuring neonatal glucose concentrations. Finally, different published opinions regarding the determination of readiness for discharge are considered. As discussed, recommendations around this issue vary. However, regardless of the strategy used, at the time of discharge important considerations should include evaluation of patient-specific factors including the history, physical examination, glucose concentration trends, and feeding pattern of each formerly hypoglycemic infant.

REFERENCES

1. Alkalay AL, Sarnat HB, Flores-Sarnat L, et al. Population meta-analysis of low plasma glucose thresholds in full-term normal newborns. Am J Perinatol 2006; 23(2):115–9.

2. Kaiser JR, Bai S, Rozance PJ. Newborn plasma glucose concentration nadirs by gestational-age group. Neonatology 2018;113(4):353–9.
3. Cornblath M, Reisner SH. Blood glucose in the neonate and its clinical significance. N Engl J Med 1965;273(7):378–81.
4. Srinivasan G, Pildes RS, Cattamanchi G, et al. Plasma glucose values in normal neonates: a new look. J Pediatr 1986;109(1):114–7.
5. Stanley CA, Rozance PJ, Thornton PS, et al. Re-evaluating "transitional neonatal hypoglycemia": mechanism and implications for management. J Pediatr 2015; 166(6):1520–5.
6. Guemes M, Rahman SA, Hussain K. What is a normal blood glucose? Arch Dis Child 2016;101(6):569–74.
7. Cornblath M, Hawdon JM, Williams AF, et al. Controversies regarding definition of neonatal hypoglycemia: suggested operational thresholds. Pediatrics 2000; 105(5):1141–5.
8. Adamkin DH. Postnatal glucose homeostasis in late-preterm and term infants. Pediatrics 2011;127(3):575–9.
9. Adamkin DH. Neonatal hypoglycemia. Curr Opin Pediatr 2016;28(2):150–5.
10. Adamkin DH, Polin R. Neonatal hypoglycemia: is 60 the new 40? The questions remain the same. J Perinatol 2016;36(1):10–2.
11. Adamkin DH, Polin RA. Imperfect advice: neonatal hypoglycemia. J Pediatr 2016; 176:195–6.
12. Harding JE, Harris DL, Hegarty JE, et al. An emerging evidence base for the management of neonatal hypoglycaemia. Early Hum Dev 2017;104:51–6.
13. Hay WW Jr, Rozance PJ. Continuous glucose monitoring for diagnosis and treatment of neonatal hypoglycemia. J Pediatr 2010;157(2):180–2.
14. McKinlay CJD, Chase JG, Dickson J, et al. Continuous glucose monitoring in neonates: a review. Matern Health Neonatol Perinatol 2017;3:18.
15. Rozance PJ, Hay WW. Hypoglycemia in newborn infants: features associated with adverse outcomes. Biol Neonate 2006;90(2):74–86.
16. Rozance PJ, Hay WW Jr. Describing hypoglycemia—definition or operational threshold? Early Hum Dev 2010;86(5):275–80.
17. Thornton PS, Stanley CA, De Leon DD, et al. Recommendations from the Pediatric Endocrine Society for evaluation and management of persistent hypoglycemia in neonates, infants, and children. J Pediatr 2015;167(2):238–45.
18. McKinlay CJ, Alsweiler JM, Ansell JM, et al. Neonatal glycemia and neurodevelopmental outcomes at 2 years. N Engl J Med 2015;373(16):1507–18.
19. McKinlay CJD, Alsweiler JM, Anstice NS, et al. Association of neonatal glycemia with neurodevelopmental outcomes at 4.5 years. JAMA Pediatr 2017;171(10):972–83.
20. Rozance PJ, Hay WW Jr. New approaches to management of neonatal hypoglycemia. Matern Health Neonatol Perinatol 2016;2:3.
21. Boardman JP, Wusthoff CJ, Cowan FM. Hypoglycaemia and neonatal brain injury. Arch Dis Child Educ Pract Ed 2013;98(1):2–6.
22. American Academy of Pediatrics Committee on Fetus and Newborn: routine evaluation of blood pressure, hematocrit, and glucose in newborns. Pediatrics 1993; 92(3):474–6.
23. Boluyt N, van KA, Offringa M. Neurodevelopment after neonatal hypoglycemia: a systematic review and design of an optimal future study. Pediatrics 2006;117(6): 2231–43.
24. Hay WW Jr, Raju TN, Higgins RD, et al. Knowledge gaps and research needs for understanding and treating neonatal hypoglycemia: workshop report from Eunice

Kennedy Shriver National Institute of Child Health and Human Development. J Pediatr 2009;155(5):612–7.

25. Harris DL, Weston PJ, Signal M, et al. Dextrose gel for neonatal hypoglycaemia (the Sugar Babies Study): a randomised, double-blind, placebo-controlled trial. Lancet 2013;382(9910):2077–83.

26. Harris DL, Alsweiler JM, Ansell JM, et al. Outcome at 2 years after dextrose gel treatment for neonatal hypoglycemia: follow-up of a randomized trial. J Pediatr 2016;170:54–9.

27. Glasgow MJ, Harding JE, Edlin R. Cost analysis of treating neonatal hypoglycemia with dextrose gel. J Pediatr 2018;198:151–5.

28. Weston PJ, Harris DL, Harding JE. Dextrose gel treatment does not impair subsequent feeding. Arch Dis Child Fetal Neonatal Ed 2017;102(6):F539–41.

29. Brown LD, Rozance PJ. A sweet addition for the treatment of neonatal hypoglycemia. J Pediatr 2016;170:10–2.

30. Weston PJ, Harris DL, Battin M, et al. Oral dextrose gel for the treatment of hypoglycaemia in newborn infants. Cochrane Database Syst Rev 2016;(5):CD011027.

31. Rawat M, Chandrasekharan P, Turkovich S, et al. Oral dextrose gel reduces the need for intravenous dextrose therapy in neonatal hypoglycemia. Biomed Hub 2016;1(3) [pii:448511].

32. Bennett C, Fagan E, Chaharbakhshi E, et al. Implementing a protocol using glucose gel to treat neonatal hypoglycemia. Nurs Womens Health 2016;20(1):64–74.

33. Stewart CE, Sage EL, Reynolds P. Supporting 'Baby Friendly': a quality improvement initiative for the management of transitional neonatal hypoglycaemia. Arch Dis Child Fetal Neonatal Ed 2016;101(4):F344–7.

34. Harris DL, Gamble GD, Weston PJ, et al. What happens to blood glucose concentrations after oral treatment for neonatal hypoglycemia? J Pediatr 2017;190: 136–41.

35. Brown LD, Cavalli C, Harwood JE, et al. Plasma concentrations of carbohydrates and sugar alcohols in term newborns after milk feeding. Pediatr Res 2008;64(2): 189–93.

36. Chantry CJ, Dewey KG, Peerson JM, et al. In-hospital formula use increases early breastfeeding cessation among first-time mothers intending to exclusively breastfeed. J Pediatr 2014;164(6):1339–45.

37. Breastfeeding and the use of human milk. Pediatrics 2012;129(3):e827–41.

38. Beardsall K. Measurement of glucose levels in the newborn. Early Hum Dev 2010; 86(5):263–7.

39. Glasgow MJ, Harding JE, Edlin R. Cost analysis of cot-side screening methods for neonatal hypoglycaemia. Neonatology 2018;114(2):155–62.

40. Woo HC, Tolosa L, El-Metwally D, et al. Glucose monitoring in neonates: need for accurate and non-invasive methods. Arch Dis Child Fetal Neonatal Ed 2014; 99(2):F153–7.

41. Nuntnarumit P, Chittamma A, Pongmee P, et al. Clinical performance of the new glucometer in the nursery and neonatal intensive care unit. Pediatr Int 2011;53(2): 218–23.

42. Seley JJ, Diaz R, Greene R. Blood glucose meters in ICUs. Am J Nurs 2016; 116(4):46–9.

43. Tendl KA, Christoph J, Bohn A, et al. Two site evaluation of the performance of a new generation point-of-care glucose meter for use in a neonatal intensive care unit. Clin Chem Lab Med 2013;51(9):1747–54.

44. Agus MS, Wypij D, Hirshberg EL, et al. Tight glycemic control in critically ill children. N Engl J Med 2017;376(8):729–41.

Neonatal Thyroid Disease
Testing and Management

Paul B. Kaplowitz, MD, PhD

KEYWORDS

- Congenital hypothyroidism • Newborn thyroid screening
- Neonatal hyperthyrotropinemia • Delayed TSH elevation • Neonatal hyperthyroidism

KEY POINTS

- Newborn thyroid screening identifies infants who have congenital hypothyroidism and need prompt initiation of thyroid hormone replacement. With the adoption of lower cutoffs by many screening programs, more infants are being identified, although it is not clear if the milder cases benefit from long-term therapy.
- Thyroid testing obtained in the first 1 to 2 days after birth often leads to elevated total T4, free T4, and/or thyroid-stimulating hormone (TSH) levels. This occurs as a result of the normal surge in TSH after birth and no treatment is required.
- Very premature and sick neonates often have low total and free T4 levels with normal TSH levels. The reasons for this are not clear and treatment is rarely necessary, as total and free T4 levels typically normalize in 6 to 10 weeks.
- Infants identified with normal free T4 and mildly elevated TSH levels in the newborn period need close follow-up but not all require treatment; the elevated TSH will prove to be transient in approximately half the cases.
- Multiple studies have shown that in sick low birthweight infants, especially those less than 1500 g and those born before 30 weeks' gestation, there may be a delayed elevation of TSH, possibly related to an immaturity of the hypothalamic-pituitary-thyroid axis. Retesting such infants at 3 to 4 weeks of age or before discharge from the hospital in the state newborn screening laboratory is suggested.

INTRODUCTION

Thyroid dysfunction that requires prompt diagnosis and treatment often becomes evident in the newborn period, in large part because of testing that is done as part of universal newborn screening, typically done at 2 to 4 days of age. Although primary congenital hypothyroidism is clearly a condition requiring urgent action to prevent

The author has no commercial or financial conflicts of interest and no source of funding for this work.
Division of Endocrinology, Children's National Health System, George Washington University School of Medicine and the Health Sciences, 111 Michigan Avenue Northwest, Washington, DC 20010, USA
E-mail address: pkaplowi@childrensnational.org

Pediatr Clin N Am 66 (2019) 343–352
https://doi.org/10.1016/j.pcl.2018.12.005   **pediatric.theclinics.com**
0031-3955/19/© 2018 Elsevier Inc. All rights reserved.

developmental delays, many of the abnormal thyroid test results, both on newborn screening and thyroid hormone testing in the newborn nursery or neonatal intensive care unit (NICU) are difficult to interpret, with a need for repeat testing and careful follow-up before initiation of treatment. This article reviews both situations with the goal of advising the reader how to effectively manage a variety of scenarios that may occur during the first month after birth.

Thyroid hormones have effects on most tissues and organs, but most critically, they stimulate many developmentally regulated nervous tissue genes during the prenatal and newborn periods. Starting in the third trimester, thyroid hormone begins to act on processes controlling neuronal differentiation, neuronal arborization, and synaptogenesis. This explains why it is so critical to identify and treat significant thyroid hormone deficiencies in the first weeks after birth to avoid developmental delays.[1]

There are 2 active thyroid hormones, L-thyroxine, also known as T4, and triiodothyronine, also known as T3. The thyroid gland secretes both T4 and T3, but much of the circulating T3 is derived from peripheral conversion of T4 to T3. Circulating levels are maintained within the desired range by the hypothalamic-pituitary-thyroid (HPT) axis. The hypothalamus produces thyrotropin-releasing hormone (TRH), which stimulates the pituitary to produce thyroid-stimulating hormone (TSH). TSH stimulates thyroid follicular cell activity and rises when the pituitary and hypothalamus sense that T4/T3 levels are too low.

In the first trimester, most of the fetal thyroid hormone comes from the pregnant woman across the placenta. By 18 weeks' gestation, the fetal HPT axis becomes functional and T4 levels rise steadily from 18 weeks on, whereas T3 levels start to rise after 30 weeks' gestation.[1] Shortly after birth, cold exposure triggers a surge in TRH and TSH production, with a significant rise in both T4 and T3 levels, which peak by 1 to 2 days of age. It is important to be aware of these changes when trying to interpret free T4 and TSH levels obtained in the first few days after birth. **Table 1** provides normal values for total T4, free T4, and TSH in term infants during the first month of age.[2]

NEWBORN THYROID SCREENING

All infants are screened for congenital hypothyroidism as part of universal thyroid screening, typically before discharge from the hospital at 2 to 4 days of age. The goal of this screening is to identify cases and initiate treatment as early as possible, ideally in the first week after birth, to minimize or eliminate effects on brain development. The most recent American Academy of Pediatrics guidelines on newborn

Table 1
Normal values for total T4, free T4, and thyroid-stimulating hormone (TSH) in term infants during the first month of age

Age	T4, µg/dL	Free T4 Range, µg/dL	TSH Range, mIU/L
Cord blood	9.2 ± 1.9	1.4 ± 0.4	6.7 ± 4.8
Day 1–3	16.5 ± 5.0	—	Up to 39
Day 7	12.7 ± 2.9	2.7 ± 0.6	2.6 ± 1.8
Day 14	10.7 ± 1.4	2.0 ± 0.3	2.5 ± 2.0
Day 28	9.7 ± 2.1	1.6 ± 0.3	1.8 ± 0.9

Data from Williams FLR, Simpson J, Celauhunty C, et al. Developmental trends in cord and postpartum serum thyroid hormones in preterm infants. J Clin Endocrinol Metab 2004;89:5314–20.

thyroid screening[3] reviewed different methodologies that states use for detecting cases. Highlights include the following:

1. Many states perform primary total T4 screening with back-up TSH if the T4 falls in the lowest 10% of test results for a given day. This method is the least expensive and works well, although on rare occasions, cases with a low-normal T4 and a high TSH will be missed because the TSH was not tested.
2. Some states obtain only TSH levels, which will detect all cases of primary congenital hypothyroidism but may miss rarer cases of secondary (pituitary) hypothyroidism in which the total T4 is low but the TSH is normal. Because of the surge of TSH in the first day after birth, programs using this method also need to adjust their TSH cutoffs based on patient age to avoid a large number of false-positives.
3. Some states test all infants for both total T4 and TSH, which is more expensive but identifies all cases of primary and secondary hypothyroidism.

A recent article analyzed the variation in thyroid screening protocols in the 51 newborn screening programs in the United States.[4] The investigators concluded that because of differences in whether a second screening is done routinely (14 states), is done when TSH is above the cutoff but <50 mIU/L (28 states), or whether age-adjusted TSH cutoffs are used for second testing, children with mild persistent TSH elevation may be missed (see later in this article).

Regardless of the method used, any abnormal newborn screen performed at a state laboratory on filter paper spots needs confirmation in a hospital or commercial laboratory. This testing should include a TSH and either a total T4 (which is less expensive and typically can be reported within hours) or free T4 (which has the advantage of being less affected by changes in thyroid binding proteins). **Table 2** summarizes some of the laboratory abnormalities found in neonates and interpretations of these results. Pediatric endocrinology should be consulted promptly if the results are abnormal and, especially if the TSH is markedly elevated (>100 mIU/L). In this latter case, the endocrinologists may recommend starting thyroid hormone supplementation while the confirmatory T4 and TSH are pending. Recommended starting doses of L-thyroxine range from 8 to 15 μg/kg, so that full-term infants will generally receive 37.5 to 50.0 μg per day. One group recommended an initial dose of 50 μg/d (12–17 μg/kg) because this led to normalization of TSH levels within 2 weeks, albeit with elevated total/free T4 levels.[5] Another study reported that doses of 10 to 12 μg/kg were sufficient and even at that lower dose, sometimes resulted in overtreatment.[6] A systematic review of 14 studies that examined the effects of different starting doses on cognitive development, growth, and behavior found no evidence to justify a high dose versus a standard dose and suggested that further studies were needed.[7] Thus, a starting dose of close to 10 μg/kg is reasonable. Although thyroid tests start to normalize within a week after treatment, it is generally not necessary to retest until the child has been treated for 3 to 4 weeks, by which time total/free T4 and TSH levels should have stabilized, and the dose can be adjusted if needed.

The appropriate cutoff for when a screening TSH is considered elevated is the subject of much debate. In the past, many states used a cutoff of 40 mIU/L and the incidence of congenital hypothyroidism was reported to be in the range of 1 in 4000. More recently, due to concerns that some cases were being missed with the cutoff of 40 mIU/L, different states have lowered the TSH cutoff to between 15 and 25 mIU/L. As a result, the incidence of congenital hypothyroidism has been reported more recently to be in the range of 1 in 2000 to 3000. Although many of the milder cases being identified as a result of the lower cutoffs for TSH appear to be consistent with hypothyroidism, the benefit of treating infants with even lower TSH cutoffs (5–15 mIU/L)

Table 2
Interpretation of thyroid laboratory testing in newborns

Total T4	Free T4	TSH	Interpretation
Increased	Increased	Increased	Testing obtained in first day after birth at time of postnatal TSH surge leading to confusing results
Decreased	Decreased	Increased	Primary congenital hypothyroidism
Decreased	Decreased	Normal	Central (pituitary) hypothyroidism
Decreased	Slightly decreased to normal	Normal	Thyroid binding globulin deficiency Extreme prematurity and non-thyroid illness, for example, respiratory distress syndrome
Normal	Normal	Increased	Neonatal hyperthyrotropinemia Immaturity of the hypothalamus-pituitary-axis

Abbreviation: TSH, thyroid-stimulating hormone.

despite normal total or free T4 is still unresolved.[8] A recent article[9] presented both sides of this debate, including the economic implications of lower TSH cutoffs leading to increased costs for retesting as well as treatment and further testing of infants with mild TSH elevation. There is a tendency among many endocrinologists to treat border-line cases at least until age 3 years. However, it has not been established that normal brain development, which clearly requires normal levels of free T4 and T3, would be impaired by a slight and persistent elevation of TSH.

WHAT ARE THE CONSEQUENCES OF THE NEWBORN SURGE OF THYROID-STIMULATING HORMONE?

Case: A 2-day-old infant transferred to the NICU for intestinal obstruction had thyroid tests done in the hospital laboratory at 24 hours of age, which showed a total T4 of 19 μg/dL and a TSH of 22 mIU/L. The laboratory reports these results to the neonatol-ogist who is concerned about the possibility of both hypothyroidism and hyperthyroid-ism. How should this infant be managed?

Newborn screening is typically done at 2 to 4 days of age before discharge from the hospital; however, it is not uncommon for healthy infants to be discharged at 24 hours of age, when T4 levels can be as high as 21.5 μg/dL and TSH levels can be as high as 39 mIU/L. For programs that use primary TSH screening, this creates a problem of many false-positives, unless the cutoffs for TSH are adjusted according to postnatal age, as they are in some states. However, when early thy-roid testing is performed by the hospital laboratory, the results often appear abnormal, because due to the neonatal TSH surge, T4, free T4, and TSH may all be elevated based on hospital normal ranges for older infants but are actually appropriate considering the age of the child.[3] The provider can be reassured that for a child younger than 24 hours of age, these elevated values are normal. The ideal time for newborn thyroid testing is 2 to 4 days of age at which time total and free T4 are still elevated but TSH will have declined to levels close to what is normal in the first year of age.

WHEN SHOULD PROVIDERS BE CONCERNED ABOUT A LOW TOTAL T4 WITH NORMAL THYROID-STIMULATING HORMONE LEVELS IN TERM INFANTS?

Case: A 4-day old term male infant with a birth weight of 3.0 kg is transferred to the NICU because of persistent hypoglycemia. His examination is notable for jaundice and micropenis. The newborn screening laboratory reports a low total T4 of 3.5 μg/dL (normal for age is 10–16 μg/dL) with a TSH of 3.7 mIU/L (normal for age). What might be the significance of this infant's low total T4 level?

This case is very suggestive of central (pituitary) hypothyroidism, where there is a low total T4 with nonelevated (or borderline high) TSH. The free T4 if measured is also low. The frequency of this condition is 1:25,000 to 1:50,000. Most cases involve multiple pituitary deficiencies (TSH, ACTH [adrenocorticotrophic hormone], growth hormone [GH], luteinizing hormone [LH]) but an entity called isolated TSH deficiency does exist. If there is evidence of other deficiencies (eg, micropenis often due to LH deficiency, hypoglycemia that can be due to low cortisol and GH), endocrinology should be consulted promptly. A brain MRI will often show an abnormal pituitary and/or pituitary stalk, an ectopic posterior pituitary, or evidence of septo-optic dysplasia (optic nerve hypoplasia and/or absence of the septum pellucidum).[3]

A low total T4 level with normal TSH levels in an otherwise normal healthy newborn may also indicate thyroid binding globulin (TBG) deficiency. It is important to obtain a free T4, which will usually be normal or low-normal, and a TBG level, which will be low. This X-linked disorder is mostly found in male infants, with an incidence of approximately 1:10,000. Because free T4 is usually normal (especially if done by the equilibrium dialysis method), there is no true deficiency and treatment is not needed, but the family needs to be aware so that any future thyroid testing will not be misinterpreted.

HOW DOES PREMATURITY AND CRITICAL ILLNESS AFFECT THYROID FUNCTION?

Case: A 28-week gestation infant with a birthweight of 1.2 kg is requiring ventilator support for respiratory distress syndrome and having difficulty tolerating feedings. His newborn screening test done at 7 days of age shows a low total T4 of 3.0 μg/dL (normal 9.8–15.6 μg/dL) and a normal TSH of 2.5 mIU/L (normal 0.8–4.4 mIU/L). A free T4 is then ordered and is 2.0 ng/dL (normal 2.1–3.3 μg/dL). What action should be taken?

Approximately 50% of extremely premature newborns have a low total T4 with normal TSH levels.[10] This is thought to be due to immaturity of the HPT axis and is often associated with a low free T4 as well.

Premature infants also can have a low total T4 with a normal TSH because of low thyroid-binding proteins. This typically affects total T4 more than free T4 by direct immunoassay. If the free T4 level is measured in a premature infant by equilibrium dialysis (a method that is more expensive but is done now in many hospitals), the free T4 result is more likely to be normal, as this testing is minimally affected by low binding proteins. The reliability of measuring free T4 by equilibrium dialysis, instead of by non-dialysis methods, is especially notable in infants born at less than or equal to 27 weeks' gestation.[11] Thyroid hormone levels typically spontaneously normalize by 6 to 10 weeks after birth and, except in the most severe cases, treatment is not considered necessary. One controlled trial of thyroid hormone supplementation to infants born at less than 30 weeks' gestation did not show long-term benefit on Intelligence Quotient by age 10.[12]

WHAT DO WE KNOW ABOUT INFANTS WITH MILD THYROID-STIMULATING HORMONE ELEVATION IDENTIFIED IN THE NEWBORN PERIOD?

A common and challenging scenario is when an infant has a normal free T4 but a mildly elevated TSH (also referred to as neonatal hyperthyrotropinemia or HT). Conservative management is to treat all such infants, although the condition is often transient, with normal tests often found when children are withdrawn from therapy at a later time, typically at 2 to 3 years of age, when brain development is no longer thyroid hormone dependent. Some of the most recent studies about long-term findings in neonates with HT are summarized as follows:

- A 2010 study of 43 patients with neonatal HT found that nearly half of those treated were able to come off treatment with normal testing after approximately 2.5 years, but those with persistent HT were more likely to have abnormal thyroid imaging.[13]
- A study of 103 patients with mild neonatal HT found that although most patients were treated, half showed overtreatment at some point, and a trial off treatment was successful in approximately half of the cases.[14] No predictors of success of a trial off therapy were found.[14]
- A study with long-term follow-up of 76 infants with neonatal HT (55% had endocrinology consults in the NICU) reported that half were never treated, and of those who were treated, 40% were successfully taken off medications at a later time with normal follow-up thyroid testing.[15] Male sex, cesarean delivery, and retinopathy of prematurity were predictors of resolution of elevated TSH levels,[15] suggesting that sicker infants are more likely to have HT that is transient.

DOES TOPICAL IODINE EXPOSURE IN THE NEONATAL INTENSIVE CARE UNIT CAUSE TRANSIENT HYPOTHYROIDISM?

- A 1978 paper from France described 5 NICU infants (of 30 tested) with a birth weight between 2200 and 3300 g who had extensive skin prepping with iodine-alcohol and had low total T4 levels and elevated TSH levels. The investigators proposed that overloading the thyroid gland with iodine shuts off intrinsic thyroid hormone production, leading to transient hypothyroidism.[16]
- A 1995 article reviewed 47 infants who had povidone-iodine applications in preparation for invasive/surgical procedures.[17] Despite very high urinary iodine levels, none of the infants had abnormal thyroid tests when measured 7 to 10 days later.[17]
- The most recent study (2017) looked retrospectively at 186 neonates undergoing cardiac catheterization (and in some cases, cardiac surgery) over a 3-year period.[18] Forty-six (25%) had a high TSH level (defined as >9–20 mIU/L depending on postnatal age) of which 18 had a TSH level greater than 20 mIU/L. The infants with the highest TSH levels were those who had 3 or more procedures or a creatinine greater than 0.9 mg/dL. The investigators recommended serial monitoring of thyroid function in neonates exposed to excess iodine.[18]

HOW COMMON IS A DELAYED RISE IN THYROID-STIMULATING HORMONE AND WHAT ARE THE RISK FACTORS?

Many studies have examined the situation in which TSH levels shortly after birth are normal but increase when repeated at a later time, especially in infants being cared for in an NICU. Some of the key studies are summarized below.

- Larson and colleagues[19] reviewed the experience of the New England Newborn Screening program from 1989 to 2002. Of 19,000 very low birth weight (VLBW) infants, defined as birth weight less than 1500 g, the investigators identified 47 cases with a delayed rise in TSH levels at a mean age of 30 days, leading to an incidence of 1:400. In comparison, the incidence of a delayed TSH rise in non-VLBW infants was only 1:75,000 (22 cases of 1,655,000). Half of the VLBW infants with a delayed TSH rise had a maximum TSH of greater than 100 mIU/mL. Of the many risk factors examined, 23% of the affected infants were exposed to topical iodine, as were 14% of the non-VLBW infants. Cardiac disease and dopamine infusion were risk factors for a delayed TSH rise in non-VLBW infants. The investigators recommended routine rescreening of infants with VLBW and sick non-VLBW infants in the NICU, especially those with cardiac disease, to identify infants who may require thyroid hormone replacement despite initial normal screening.
- A study from Rhode Island[20] reported delayed TSH elevation in 1:58 extremely low birthweight infants and in 1:95 VLBW infants but this occurred in only 1:30,000 infants weighing more than 1500 g at birth.
- A more recent study from Israel[21] reviewed data from a cohort of 13,000 newborns admitted to the NICU over a 6-year period. They found 1:40 had an elevated TSH identified on the second screen with 66% having a birthweight of greater than 1500 g, and reported that 58% received thyroid hormone replacement.
- In a recent study from Iowa,[22] 280 infants born at less than 30 weeks' gestation were routinely retested at 30 days of age. The investigators identified 26 patients (9.1%) with thyroid dysfunction, of whom 20 were eventually started on L-thyroxine therapy; however, 18 had borderline TSH elevation (between 7 and 15 mIU/L) and only 2 had TSH greater than 15 mIU/L (specific levels not reported). Whether those patients would have had their TSH levels normalize with further monitoring was not clear, but the investigators recommended measurement of free T4 and TSH on 30 days of age in all infants born at less than 30 weeks' gestation.

MANAGEMENT OF NEONATES WITH POSSIBLE HYPERTHYROIDISM

Case: A 3-day-old male infant with extreme tachycardia and restlessness is transferred to the NICU from an outside hospital. The infant's heart rate was between 180 and 200 beats per minute and he has not been feeding well. You learn that his mother has been treated in the past for hyperthyroidism, had radioiodine ablation, and is on L-thyroxine; her thyroid function tests are currently normal. How would you evaluate this infant and does he require antithyroid medication?

Newborns at risk for developing hyperthyroidism are those born to mothers with Graves disease, due to transplacental passage of TSH receptor stimulating antibodies. Although transient, usually resolving in 1 to 2 months, some infants are symptomatic enough to require treatment and close follow-up. Different studies suggest that the incidence of hyperthyroidism in infants born to mothers with Graves disease varies between 2% and 20%. Symptoms of hyperthyroidism in newborns are diverse and may include low birth weight, tachycardia, hypertension, stare, diarrhea, irritability, poor feeding, and poor weight gain. Goiter is often present and may be large enough to compress the trachea.

In a recent review of this topic,[23] the investigators highlighted that measurement of free T4 and TSH in cord blood or on the first day after birth is not reliable if the infant's mother has been taking antithyroid medication (methimazole or propylthiouracil) during the pregnancy, as these compounds cross the placenta and can suppress fetal thyroid function for the first 2 to 3 days after birth. On the other hand, measurement of TSH receptor antibodies in the pregnant woman during the second or third trimester, in cord blood, or on the first day after birth can be helpful, because if these antibodies are not present, the infant is not at risk of neonatal hyperthyroidism. However, the turn-around time for TSH receptor antibodies is such that results may not be available until after the infant is discharged from the hospital. Measurement of free T4 and TSH at 1 to 3 days in infants whose mothers are untreated or symptomatic, or at 3 to 5 days if the mother is taking antithyroid medication, is recommended. A recent multicenter study of 23 hyperthyroid infants born to 415 women with Graves disease and positive TSH receptor antibodies reported that a TSH of less than 0.90 mIU/L at 3 to 7 days of age predicted neonatal hyperthyroidism with a sensitivity of 78% and a specificity of 99%.[24] Those with abnormal results can be referred to endocrinology. Therapy for symptomatic infants includes methimazole to block new thyroid hormone synthesis, beta blockers to slow heart rate and reduce the risk of heart failure, and sometimes Lugol iodine.

SUMMARY

1. Newborn thyroid screening identifies infants who have congenital hypothyroidism and need prompt initiation of thyroid hormone replacement. However, with lower cutoffs adopted by many screening programs (TSH between 15 and 25 mIU/L), more infants are being identified, although it is not clear if the milder cases benefit from long-term therapy. Consultation with pediatric endocrinology is needed to either initiate therapy or track these infants following discharge from the hospital, as many TSH levels normalize over time and treatment can be withheld.
2. Thyroid testing obtained in the first 1 to 2 days after birth often leads to elevated total T4, free T4, and/or TSH levels. This occurs as a result of the normal surge in TSH after birth and no treatment is required.
3. Very premature and sick neonates often have low total and free T4 levels with normal TSH levels. The reasons for this are not clear but checking free T4 by equilibrium dialysis is a more accurate way of assessing thyroid function in such infants. Treatment is rarely necessary, and total and free T4 levels typically normalize in 6 to 10 weeks.
4. Infants identified with normal free T4 and mildly elevated TSH (eg, 5–30 mIU/L) levels in the newborn period need close follow-up but not all require treatment; if treated, the condition will prove to be transient in approximately half the cases.
5. Multiple studies have shown that in sick low birthweight (LBW) infants, especially those less than 1500 g and those born before 30 weeks' gestation, there may be a delayed elevation of TSH, possibly related to an immaturity of the HPT axis. It is not clear whether these infants should receive thyroid hormone replacement and if so, for how long. It seems reasonable to routinely retest such infants at 3 to 4 weeks of age or before discharge from the hospital, which can be done by the state newborn screening laboratory rather than in the hospital. If the repeated results are abnormal, consultation with endocrinology is recommended and additional testing and follow-up may be needed.
6. Infants exposed to topical iodine before surgery or procedures are at increased risk of developing hypothyroidism as a result of iodine overload. In most cases, this is transient, although short-term treatment may be needed in some cases.
7. Infants born to mothers with a history of Graves disease are at risk for transient neonatal hyperthyroidism. If maternal TSH receptor antibodies have not been measured during the second or third trimester to identify those infants at risk,

checking the cord blood or the newborn for such antibodies is the best approach to identifying those at risk who will need close follow-up and possible treatment.

REFERENCES

1. Polak M. Human fetal thyroid function. Endocr Dev 2014;26:17–25.
2. Williams FLR, Simpson J, Celauhunty C, et al. Developmental trends in cord and postpartum serum thyroid hormones in preterm infants. J Clin Endocrinol Metab 2004;89:5314–20.
3. American Academy of Pediatrics, the AAP Section on Endocrinology, the American Thyroid Association and the Pediatric Endocrine Society, et al. Update of newborn screening and therapy for congenital hypothyroidism. Pediatrics 2006; 117:2290–303.
4. Kilberg MJ, Rasooly IR, LaFranchi SH, et al. Newborn screening in the US may miss mild persistent hypothyroidism. J Pediatr 2018;192:204–8.
5. Selva KA, Mandel SH, Rien L, et al. Initial treatment dose of l-thyroxine in congenital hypothyroidism. J Pediatr 2002;141:786–92.
6. Vaidyanathan P, Pathak M, Kaplowitz PB. In congenital hypothyroidism, an initial L-thyroxine dose of 10-12 µg/kg/day is sufficient and sometimes excessive based on thyroid tests 1 month later. J Pediatr Endocrinol Metab 2012;25:849–52.
7. Hrytsiuk I, Gilbert R, Logan S, et al. Starting dose of levothyroxine for the treatment of congenital hypothyroidism: a systematic review. Arch Pediatr Adolesc Med 2002;120:485–91.
8. Deladoey J, Ruel J, Giguere Y, et al. Is the incidence of congenital hypothyroidism really increasing? A 20-year retrospective population-based study in Quebec. J Clin Endocrinol Metab 2011;96:2422–9.
9. Lain S, Trumpf C, Grosse SD, et al. Are lower TSH cutoffs in neonatal screening for congenital hypothyroidism warranted? Eur J Endocrinol 2017;177:D1–12.
10. La Gamma EF, Paneth N. Clinical importance of hypothyroxinemia in the preterm infant and a discussion of treatment concerns. Curr Opin Pediatr 2012;24: 172–80.
11. Deming DD, Rabin CW, Hopper AO, et al. Direct equilibrium dialysis compared to two non-dialysis free T4 methods in premature infants. J Pediatr 2007;151:404–8.
12. van Wassenaer AG, Westera J, Houtzager BA, et al. Ten-year follow-up of children born at <30 weeks' gestational age supplemented with thyroxine in the neonatal period in a randomized, controlled trial. Pediatrics 2005;116:e613–8.
13. Zung A, Tenenbaum-Rakover Y, Barkan S, et al. Neonatal hyperthyrotropinemia: population characteristics, diagnosis, management and outcome after cessation f therapy. Clin Endocrinol 2010;72:264–71.
14. Oren A, Wang MK, Brnjac L, et al. Mild neonatal hyperthyrotropinemia: 10 year experience suggests the condition is increasingly common but often transient. Clin Endocrinol 2013;79:832–7.
15. Aguilar L, Garb J, Reiter E, et al. Can one predict resolution of neonatal hyperthyrotropinemia? J Pediatr 2016;174:71–7.
16. Chabrolle P, Rossier A. Goitre and hypothyroidism in the newborn after cutaneous absorption of iodine. Arch Dis Child 1978;53:495–8.
17. Gordon CM, Rowtitch DH, Mitchell ML, et al. Topical iodine and neonatal hypothyroidism. Arch Pediatr Adolesc Med 1995;149:1336–9.
18. Thaker VV, Galler MF, Marshall AC, et al. Hypothyroidism in infants with congenital heart disease exposed to topical iodine. J Endocr Soc 2017;1:1067–78.

19. Larson C, Hermos R, Delaney A, et al. Risk factors associated with delayed thyrotropin elevations in congenital hypothyroidism. J Pediatr 2003;143:587–91.
20. Woo HC, Lizarda A, Tucker R, et al. Congenital hypothyroidism with a delayed TSH elevation in very premature infants: incidence and growth and developmental outcomes. J Pediatr 2011;158:538–42.
21. Zung A, Yehieli A, Blau A, et al. Characteristics of delayed TSH elevation in neonatal intensive care unit newborns. J Pediatr 2016;178:135–40.
22. Kaluarachchi DC, Colaizy TT, Pesce LM, et al. Congenital hypothyroidism with delayed TSH elevation in premature infants born at less than 30 weeks gestation. J Perinatol 2017;37:277–82.
23. Van der Kaay DCM, Wasserman JD, Palmert M. Management of neonates born to mothers with Graves' disease. Pediatrics 2016;137:e20151878.
24. Banige M, Polak M, Luton D. and the Research Group for Perinatal Dysthyroidism. Prediction of neonatal hyperthyroidism. J Pediatr 2018;197:249–54.

Neonatal Abstinence Syndrome

Lauren M. Jansson, MD[a],*, Stephen W. Patrick, MD, MPH, MS[b]

KEYWORDS

- Neonatal abstinence syndrome • Substance-exposed infant
- Maternal substance use disorder • Neonatal opioid withdrawal syndrome

KEY POINTS

- Neonatal abstinence syndrome (NAS) is a complex and variable disorder of neuroregulatory dysfunction in the infant; no one common problem can explain all signs.
- Primary management of NAS should be nonpharmacologic assessment and care, which begins prenatally or at birth and continues throughout the infant's hospitalization, regardless of the requirement for pharmacologic treatment for NAS.
- Treatment of NAS necessitates assessment of and treatment for the mother.

EPIDEMIOLOGY

Over the previous 2 decades, use of opioids grew dramatically across the United States. In 2015, 37% of American adults were prescribed at least one opioid pain reliever (OPR)[1]—3 times as many as in 1999.[2] Although OPR use remains elevated across the United States, more recently consumption of heroin and fentanyl and deaths from overdose of these drugs increased substantially.[3] Rising opioid use across the United States has been associated with complications among many populations, including pregnant women and infants.[4] Neonatal abstinence syndrome (NAS) is a postnatal withdrawal syndrome that manifests shortly after birth in infants born to women with opioid use (including heroin, use or misuse of prescription painkillers, or maternal treatment medications such as methadone or buprenorphine) during pregnancy. Concurrent with the increase in opioid use among pregnant women, the number of infants diagnosed with NAS grew nearly 7-fold from 2000 to 2014.[4–6] By 2014, more than 30,000 infants were diagnosed with the syndrome, accounting

Disclosures: Research reported in this publication was supported by the National Institute on Drug Abuse of the National Institutes of Health under award number RO1DA0413671 (Jansson) K23DA038720 (Patrick), R01DA045729 (Patrick), The content is solely the responsibility of the authors and does not necessarily represent the official views of the National Institutes of Health.
[a] The Center for Addiction and Pregnancy, Johns Hopkins Bayview Medical Center, 4940 Eastern Avenue, D4E, Baltimore, MD 21224, USA; [b] Vanderbilt Center for Child Health Policy, 2525 West End Avenue, Suite 1200, Nashville, TN 37027, USA
* Corresponding author.
E-mail address: ljansson@jhmi.edu

Pediatr Clin N Am 66 (2019) 353–367
https://doi.org/10.1016/j.pcl.2018.12.006
0031-3955/19/© 2018 Elsevier Inc. All rights reserved.

for more than $500 million in hospitalization costs.[6] Increases in NAS occurred disproportionately in rural areas[7] and in US states with high rates of other opioid-related complications including overdose death.[8]

NAS is a complex disorder that is variably expressed, both in types of signs and severity, among different infants, and in the same infant over time. Every opioid-exposed infant is unique and resides along a continuum of signs of withdrawal.[9] Currently, there is no way to accurately predict the severity of NAS expression in any given infant. NAS is typically associated with maternal use or misuse of opioids (heroin, prescription painkillers), or with maternal treatment medications such as methadone or buprenorphine. However, its expression can be modified by many maternal, infant, and environmental factors (**Table 1**).[10–27] Timing of exposure during gestation, maternal

Table 1
Maternal, infant, and/or environmental factors that can alter infant neonatal abstinence syndrome expression

Maternal Factors	
Illicit substance use: heroin, cocaine, marijuana	In general, polysubstance exposure alters NAS expression by increasing its severity, or causes neurobehavioral signs consistent with a withdrawal phenomenon.[10]
Licit substance use/misuse: oxycodone, benzodiazepines, gabapentin, nicotine	Oxycodone and benzodiazepines increase NAS expression.[11–13] Gabapentin produces an atypical NAS display.[14] Cigarette smoking can increase NAS severity.[15,16]
Licit medications: psychotropics, OUD treatment medications (eg, methadone, buprenorphine)	Psychotropic exposure can alter or increase NAS display.[17] OUD treatment medications can predispose the exposed infant to NAS, but benefits associated with maternal comprehensive treatment that includes medications for OUD are paramount for the dyad.
Genetics/epigenetics	Infants with particular genotypes (SNPs) at the OPRM1 and COMT gene sites had less severe NAS expression.[18] Hypermethylation at the same sites was associated with more severe NAS, consistent with gene silencing.[19]
Breastfeeding	Can reduce NAS severity.[20]
Infant factors	
Sex	Male infants have been reported to have more severe NAS expression.[21,22]
Gestational age	Preterm infants have less severe expression of NAS (notably, NAS measurement tools were designed for term infants. As such, NAS may not be adequately assessed in preterm infants).[23]
Fetal programming	The fetus adapts to an unfavorable intrauterine environment by altering ANS set points. These changes can be adaptive in utero and maladaptive ex utero and may be expressed as NAS.[22] Alterations from these changes may not be evident until the affected neurosystem matures, potentially later in life.[24]
Environmental factors	
Physical environment	NICU care can exacerbate NAS severity, while maternal rooming-in can reduce NAS severity.[25,26]
Caregiver (parent or medical staff) handling and communication	Misinterpretation of or inappropriate responses to infant cues or insensitive handling can exacerbate NAS expression.[27]

Abbreviations: ANS, autonomic nervous system; NICU, newborn intensive care unit; OUD, opioid use disorder; SNP, single nucleotide polymorphism.

stress associated with opioid use disorder (OUD), poor maternal nutrition, or lack of medical or obstetric care can affect the fetus and the intrauterine environment. Infant co-morbid medical conditions can also complicate the postnatal picture of NAS.

SIGNS OF NEONATAL ABSTINENCE SYNDROME

NAS is a disorder of neurobehavioral dysregulation; hence, it is important to consider the development of regulatory capacity in understanding this disorder. Each infant has a specific functional repertoire and neurobehavioral competencies that are unique. According to Als' Model of Synactive Organization of Behavioral Development,[28] development fundamentally represents the emergence of more complex and integrated forms of self-regulation over the lifespan. This self-regulatory capacity serves to regulate the infant's own functioning as well as caregiver behaviors and responses. Each of 4 behavioral subsystems (autonomic control, motor and tone control, state control and attention, and sensory processing) supports the others and interacts with the infant's environment. When newborn development is disturbed, as with substance exposure or inappropriate caregiver responses, disturbances in self-regulation and altered trajectories of development may occur.[29] For example, an opioid-exposed infant who spends an exorbitant amount of energy in one subsystem, such as tone in hypertonic infants, may have little energy to spend in other subsystems, such as attention/interaction. This dysregulatory imbalance is the hallmark of infants affected by NAS.

The signs of NAS can be thought of as arising from dysregulation in these 4 behavioral domains. Dysfunction in one domain can influence regulation in another domain (**Fig. 1**).[27] Specific symptoms include irritability and crying; poor state control;

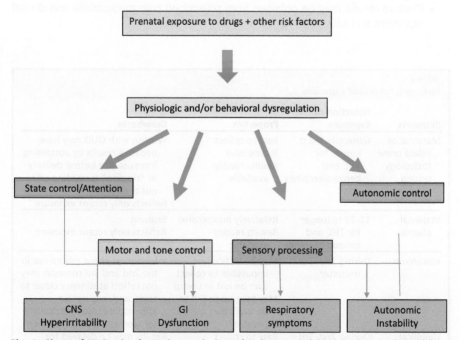

Fig. 1. Signs of NAS arise from dysregulation of 4 domains of functioning. (*Adapted from* Velez M, Jansson LM. Non-pharmacologic care of the opioid dependent mother and her newborn. J Addiction Med 2008;2:113–20.)

hypertonicity; tremors and jitteriness and accompanying skin breakdown; failure to thrive; hyper- or hyposensitivity to ordinary stimuli; vomiting/diarrhea; and autonomic signs such as hiccups, gagging, color changes, tachypnea, or fever. For example, an infant who is hypersensitive to stimuli may have problems with state control and difficulties achieving a quiet alert state necessary for feeding, leading to weight loss (**Fig. 2**).[27]

IDENTIFICATION OF NEONATAL ABSTINENCE SYNDROME AND DIFFERENTIAL DIAGNOSIS

Identifying the infant at risk for NAS is important for initiating nonpharmacologic care, scoring for NAS, and maternal treatment and is not intended to subject the mother to punitive action. Screening for opioid use or misuse in all pregnant women should be performed periodically and can be done by using one of many available screening instruments[30] (eg, 4Ps Plus tool).[31] Ideally, the infant presenting with signs of NAS has a clear and defined history of opioid exposure, and the mother is receiving comprehensive care and maintenance treatment with methadone or buprenorphine for an OUD. The utility of universal infant urine toxicologic screening for maternal substance use or misuse is debated today.

If an infant born to a mother who denies opioid use or misuse exhibits signs of NAS, toxicology screening using urine (infant or maternal), meconium, umbilical cord blood, or maternal plasma may be necessary. There are drawbacks to each method, which are summarized in **Table 2**. Drawbacks common to all include the following:

- Negative results do not rule out an OUD.
- Positive results may be obtained from prescribed pain medications and do not represent an OUD.

Table 2
Screening for opioid exposure

Biomatrix	Detection of Exposure	Properties	Drawbacks
Maternal or infant urine toxicology testing	Generally 1–3 d; longer for THC and benzodiazepines	Easy to collect Inexpensive Results readily available	Women with OUD may have negative results by abstaining from use just before delivery or "rigging" (providing urine not their own) Reflects only recent exposure
Maternal plasma	12–72 h; longer for THC and benzodiazepines	Relatively inexpensive Results readily available	Bruising Reflects only recent exposure
Meconium	During 2nd–3rd trimester	May be difficult or impossible to collect (can be lost in utero) May take up to 5 d to be available Expensive	Information about opioid use in the 2nd and 3rd trimester may not reflect abstinence closer to term, and may not be appropriate tests, particularly for women in OUD treatment
Umbilical cord	During 2nd–3rd trimester	Easy to collect Expensive	Results may be delayed for several days

Abbreviation: THC, tetrahydrocannabinol.

- Positive results do not quantify use; alcohol, which arguably has the greatest impact on the fetus, is not detected due to a short half-life.
- Detection of OUD at birth has no value in mitigating teratogenic effects in early pregnancy.

NAS should be a considered a diagnosis of exclusion, and considering other diagnoses is important, because many infants with NAS are at elevated risk for infections and other comorbidities (**Table 3**). Further, some clinical signs of NAS (eg, irritability) can be present with other conditions, including sepsis. It is also important to avoid attributing every aspect of infant adaptation in the early postnatal period to NAS. Insensitive handling, pain, toxidromes related to substance or medication exposures, hunger, suboptimal physical environments, and transient tachypnea of the newborn are factors that may be misinterpreted as signs of NAS; however, all can occur concomitantly in an infant experiencing NAS.

The onset of signs of NAS varies with the maternal substance used and its half-life. Heroin-exposed infants exhibit signs of withdrawal the earliest, typically at 12 to 24 hours of age[32]; whereas, methadone- and buprenorphine-exposed infants begin to show symptoms at 48 to 72 hours of age.[33] The onset of NAS can be delayed in some infants, beginning at 5 to 7 days of age, sometimes after the infant has been discharged from the hospital.[34]

Table 3	
Neonatal abstinence syndrome differential diagnosis	
Specific NAS Sign	**Differential Diagnosis**
Irritability	GE reflux
	Pain/discomfort
	Sepsis
	Brain injury
Fever	Sepsis (especially herpes simplex virus)
	Hyperthyroidism
Feeding problems	Oromotor dysfunction
	Anomalies (eg, cleft palate, micrognathia, Pierre Robin sequence, genetic syndromes such as Prader Willi)
	Polycythemia
	Immaturity, including late preterm birth
	Brain injury
	Sepsis
Jitteriness	Hypoglycemia
	Hypocalcemia
	Immaturity
	Injury of the nervous system
Myoclonic jerking[a]	Not uncommon in opioid-exposed infants and can be mistaken for seizure activity
Seizures (rare in infants with NAS)	Hypocalcemia
	Hypoglycemia
	Hypoxic-ischemic encephalopathy
	Brain hemorrhage/stroke

Abbreviation: GE, gastroesophageal.

[a] Myoclonic jerks can be unilateral or bilateral, occur during sleep, and do not stop when the extremity or affected body part is held. They may be medication related. Electroencephalograms are not warranted in infants with myoclonic jerks. They generally do not respond to medications used to treat NAS.

ASSESSMENT FOR NEONATAL ABSTINENCE SYNDROME

Periodic and frequent assessment of the infant with NAS using standardized assessment tools, such as a modification of the Finnegan scale, is currently the standard of care in the United States. There are no empirically derived data to inform the use of any one tool as superior, and there is wide variation in tools used today. These tools are designed to frequently assess/reassess the infant and to determine whether initiation of medication therapy is needed (in approximately 50%–60% of opioid-exposed infants), dosing parameters, and eligibility for weaning. Ideally, infant scoring should include maternal input when appropriate. Drawbacks of these tools are the subjective reporting of signs/symptoms by caregivers; therefore, it is recommended that periodic interrater reliability training occur. Further, assessment tools do not consider dyadic communication and synchrony (ie, the mother's ability to read, interpret, and respond appropriately to infant cues and the ability of the infant to effectively relay needs to the mother), which can be an important aspect of the infant's functioning in the immediate postnatal period and beyond.

In general, the infant at risk for experiencing NAS is assessed with a score every 3 to 4 hours during the entire hospital stay, with the score representing the period since the last evaluation. A rescore is recommended for the institution or escalation of medication for NAS, to allow for assessment of the infant's external (ie, soiled diapers, improper handling) or internal (ie, hunger) environments and their potential contribution to the infant's display. In these cases, the infant is rescored within the 4-hour time frame after care for the noxious stimuli has been completed. When short-acting medications such as morphine are used for treatment, scoring intervals longer than 4 hours can result in more severe or rebound NAS expression as the medication is metabolized.[35] Therefore, it is recommended to start scoring the infant at closer to 3 hours, when warranted, to avoid going beyond the 4-hour treatment window.

Scoring may need to be adjusted for older infants to reflect their progress developmentally. For example, the sleep item may be eliminated to allow the older infant to sleep for shorter periods between feedings so it does not "count against" the infant and result in a higher score than necessary. Recently, the Eat, Sleep, Console method for evaluation and treatment has resulted in less medication and shorter hospitalizations for infants with NAS.[36] However, it remains to be seen if less appreciation for the widely variable infant expression of NAS, as would occur with assessment reduced to only 3 infant functions, will result in improved care. The impact of this approach on maternal comprehension of the infant and her ability to deliver appropriate care and on infant development, which should be the paramount goal of any intervention (instead of shorter hospitalization), is also unknown.

MANAGEMENT OF NEONATAL ABSTINENCE SYNDROME

Optimal management of the infant with NAS includes the following:

- Nonpharmacologic management of the infant, beginning at birth and continuing throughout hospitalization and after discharge
- Pharmacologic treatment for the subset of infants that cannot thrive with nonpharmacologic care alone
- Comprehensive care of the mother

Nonpharmacologic Care

This has traditionally been thought of as dimming lights, swaddling, pacifier use, and gentle handling. However, it is actually more complex, requiring a focus on each

Table 4 Nonpharmacologic care of the maternal-infant dyad affected by neonatal abstinence syndrome	
Assessment Functioning of the:	With the Goal of:
Infant	Implementing comforting techniques and environmental modifications that decrease signs of neurobehavioral dysregulation Promoting the infant's self-regulation Nurturing healthy development and interactive capabilities
Mother	Promoting maternal self-regulation Encouraging and supporting parenting confidence Fostering maternal ability to support her child's healthy development and to maximize her interactional capacity
Dyad	Bidirectional communication and dyadic synchrony

Data from Velez M, Jansson LM. The opioid dependent mother and her newborn. J Addiction Med 2008;2:113–20.

unique mother-infant dyad and, when effectively implemented, can reduce or eliminate the need for medication for NAS treatment. Nonpharmacologic care is a set of interventions, ideally applied prenatally as well as in the postpartum period, which leads to a thorough understanding of the infant, the mother, and their interaction, resulting in modifications to care and the environment to optimize regulation of the dyad (**Table 4**).[27] Nonpharmacologic care is provided to the infant and mother at all times, independent of initiation of medication, during the postnatal period and beyond.

Additional aspects of nonpharmacologic care include education of physicians, nurses, therapists, and the infant's care providers regarding the unique features of NAS in the infant. Systematic observation of the newborn before, during, and after interventions can help to define these features, as well as differentiating them from typical competencies of infants of different gestational and chronologic ages. Based on the observed infant's cues and behaviors, an approach is developed that includes modification of the environment and caregiver (mother, nurses, doctors) interactions to support the infant's self-regulation.[27]

Observing the infant's capacities in the 4 domains (see **Fig. 2**) and how they interact with each other, as well as how the infant responds to environmental and handling modifications, will help to guide nonpharmacologic interventions.[27] For infants who display problems with sensory integration (ie, those infants who become dysregulated with ordinary stimuli), observing the infant's responses (eg, changes in tone, autonomic function, etc) to careful introduction of visual, auditory, and touch stimuli can help to guide nonpharmacologic interventions. For example, if an infant becomes easily overstimulated to auditory but not visual stimuli, a provider might make the environment quiet, but not necessarily dim the lights. Swaddling is helpful for infants with hypertonicity, but may need to be modified for infants who have more autonomic features, such as fever. Teaching the handler to recognize infant signs that signal dysregulation (eg, signs of stress, such as color changes, hiccups, mottling, gas, vomiting, tachypnea, etc.) and ways to intervene to allay those symptoms, such as eliminating or reducing the stimuli that caused the signs, can be simple but important information to relay.

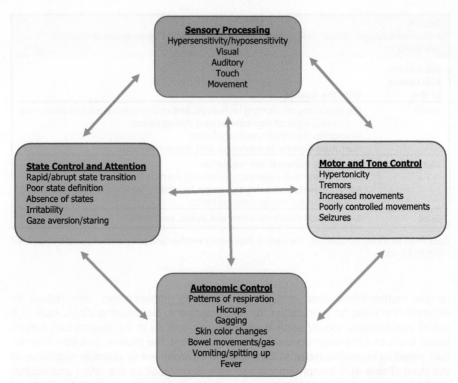

Fig. 2. Signs of NAS expression in each of the 4 domains of functioning can influence expression in other domains. (*Adapted from* Velez M, Jansson LM. Non-pharmacologic care of the opioid dependent mother and her newborn. J Addiction Med 2008;2:113–20.)

State control issues are common in infants with NAS, and can be reflected as poorly defined or absent states (**Table 5**). Infants with difficulties with state control can fluctuate between crying and sleeping, which can be problematic because a state 4 is necessary for feeding and interaction.[37] Helping the infant to achieve both quiet sleep (state 1) and a quiet alert state (state 4) is important for the regulation of infant functioning in all domains. To attain this goal, caregivers need to be taught how to gently move the infant from sleep to awake states by eliminating all triggers of dysregulation and keeping the infant from stressful stimuli that will cause the infant to go directly to a state 5 or 6. Similarly, allowing the infant to fall back to a sleep state by reducing the same stimuli can promote more regular and prolonged sleep. Failing to intervene for early neuroregulatory problems can result in altered trajectories of development that can affect the child's behavioral, cognitive, emotional, and social capacities later in life.

Pharmacologic Care

Medication used to treat more severe NAS expression generally begins when the infant reaches a certain numerical score based on a scoring tool, indicating that the infant is not thriving with nonpharmacologic care alone. Although optimal scoring and treatment paradigms have not been scientifically defined, there are 2 general methods of approach, symptom-based and weight-based treatment algorithms. The weight-based approach treats infants on an mg per kg basis, providing higher initial doses of medication and higher doses to infants of larger weight. In the symptom-based

Table 5
Infant sleep-wake states

Infant State	Description
1. Quiet sleep	Nearly still, with the occasional startle or twitch
2. Active sleep	Some body movements Rapid eye movements May smile or make fussy sounds
3. Drowsy	Variable activity level; the infant may startle and open and close eyes
4. Quiet alert	Attentive with eyes wide and bright Regular breathing
5. Active alert	Variable activity Eyes open but dull or glazed Irregular breathing May have periods of fussiness
6. Crying	Increased activity Skin color changes present Eyes tightly closed or open Responsive to stimuli

Adapted from Brazelton TB. Neonatal behavioral assessment scale. Clinics in developmental medicine No 50, 1973. p. 5–8. with permission. Available at: http://nidcap.org/wp-content/uploads/2013/12/Brazelton-1973-BNBAS.pdf.

approach, lower starting doses can be administered to infants with less severe expression, theoretically allowing mildly affected infants to be treated with less medication and to be discharged sooner from the hospital. Conversely, infants with more significant symptoms of NAS receive higher initial doses. One example of a symptom-based approach has been published previously.[38]

Optimal medications for NAS have not been defined, although first-line medications for opioid-induced abstinence should consist of opioids, such as morphine or methadone.[39] Clonidine in combination with an opioid[40] or as monotherapy[41] may be as effective, but clinical trials are needed. Buprenorphine has been suggested as a first-line medication, and recent data for this medication are promising.[42] Second-line medication use is reserved for those cases of severe or complex (usually polysubstance-induced) abstinence and is instituted when the infant is unable to be managed by one medication alone. These medications are usually clonidine or phenobarbital. Medications no longer used include paregoric, diazepam, or chlorpromazine.

Weaning an infant from medications used to treat NAS is done in a step-wise fashion, slowly over time, with an observation period at the end, before discharge. Occasionally, an infant who is undergoing weaning from medication experiences an escalation of signs of NAS, necessitating an increase in medication. These increases are generally at lower doses than initial escalation dosing (see **Table 4**). Some institutions have elected to discharge home infants on medication weans; however, although this practice does shorten hospital stays, it is associated with prolonged lengths of treatment that may not be necessary and potentially have a negative effect on development.[43] In general, home medication weans should be avoided unless in a rigorous, closely monitored, and comprehensive program for infants with NAS.

CARE OF THE MOTHER AND BREASTFEEDING

Although maternal care is often not provided by pediatric providers, it is important to recognize that the mother's well-being for the high-risk opioid-exposed dyad is imperative for the infant to thrive and develop optimally. Women with OUDs are at high risk for psychiatric comorbidities, most often depression but also anxiety, posttraumatic stress disorder and attention deficit hyperactivity disorder, abuse (physical, sexual, and emotional),[44] and medical concerns (related to substance use, prostitution, or other factors associated with lifestyles of women with substance use disorders). Pediatricians are well-positioned to evaluate the dyad and to observe difficulties that interfere with the well-being of both mother and infant (**Table 6**).[45,46] Providers should never assume that all family members or significant others are aware of maternal OUD or methadone or buprenorphine treatment and maternal confidentiality should be strictly maintained at all times. Judgmental or punitive attitudes have no place in the care of the woman with OUD. Pediatric providers may also provide the only link to any type of care for the dyad once the infant is discharged from the hospital. As such, the responsibility of care for the at-risk dyad as opposed to only the pediatric patient should be paramount. Pediatric providers should be able to provide links to appropriate maternal OUD treatment (ideally gender specific, comprehensive care programs that accept the infant's presence) and psychiatric care if necessary.

Breastfeeding may provide particular benefit for the opioid-exposed dyad and is not contraindicated in most women with OUD[47]; formula feeding should not be the default choice. Medications used to treat maternal OUD (such as methadone, buprenorphine, and some psychiatric medications) are not incompatible with breastfeeding. In general, breastfeeding is recommended for women who are not in active use patterns for any substance of abuse or misuse (including marijuana) and who have maintained abstinence from substance use for a period of time before delivery.[48] Similar to other breastfeeding women in the United States, breastfeeding is contraindicated for women who are positive for human immunodeficiency virus or are hepatitis C virus positive with cracked or bleeding nipples.[49] Breastfeeding an infant with NAS can be affected by the infant's signs and maternal appreciation of these signs, and women should receive support from an experienced lactation specialist.

FOLLOW-UP CARE FOR THE INFANT WHO EXPERIENCES NEONATAL ABSTINENCE SYNDROME

It is important to recognize that the infant affected by NAS, regardless of the need for pharmacotherapy for NAS, will be discharged from the hospital with residual signs that may last for months. In addition, in some instances, late-onset signs of abstinence can occur (particularly for opioid- and benzodiazepine-exposed infants), necessitating rehospitalization.[50] As such, reliable, timely, and knowledgeable pediatric care should be instituted before delivery. This care should be accessible to the mother, who may not have transportation or who has programmatic obligations to receive medications daily. In addition, this pediatric care should be instituted immediately after hospital discharge to avoid complications of NAS that may include rehospitalization. The woman should be satisfied with their provider, because many women with OUD may have issues trusting medical professionals due to harmful past experiences, and providers not infrequently possess biases against this group of mothers. Ideally, this relationship should develop before hospital discharge, and the mother should be provided with information to be able to access care when she needs it.

Federal law requires that Plans of Safe Care be created for substance-exposed infants who should include ensuring a safety plan for the infant as well as connection of the mother with treatment resources. It is important to know your state's reporting requirements for substance-exposed infants. Although the goal of child welfare involvement is to provide services to allow the family to stay together, sometimes

Table 6
The role of the pediatrician in the care of the mother with an opioid use disorder as part of an at-risk dyad

Recommendation	Things to Consider	Actions
Think outside of the box	Consider the mother and her unique needs	Refer to comprehensive OUD treatment program that will accept the infant's presence, if needed Refer for trauma informed care, if warranted Refer for psychiatric care, when warranted
	Consider the environment in which the dyad resides	Discuss the needs of significant others (eg, substance use disorder treatment) and physical needs of the mother (eg, legal, housing, etc.)
Provide multidisciplinary care, which is the gold standard for opioid-exposed dyads	Discuss dyadic care with obstetric providers Discuss the dyad with substance use treatment providers, if present (with maternal written consent)	Ensure appropriate postpartum care, including contraceptive services, if desired All women on methadone or buprenorphine for OUD treatment have an addiction treatment provider and a written care plan. Discuss necessary and specific care of the infant as part of comprehensive care for the mother
Beware of overtly or covertly undermining dyadic attachment and communication, both within the dyad and with caregivers	Recognize that language and terms used are important	Avoid use of stigmatizing terms such as "addicted newborn," "NAS baby," "methadone baby," "withdrawal baby," "if your baby were a normal baby," etc. All of these terms are pejorative and can negatively affect the interest of the mother with OUD to seek and engage in necessary medical and psychosocial treatment for herself and her infant
Provide trauma-informed care	Be aware that sexual, physical, and emotional trauma are common in women with OUD and are often not diagnosed before delivery	Refer for specialized psychiatric care as soon as a history of trauma is suspected Modify the environment and care to assure the comfort of the mother based on her unique experiences. This may include only female nursing staff, no nighttime visitors, being aware of exposing the mother's body, avoiding standing IVs that "tether" her to the bed Recognize that there may be obstacles to breastfeeding,[45] including early cessation[46]

Abbreviation: IV, intravenous.

alternative custody arrangements are needed. Communications about child welfare are stressful to the mother who is likely dealing with an infant experiencing NAS, causing additional guilt and anxiety. It is important to provide information to mothers in clear and consistent, nonthreatening language, while maintaining her confidentiality (other family members may not know about methadone maintenance, OUD treatment, etc.). It is important to provide mothers with follow-up care for OUD, including medication-assisted treatment, trauma services, psychiatric care, contraceptive services, and any other interventions that she needs, regardless of infant custody.

Pediatric care for opioid-exposed children should be frequent (ie, monthly in the first 6 months, every 1–2 months until 1 year, every 3 months in the second year, and biannually or more frequently afterward as needed) to enhance detection of failures of communication or outstanding needs of the mother. It should include periodic developmental assessment to allow for early detection of problems that warrant intervention, such as expressive language concerns, common in this population of children. A good rapport with the mother and a trusting mother-provider relationship is important to be able to discuss issues about maternal OUD treatment, violence exposure, or relapse that are multiply important for child health and development. Child welfare services should be used when warranted (such as in cases of child maltreatment, neglect, or harm) but not automatically for instances of maternal relapse or psychiatric concerns, where the more appropriate response is maternal engagement in or enhancement of services. Engagement of significant others can also be important, if appropriate. Asking about maternal OUD treatment, exposure to violence, contraceptive care, and medical and psychiatric health care should all be a part of these visits. A current list of referrals for treatment in any arena should be available, and close follow-up to assure that the mother is able to obtain this treatment is important. The dyad affected by opioid exposure is often challenging for the pediatric provider but should be considered among the highest risk children for myriad reasons; as such, these children should receive pediatric care of the highest quality with compassionate consideration for the mother and the environment. Pediatricians play a large role in addressing the opioid epidemic faced by the United States today by providing comprehensive care to affected children and their families.

SUMMARY

NAS is not simply a complex array of clinical signs expressed by a substance-exposed infant. It also represents complicated social, physical, and psychological stressors for the mother-infant dyad. Optimal care for the at-risk infant must be inclusive of the mother's needs, beginning with standardized approaches to diagnosis and treatment, and emphasizing the importance of nonpharmacologic care and ensuring adequate follow-up for the child and the mother after hospital discharge.

REFERENCES

1. Han B, Compton WM, Blanco C, et al. Prescription opioid use, misuse, and use disorders in U.S. adults: 2015 national survey on drug use and health. Ann Intern Med 2017;167:293–301.
2. Guy GP, Zhang K, Bohm MK, et al. Vital signs: changes in opioid prescribing in the United States, 2006-2015. MMWR Morb Mortal Wkly Rep 2017;66:697–704.
3. Hedegaard H, Warner M, Minino AM. Drug overdose deaths in the United States, 1999-2016. NCHS Data Brief 2017;294:1–8.

4. Patrick SW, Schumacher RE, Benneyworth BD, et al. Neonatal abstinence syndrome and associated health care expenditures: United States, 2000-2009. JAMA 2012;307:1934–40.

5. Patrick SW, Davis MM, Lehmann CU, et al. Increasing incidence and geographic distribution of neonatal abstinence syndrome: United States 2009 to 2012. J Perinatol 2015;35:650–5.

6. Winkelman TNA, Villapiano N, Kozhimannil KB, et al. Incidence and costs of neonatal abstinence syndrome among infants with medicaid: 2004-2014. Pediatrics 2018;141(4) [pii:e20173520].

7. Villapiano NL, Winkelman TN, Kozhimannil KB, et al. Rural and urban differences in neonatal abstinence syndrome and maternal opioid use, 2004 to 2013. JAMA Pediatr 2017;171:194–6.

8. Ko JY, Patrick SW, Tong VT, et al. Incidence of neonatal abstinence syndrome - 28 States, 1999-2013. MMWR Morb Mortal Wkly Rep 2016;65:799–802.

9. Jansson LM, Velez M. Neonatal abstinence syndrome. Curr Opin Pediatr 2012; 24:252–8.

10. Hudak ML, Tan RC, AAP The Committee on Drugs, Committee on fetus and newborn. Neonatal drug withdrawal. Pediatrics 2012;129(2):e540–60.

11. Seligman NS, Salva N, Hayes EJ, et al. Predicting length of treatment for neonatal abstinence syndrome in methadone-exposed neonates. Am J Obstet Gynecol 2008;199:396.e1–7.

12. Wachman EM, Newby PK, Vreeland J, et al. The relationship between maternal opioid agonists and psychiatric medications on length of hospitalization for neonatal abstinence syndrome. J Addict Med 2011;5:293–9.

13. Pritham UA, Paul JA, Hayes MJ. Opioid dependency in pregnancy and length of stay for neonatal abstinence syndrome. J Obstet Gynecol Neonatal Nurs 2012; 41:180–90.

14. Loudin S, Murray S, Prunty L, et al. An atypical withdrawal syndrome in neonates prenatally exposed to gabapentin and opioids. J Pediatr 2017;37:1108–11.

15. Jones HE, Heil SH, Tuten M, et al. Cigarette smoking in opioid-dependent pregnant women: neonatal and maternal outcomes. Drug Alcohol Depend 2013;131: 271–7.

16. Kaltenbach K, Holbrook AM, Coyle MG, et al. Predicting treatment for neonatal abstinence syndrome in infants born to women maintained on opioid agonist medication. Addiction 2012;107(Suppl 1):45–52.

17. Huybrechts KF, Bateman BT, Desai RJ, et al. Risk of neonatal drug withdrawal after intrauterine co-exposure to opioids an psychotropic medications: cohort study. BMJ 2017;358:j3326.

18. Wachman EM, Hayes MJ, Brown MS, et al. Association of OPRM1 and COMT single-nucleotide polymorphisms with hospital length of stay and treatment of neonatal abstinence syndrome. JAMA 2013;309:1821–7.

19. Wachman EM, Hayes MJ, Lester BM, et al. Epigenetic variation in the mu-opioid receptor gene in infants with neonatal abstinence syndrome. J Pediatr 2014;165: 472–8.

20. Welle-Strand GK, Skurtveit S, Jansson LM, et al. Breastfeeding among women in opioid maintenance treatment in Norway and it's influence on neonatal abstinence syndrome. Acta Paediatr 2013;102:1060–6.

21. Charles MK, Cooper WO, Jansson LM, et al. Male sex associated with increased risk for neonatal abstinence syndrome. Hosp Pediatr 2017;7:328–34.

22. Jansson LM, DiPietro JA, Elko A, et al. Maternal vagal tone change in response to methadone is associated with neonatal abstinence syndrome severity in exposed neonates. J Matern Fetal Neonatal Med 2007;20:677–85.

23. Gibson KS, Stark S, Kumar D, et al. The relationship between gestational age and the severity of neonatal abstinence syndrome. Addiction 2017;112:711–6.

24. Barker DJ. In utero programming of chronic disease. Clin Sci (Lond) 1998;95: 115–28.

25. Abrahams RR, Kelly SA, Payne S, et al. Rooming-in compared with standard care for newborns of mothers using methadone or heroin. Can Fam Physician 2007;53: 1722–30.

26. MacMillan KDL, Rendon CP, Verma K, et al. Association of rooming-in with outcomes for neonatal abstinence syndrome: a systematic review and meta-analysis. JAMA Pediatr 2018. https://doi.org/10.1001/jamapediatrics.2017.5195.

27. Velez M, Jansson LM. Non-pharmacologic care of the opioid dependent mother and her newborn. J Addict Med 2008;2:113–20.

28. Als H. Toward a synactive theory of development: promise for the assessment and support of infant individuality. Infant Ment Health J 1982;3:229–43.

29. Als H. Neurobehavioral organization of the newborn: opportunity for assessment and intervention. NIDA Res Monogr 1991;114:106–16.

30. World Health Organization. Guidelines for the Identification and Management of Substance Use and Substance Use Disorders in Pregnancy. (Annex 3 Screening instruments for substance use in prenatal or pregnant women). Switzerland (Geneva): WHO Document Production Services; 2014. Available at: http://apps.who.int/iris/bitstream/handle/10665/107130/9789241548731_eng. pdf;jsessionid=AC00997ED4A94B7074D04344600E7A00?sequence=1.

31. Chasnoff IJ, McGourty RF, Bailey GW, et al. The 4P's Plus screen for substance use in pregnancy: clinical application and outcomes. J Perinatol 2005;25:368–74.

32. Zelson C, Rubio E, Wasserman E. Neonatal narcotic addiction: 10 year observation. Pediatrics 1971;48:178–89.

33. Gaalema DE, Heil SH, Badger GJ, et al. Time to initiation to treatment for neonatal abstinence syndrome in neonates exposed in utero to buprenorphine or methadone. Drug Alcohol Depend 2013;133:266–9.

34. Kandall SR, Gartner LM. Late presentation of drug withdrawal symptoms in newborns. Am J Dis Child 1974;127:58–61.

35. Jones HC. Shorter dosing interval for opiate solution shortens hospital stay for methadone babies. Fam Med 1999;31:327–30.

36. Grossman MR, Lipshaw MJ, Osborn RR, et al. A novel approach to assessing infants with neonatal abstinence syndrome. Hosp Pediatr 2017;8(1). https://doi.org/10.1542/hpeds.2017-0128.

37. Als H, Tronick E, Lester BM, et al. The Brazelton neonatal behavioral asssssment scale. J Abnorm Child Psychol 1977;5:215–31.

38. Jansson LM, Velez M, Harrow C. The opioid exposed newborn: assessment and pharmacologic management. J Opioid Manag 2009;5(1):47–58.

39. Osborn DA, Jeffery HE, Cole MJ. Opiate treatment for opiate withdrawal in newborn infants. Cochrane Database Syst Rev 2005;(3):CD002059.

40. Agthe AG, Kim GR, Mathias KB, et al. Clonidine as an adjunct therapy to opioids for neonatal abstinence syndrome: a randomized controlled trial. Pediatrics 2009; 123:e849–56.

41. Streetz VN, Gildon BL, Thompson DF. Role of clonidine in neonatal abstinence syndrome: a systematic review. Ann Pharmacother 2016;50:301–10.

42. Kraft WK, Adeniyi-Jones SC, Chernova I, et al. Buprenorphine for the treatment of neonatal abstinence syndrome. N Engl J Med 2017;377:997–8.
43. Maalouf FI, Cooper WO, Slaughter JC, et al. Outpatient pharmacotherapy for neonatal abstinence syndrome. J Pediatr 2018;141(4) [pii:e20173520].
44. Velez ML, Montoya ID, Jansson LM, et al. Exposure to violence among substance-dependent pregnant women and their children. J Subst Abuse Treat 2006;30:31–8.
45. Kendall Tackett K. Breastfeeding and the sexual abuse survivor. Unit 10 lactation consultant series two. North Carolina (US): La Leche League International publication; 2003. No. 1561. Available at: http://breastfeedingmadesimple.com/wp-content/uploads/2016/02/LCSA.pdf.
46. Sorbo MF, Lukasse M, Brantsaeter AL, et al. Past and recent abuse is associated with early cessation of breastfeeding: results from a large prospective cohort in Norway. BMJ Open 2015;5(12):e009240.
47. Jansson LM, Velez M. Lactation and the substance-exposed dyad. J Perinat Neonatal Nurs 2015;29:277–86.
48. Jansson LM. Academy of breastfeeding medicine protocol #21: guidelines for breastfeeding and the drug-dependent woman. Breastfeed Med 2009;4:225–8.
49. Jansson LM, Patrick SW. Breastfeeding and the substance-exposed dyad. In: Wright TE, editor. Opioid use disorders in pregnancy: management guidelines for improving outcomes. Cambridge (United Kingdom): Cambridge University Press; 2018. p. 127–38.
50. Patrick SW, Burke JF, Biel TJ, et al. Risk of hospital readmission among infants with neonatal abstinence syndrome. Hosp Pediatr 2015;5:513–9.

The Current State of Newborn Screening in the United States

Noelle Andrea V. Fabie, MD[a,b], Kara B. Pappas, MD[a,c,*],
Gerald L. Feldman, MD, PhD[a,c,d]

KEYWORDS

- Newborn screening • Inborn errors of metabolism • Tandem mass spectroscopy
- Dried blood spot • ACMG ACT sheets

KEY POINTS

- Newborn screening is performed in all states, and a panel of disorders has been recommended for all states to follow.
- Newborn screening for inborn errors of metabolism includes collection of blood sample on a filter paper card, transportation of sample to a central laboratory, and testing for specific disorders.
- Disorders tested for can have significant morbidity and/or mortality if not treated early.
- Neonatal and maternal factors may affect results of the newborn screen.
- New disorders continue to be added as technology advances and new treatment options become available.

Funding Source: Drs K.B. Pappas and N.A.V. Fabie are recipients of the 2017 ACMG Foundation/
Shire Medical Biochemical Genetics Subspecialty Fellowship Award. Gerald Feldman was supported in part through funding provided by the State of Michigan/Michigan Department of Health and Human Services Metabolic Clinic Grant.
Financial Disclosure: None.
Conflict of Interest: None.
Clinical Trial Registration: None.
[a] Division of Genetics, Genomics and Metabolic Disorders, Children's Hospital of Michigan, 3950 Beaubien Street, Detroit, MI 48201, USA; [b] Department of Medical Genetics and Genomics, Children's Hospitals and Clinics of Minnesota, 2545 Chicago Avenue, South MDB 17-700, Minneapolis, MN 55404, USA; [c] Department of Pediatrics, Wayne State University School of Medicine, 540 E Canfield #2375, Detroit, MI 48201, USA; [d] Center for Molecular Medicine and Genetics and Department of Pathology, Wayne State University School of Medicine, 2375 Scott Hall, 540 East Canfield, Detroit, MI 48201, USA
* Corresponding author. Division of Genetics, Genomics and Metabolic Disorders, Children's Hospital of Michigan, 3950 Beaubien Street, Detroit, MI 48201.
E-mail address: kpappas@dmc.org

Pediatr Clin N Am 66 (2019) 369–386
https://doi.org/10.1016/j.pcl.2018.12.007
0031-3955/19/© 2018 Elsevier Inc. All rights reserved.

INTRODUCTION

The goal of newborn screening is the diagnosis of treatable disorders early enough to provide an intervention that will improve outcome. Newborn screening in the United States consists of point-of-care tests (for hearing loss and congenital heart disease), as well as screening on dried blood spots for a variety of other disorders. In this review, the authors describe how disorders are selected for newborn screening, the process of newborn screening as well as the disorders that are currently screened for in the United States. They also discuss some special considerations for newborn screening, especially for patients in the neonatal intensive care unit (NICU) and some of the ethical debates that surround newborn screening. Finally, future directions of newborn screening from both a disease perspective and from a technology driven perspective are also discussed.

Selection of Disorders for Newborn Screening

The selection of disorders for newborn screening remains a subject of much discussion, especially in recent times with the advancement of genetic technologies. Clinical disease characteristics must considered, such as incidence, clinical manifestations, and outcome if not treated. Then one must consider the feasibility of screening, such as how to screen, the cost of screening, and the turnaround time of testing. Finally, the availability and efficacy of treatment must be considered, because one might question whether there is value in screening if there is no effective treatment. In 2006, the American College of Medical Genetics and Genomics (ACMG) published a summary that outlined a process of standardization of the newborn screening process, which included recommendations for a uniform panel. These guidelines outlined "primary" or "core" disorders that newborn screening should include. "Secondary" disorders were also recommended; most of these are disorders that are screened for as a by-product of screening for primary disorders and may have clinical consequences.[1]

The Department of Health and Human Services maintains the Recommended Uniform Screening Panel (RUSP). The RUSP currently includes 35 primary and 26 secondary disorders (**Table 1**). Individual states have the final authority to choose which disorders to screen for and what methods they use to screen for each disorder—for example, states may have different cut-offs or use different analytes. States can add additional disorders beyond the RUSP if they choose. For example, infants in Illinois are screened for Fabry and Gaucher diseases, whereas Michigan recently approved adding testing for guanidinoacetate methyltransferase (GAMT) deficiency, a disorder of creatine metabolism.

The Process of Newborn Screening

The dried blood card

The newborn screen is obtained on filter paper, via a heel stick, typically between 24 and 48 hours after birth. The newborn screen is generally obtained by hospital personnel such as a nurse or in the case of a home birth, the midwife. Some states require a second newborn screen at 1 to 2 weeks of age, which is often obtained by the pediatrician if the child is at home. If a child is in the NICU, some states require further testing during hospitalization, as well as an additional newborn screen before discharge.

Parents must fill out information to accompany the newborn screen. Generally, this includes their contact information as well as the contact information for their pediatrician. The dried blood spot card then must be transported or mailed to the state or regional laboratory. Many laboratories use couriers to pick up and deliver newborn screens. This means that the distance between the hospital and the state laboratory may influence when the newborn screen is received.

Table 1
Disorders in the recommended uniform screening panel as of July, 2018

Primary	Secondary
Organic acidemias	
Propionic academia	Methylmalonic academia with homocystinuria
Methylmalonic academia	Malonic academia
Isovaleric academia (IVA)	Isobutyrylglycinuria
Glutaric academia type I (GA-I)	2-Methylbutyrylglycinuria
3-Methylcrotonyl-CoA carboxylase	3-Methylglutaconic aciduria
deficiency (3-MCC)	2-Methyl-3-hydroxybutyric aciduria
3-Hydroxy-3-methylglutaric aciduria	
Holocarboxylase deficiency	
β-Ketothiolase deficiency	
Fatty acid oxidation disorders	
Carnitine uptake defect/carnitine	Short-chain acyl-CoA dehydrogenase deficiency
transport defect (CUD/CTD)	(SCAD)
Medium-chain acyl-CoA	Medium/short-chain L-3-hydroxyacyl-CoA
dehydrogenase (MCAD) deficiency	dehydrogenase deficiency (M/SCHAD)
Very long-chain acyl-CoA	Glutaric academia type II (GA-II)
dehydrogenase (VLCAD) deficiency	Medium-chain ketoacyl-CoA thiolase deficiency
Long-chain L-3 hydroxyacyl-CoA	2,4-Dienoyl-CoA reductase deficiency
dehydrogenase (LCHAD) deficiency	Carnitine palmitoyltransferase type I (CPT-I)
	deficiency
	Carnitine palmitoyltransferase type II (CPT-II)
	deficiency
	Carnitine acylcarnitine translocase (CACT)
	deficiency
Amino acid disorders	
Argininosuccinic aciduria	Argininemia
Citrullinemia type I	Citrullinemia, type II
Maple syrup urine disease	Hypermethioninemia
Homocystinuria	Benign hyperphenylalaninemia
Classic phenylketonuria	Biopterin defect in cofactor biosynthesis
Tyrosinemia type I	Biopterin defect in cofactor regeneration
	Tyrosinemia type II
	Tyrosinemia, type III
Hemoglobinopathies	
Sickle cell disease	Various other hemoglobinopathies
Sickle beta thalassemia	
Sickle cell–hemoglobin C disease	
Other disorders	
Biotinidase deficiency	Galactoepimerase deficiency
Cystic fibrosis	Galactokinase deficiency
Classic galactosemia	T-cell–related lymphocyte deficiencies
Glycogen storage disease type II (Pompe)	
Severe combined immunodeficiencies	
Mucopolysaccharidosis type I (MPS-I)	
X-linked adrenoleukodystrophy (X-ALD)	
Spinal muscular atrophy (SMA)	

Once in the state laboratory, the newborn screen must be processed. Generally, small samples are taken from the dried blood spots for the various tests. Scientists in the newborn screening laboratory then review the newborn screening results. Any abnormal result must be communicated to the designated personnel responsible for follow-up. In many states, the abnormal results are communicated to the pediatrician listed on the newborn screen. The pediatrician is then responsible for calling the family and arranging follow-up, involving local specialists if relevant. Other states have designated follow-up centers, where highly trained personnel inform the family of results and directly arrange management.

The urgency of follow-up depends on the disorder. Because of the severity of some disorders, patients may need to be transported to a tertiary care hospital for confirmatory laboratory testing and initiation of treatment. Confirmatory tests and treatment for other disorders may be less urgent. The ACMG has published recommendations for each disorder. These include an ACTion (ACT) sheet (available at: https://www.ncbi.nlm.nih.gov/books/NBK55827/), which outlines the actions that should be taken by medical personnel following-up the child. In addition, there are diagnostic algorithms for each disorder that lists the confirmatory tests recommended to confirm the diagnosis (**Fig. 1**, Supplemental Fig. 1).

Newborn hearing screen
The US Preventive Services Task Force recommends screening for hearing loss in all newborns. Screening can be done by 1 of 2 testing methods: otoacoustic emissions (OAE) or auditory brainstem response (ABR). Some use a 2-step process, using ABR if

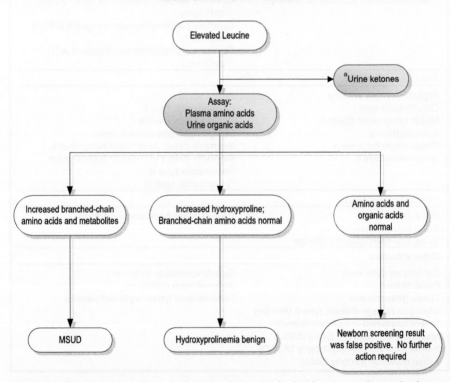

Leucine Elevated

Fig. 1. Confirmatory algorithm. Actions are shown in shaded boxes; results are in the unshaded boxes. [a] When the positive predictive values of screening are sufficiently high and the risk to the baby is high, some initiate diagnostic studies at the same time as confirmation of the screening result is done. MSUD, Maple (syrup) urine disease. (*Data from* American College of Medical Genetics. Available at: https://www.ncbi.nlm.nih.gov/books/NBK55827. Accessed August 1, 2018; with permission.)

a newborn fails OAE. It is recommended that all infants are screened before 1 month of age. If a newborn fails the hearing screen, they should have a follow-up evaluation within 3 months.[2] Please refer to the article by Stewart and Bentley on Hearing Risks for further details about hearing screens.

Critical congenital heart disease

Screening for critical congenital heart disease (CCHD) was added to the RUSP in 2011. Screening is designed to detect structural heart disorders that result in low blood oxygen saturation (**Box 1**). Screening is done by pulse oximetry after 24 hours of age but before hospital discharge. Oxygen saturation at a preductal and a postductal location is checked (typically the right hand and either foot, respectively). **Fig. 2** provides an algorithm for CCHD screening. Those infants with positive screens require further evaluation. An infant who has a negative pulse oximetry screen could still have structural heart disease. If a newborn has already had a postnatal echocardiogram, CCHD screening does not need to be done. For infants who are being treated with supplemental oxygen, oxygen must be discontinued before CCHD screening. If an infant cannot be weaned off oxygen before discharge, an echocardiogram is recommended.[3]

Inborn Errors of Metabolism Included in Newborn Screening

The expansion of newborn screening in recent years has been driven mainly by advancements in technology and new treatments for previously untreatable diseases. Tandem mass spectroscopy allows many different metabolites to be identified at once. Thus, multiple disorders can be detected through just one test. In newborn screening, tandem mass spectroscopy is used to measure amino acids and acylcarnitines in dried blood spots. Other methods are used to detect other disorders, such as biotinidase or galactosemia or lysosomal storage diseases. Some clinical features, diagnostic tests, and treatment of select groups of inborn errors of metabolism are discussed in this article. This is meant to be a brief overview and not a comprehensive review. The authors highly recommend consulting a biochemical or clinical geneticist when an inborn error of metabolism is suspected.

Box 1
Critical congenital heart disease target disorders

- Pulmonary atresia
- Tricuspid atresia
- Truncus arteriosus
- Total anomalous pulmonary venous return
- Hypoplastic left heart syndrome
- D-Transposition of the great vessels
- Double outlet right ventricle
- Ebstein anomaly
- Interrupted aortic arch
- Single ventricle complex
- Coarctation of the aorta
- Tetralogy of Fallot

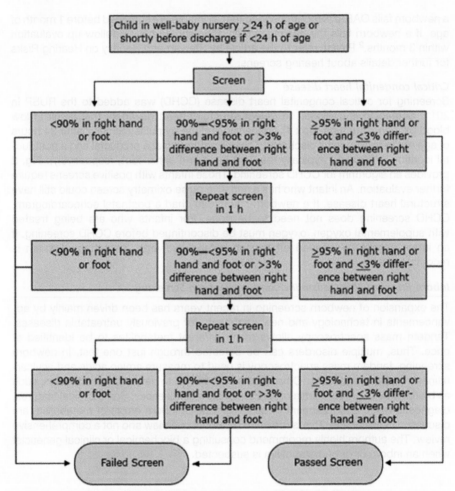

Fig. 2. Critical congenital heart disease algorithm. (*Data from* Centers for Disease Control and Prevention: congenital heart defects-information for health care providers. Available at: http://www.cdc.gov/ncbddd/heartdefects/hcp.html. Accessed August 1, 2018.)

Organic acidemias

Organic acidemias are a group of disorders primarily due to a defect in protein and/or fat metabolism that causes abnormal organic acids to accumulate. Patients may present very early in the neonatal period with feeding difficulties, changes in muscle tone, vomiting, hypoglycemia, metabolic acidosis, and/or hyperammonemia. Long-term management of a child with an organic acidemia generally consists of a protein-restricted diet with the addition of specialized metabolic formula to provide other nonoffending amino acids. Supplemental carnitine is used to treat patients with some conditions, because carnitine binds excess organic acids that can then be excreted in the urine, as well as to treat secondary carnitine deficiency (caused by the loss of the bound carnitine). Other medications may be used depending on the disorder (**Table 2**).

Amino acid disorders

Amino acid disorders are a diverse group of disorders caused by a defect in amino acid metabolism. Signs and symptoms vary widely, based on the specific disorder.

Table 2
Core recommended uniform screening panel disorders: organic acidemias

General Clinical Presentation	Disease-Specific Clinical Findings	Initial Workup	Laboratory Findings	Initial Treatment

Lethargy
Hypotonia
Feeding difficulty
Failure to thrive
Respiratory distress
Encephalopathy
Coma
Metabolic stroke
	• PA
	  Cardiomyopathy
	  Arrhythmia (QT interval prolongation)
	  Pancreatitis
	  Chronic renal failure
	• MMA
	  Cardiomyopathy
	  Pancreatitis
	  Progressive renal impairment
	• IVA
	  Odor of sweaty feet
	• GA-I
	  Macrocephaly
	  Dystonic movements
		Glucose
		Ammonia
		Electrolytes
		Blood gas
		CBC
		Liver enzymes (AST/ALT)
		Urinalysis
		Urine organic acid
		Plasma acylcarnitine profile
		Free and total carnitine
			High anion gap metabolic acidosis
			Hyperammonemia
			Lactic acidosis
			Hypoglycemia
			Ketosis
			Leukopenia
			Thrombocytopenia
			Pancytopenia
				1. Initiate high caloric supplementation to suppress catabolism. This is usually achieved by starting 10% dextrose with age-appropriate electrolytes at 1.5 the maintenance rate for patient's weight. Consider use of intralipids if higher caloric support is required by the patient.
				2. Stop protein intake.
				3. Correct metabolic abnormalities (hypoglycemia, metabolic acidosis, hyperammonemia).
				4. Identify and treat precipitating factors (illness, stress, etc.).

Abbreviations: GA-I, glutaric acidemia type I; IVA, isovaleric acidemia; MMA, methylmalonic acidemia; PA, propionic acidemia.
Data from Refs.[15–18]

Some of these disorders may present in the neonatal period similar to organic acidemias (such as maple syrup urine disease). Symptoms may develop despite treatment, such as developmental or behavioral disorders in patients with phenylketonuria. Almost all patients with these disorders will require a protein-restricted diet for life with supplemental specialized metabolic formulas. Specific treatments for each disorder, including medications, are listed in **Table 3**.

Fatty acid oxidation disorders

Fatty acid oxidation disorders are caused by a defect in fatty acid metabolism. These can be due to (1) a defect in the primary enzymes involved in beta-oxidation or (2) a defect in the carnitine cycle, because carnitine is required to shuttle long-chain fats into the mitochondria for beta-oxidation. Patients typically present in infancy/early childhood with hypoglycemia. In some of the long-chain fatty acid oxidation disorders, neonates may present with cardiomyopathy and other life-threatening conditions. Long-term management typically consists of frequent feedings, avoidance of fasting, restriction of specific types of fats, and supplemental carnitine. In patients with defects in long-chain fatty acid metabolism, supplementation of diet with medium-chain fats may be given **(Table 4)**.

Galactosemia

Galactosemia is a disorder usually caused by a deficiency of galactose-1-uridyltransferase, an enzyme that breaks down the sugar galactose. Galactose is also contained in lactose. Untreated patients with galactosemia typically present in the neonatal period with feeding intolerance, leading to failure to thrive, hepatocellular dysfunction including jaundice and bleeding diathesis, and *Escherichia coli* sepsis. Patients are treated with a galactose-restricted diet. Even with early treatment, children may still have developmental delays (especially speech issues) and motor abnormalities such as tremors and difficulties with gait and balance. Most women will develop premature ovarian insufficiency **(Table 5)**.

Biotinidase deficiency

Biotin (Vitamin B_7) is an important cofactor of carboxylase enzymes required for different intracellular processes. In biotinidase deficiency, the body is unable to (1) produce free biotin from dietary sources and (2) recycle biotin bound to intracellular enzymes. If untreated, children with profound biotinidase deficiency (10% or less enzyme activity) may develop seizures, hypotonia, hearing loss, optic nerve atrophy, and skin abnormalities. In patients with untreated partial biotinidase deficiency (10%–30% of normal enzyme activity), common problems may include alopecia, skin problems (eczemalike skin lesions), and hypotonia. Early initiation and lifelong treatment with oral biotin are usually adequate to prevent the development of these complications (see **Table 5**).

Lysosomal storage diseases

Lysosomal storage diseases (LSDs) are a heterogeneous group of disorders in which a substance accumulates in various organ tissues due to a nonworking lysosomal enzyme. LSDs typically present in older infancy/childhood with symptoms such as coarse facial features, developmental delays, musculoskeletal abnormalities, hepatosplenomegaly, and ocular changes. Some affected patients may present in the neonatal period with features such as hydrops fetalis or hypertrophic cardiomyopathy (Pompe disease). Newborn screening for 2 lysosomal storage diseases was added to the RUSP in 2016—Pompe disease and mucopolysaccharidosis type 1 (MPS-1, also known as Hurler syndrome). Some states screen for additional

Table 3
Core recommended uniform screening panel disorders: amino acid disorders

Disorder	Disease-Specific Clinical Findings	Initial Workup	Laboratory Findings	Initial Treatment
Disorders that may present with a metabolic crisis				
Argininosuccinic aciduria (ASA/ASL)	Lethargy Irritability Vomiting Encephalopathy Protein aversion	Electrolytes Blood gas Ammonia Liver function tests (AST/ALT) Plasma amino acids	Hyperammonemia Normal to increased liver enzymes	1. Initiate high caloric supplementation to suppress catabolism. 2. Stop protein intake. 3. Promote nitrogen excretion by starting nitrogen scavengers (sodium benzoate and sodium phenylacetate/buphenyl). 4. Consider starting L-arginine to enhance residual urea cycle function. 5. Identify and treat precipitating factors (illness, stress, etc.).
Citrullinemia type I (CIT-I/ASS)	Lethargy Irritability Vomiting Encephalopathy Protein aversion Liver failure	Electrolytes Blood gas Ammonia Liver function tests (AST/ALT) Plasma amino acids Urine orotic acid	Hyperammonemia Normal to increased liver enzymes	
Maple syrup urine disease (MSUD)	Lethargy Irritability Vomiting Feeding difficulty Ataxia Seizures Encephalopathy Maple syrup odor to urine, ear wax Cerebral edema	Glucose Ammonia Electrolytes Osmolality Blood gas CBC Urinalysis Plasma amino acids	High anion gap metabolic acidosis Hypoglycemia Hyperammonemia Low to normal serum osmolality Low to normal sodium	1. Initiate high caloric supplementation to suppress catabolism. 2. Stop protein intake. 3. Monitor leucine, valine, and isoleucine levels. 4. Correct metabolic abnormalities (hypoglycemia, metabolic acidosis, hyperammonemia). 5. Monitor sodium level to prevent cerebral edema. 6. Identify and treat precipitating factors (illness, stress, etc.).

(continued on next page)

Table 3
(continued)

Disorders that have an insidious onset

Disorder	Disease-Specific Clinical Findings	Initial Workup	Laboratory Findings	Initial Treatment
Homocystinuria (HCY)	Developmental delay Ectopia lentis Thromboembolism/thromboses Marfanoid appearance Osteoporosis	Plasma amino acids Plasma total homocysteine Plasma MMA	Increased methionine Increased total homocysteine	Treatment Goal Prevent HCY-associated complications. Treatment options include use of vitamin B6 (pyridoxine) therapy (if responsive), a methionine-restricted diet, folate, vitamin B12, and Betaine. Evaluate for skeletal and ophthalmologic complications.
Phenylketonuria (PKU)	Developmental delay Impaired executive function Hypopigmentation	Plasma amino acids Urine pterins Dihydropteridine reductase (DHPR) activity in RBC	Increased phenylalanine level Normal to decreased tyrosine Normal pterins and DHPR activity	Treatment Goal Maintain phenylalanine level between 120–360 µmol/L (2–6 mg/dL). Start phenylalanine-restricted diet Consider use of sapropterin (BH₄), if responsive.
Tyrosinemia type I (TYR-I)	Liver failure Chronic renal failure/tubulopathy Increased risk for hepatocellular cancer	Plasma amino acids Succinylacetone Liver enzymes Serum alpha Fetoprotein (AFP) Coagulation profile (PT, PTT, INR) Vitamin K-dependent coagulation factors Abdominal/renal ultrasound	Increased liver enzymes Prolonged (PT, PTT, INR) Elevated AFP Increased succinylacetone in blood and urine Increased plasma tyrosine, methionine, and phenylalanine	Treatment Goal Maintain tyrosine level less than 400–500 µmol/L. Prompt initiation of nitisinone [2-(2-nitro-4-trifluoro-methylbenzyol)-1,3 cyclohexanedione (NTBC)] Start phenylalanine- and tyrosine-restricted diet.

Data from Refs.[19–22]

Table 4
Primary recommended uniform screening panel disorders: fatty acid oxidation disorders

General Clinical Presentation	Disease-Specific Clinical Findings	Initial Workup	Laboratory Findings	Initial Treatment
Hypoketotic hypoglycemia Lethargy Poor feeding Hypotonia Myopathy	• CUD/CTD Cardiomyopathy Liver dysfunction Rhabdomyolysis • MCAD Sudden decrease in glucose level that may be mistaken for SIDS • LCHAD Cardiomyopathy Arrhythmia Peripheral neuropathy Liver dysfunction Pigmentary retinopathy Maternal HELLP	Glucose Ammonia Electrolytes Blood gas Liver enzymes tests (AST/ALT) Creatine kinase (CK) Urinalysis Plasma acylcarnitine profile Free and total carnitine	Hypoglycemia Hyperammonemia (especially in MCAD and LCHAD) Elevated liver enzymes	1. Initiate high caloric supplementation by starting 10% dextrose with age-appropriate electrolytes at 1.5 times the maintenance rate for patient's weight. 2. Correct metabolic abnormalities (hypoglycemia, metabolic acidosis, hyperammonemia) 3. Consider carnitine supplementation (50–100 mg/kg/d). 4. Identify and treat precipitating factors (illness, stress, etc.).

Abbreviations: CUD/CTD, carnitine uptake defect/carnitine transport defect; LCHAD, long-chain L-3 hydroxyacyl-CoA dehydrogenase deficiency; MCAD, medium-chain acyl-CoA dehydrogenase deficiency; VLCAD, very long-chain acyl-CoA dehydrogenase deficiency.
Data from Refs. [18,23,24]

Table 5
Further reading for other inborn errors of metabolism

Galactosemia	Demirbas D, Coelho AI, Rubio-Gozalbo ME, et al. Hereditary galactosemia. Metabolism 2018;83:188–96; and Welling L, Bernstein LE, Berry GT, et al. International clinical guideline for the management of clssical galactosemia: diagnosis, treatment, and follow-up. J Inherit Metab Dis 2017;40(2):171–76
Biotinidase Deficiency	Wolf B. Biotinidase deficiency. 2000 Mar 24 [Updated 2016 Jun 9]. In: Adam MP, Ardinger HH, Pagon RA, et al., editors. GeneReviews® [Internet]. Seattle (WA): University of Washington, Seattle; 1993-2018. Available at: https://www.ncbi.nlm.nih.gov/books/NBK1322/
Lysosomal Storage Disease	Kishnani PS, Steiner RD, Bali D, et al. Pompe disease diagnosis and management guideline. Genet Med 2006;8(5):267–88. Tarnopolsky M, Katzberg H, Petrof BJ, et al. Pompe disease: diagnosis and management. evidence-based guidelines from a Canadian expert panel. Can J Neurol Sci 2016;43(4):472–85. Muenzer J, Wraith JE, Clarke LA, I ICPoMaToM. Mucopolysaccharidosis I: management and treatment guidelines. Pediatrics 2009;123(1):19–29.

disorders, including mucopolysaccharidosis type 2 (MPS-2), Fabry disease, Gaucher disease, Krabbe disease, and Niemann-Pick disease type A/B. Some lysosomal storage diseases can be treated using enzyme replacement therapy, in which a synthetic version of the deficient enzyme is provided intravenously on a regular basis (see **Table 5**).

Other Newborn Screening Disorders

A variety of other types of genetic disorders are also included as part of newborn screening but are beyond the scope of this article. References are provided for further reading (**Table 6**).

Special Considerations and Issues with Newborn Screening

The premature and sick infant

All preterm and critically ill newborns must also undergo newborn screening. However, extra care must be performed in collecting samples at the right time so that reliable results are obtained. Some metabolites are greatly affected by a variety of prenatal factors, including gestational age, birth weight, and nutritional status.[4] In addition, several NICU procedures are known to interfere with the interpretation of newborn screening results, such as the use of certain antibiotics, blood transfusions, and use of total parenteral nutrition. Premature and sick infants are more likely to have a false-positive result on their initial screen due to immaturity of enzymes involved in metabolic pathways or clinical interventions received. **Table 7** shows some of the factors that may affect screening results.

In 2009, the Clinical and Laboratory Standards Institute developed Guidelines for Newborn Screening for Preterm, Low Birth Weight, and Sick Newborns. The guideline provides recommendations on NBS specimen collection in this special group of infants, with the goal of completing the screen in the shortest period of time and least number of specimens while maintaining high reliability.[5]

Maternal conditions that may affect newborn screening results

Maternal disorders and medication use may also affect newborn screening results. Some disorders, such as a previously undiagnosed maternal glutaric aciduria type

Table 6
Further reading for other newborn screening disorders

Cystic Fibrosis	Rosenfeld M, Sontag MK, Ren CL. Cystic fibrosis diagnosis and newborn screening. Pediatr Clin North Am 2016;63(4):599–615.
Severe Combined Immunodeficiency	Chinn IK, Shearer WT. Severe combined immunodeficiency disorders. Immunol Allergy Clin North Am 2015;35(4):671–94.
Congenital Hypothyroidism	Léger J, Olivieri A, Donaldson M, et al. European Society for Pediatric Endocrinology consensus guidelines on screening, diagnosis, and management of congenital hypothyroidism. J Clin Endocrinol Metab 2014;99(2):363–84.
Congenital Adrenal Hyperplasia	Nimkarn S, Lin-Su K, New MI. Steroid 21 hydroxylase deficiency congenital adrenal hyperplasia. Pediatr Clin North Am 2011;58(5):1281–300, xii.
Hemoglobinopathies	Quinn CT. Sickle cell disease in childhood: from newborn screening through transition to adult medical care. Pediatr Clin North Am 2013;60(6):1363–81.
Congenital Hearing Loss	US Preventive Services Task Force. Universal screening for hearing loss in newborns: US Preventive Services Task Force recommendation statement. Pediatrics 2008;122(1):143–8.
Critical Congenital Heart Disease	Fillipps DJ, Bucciarelli RL. Cardiac evaluation of the newborn. Pediatr Clin North Am 2015;62(2):471–89.
X-linked Adrenoleukodystrophy	Kemper AR, Brosco J, Comeau AM, et al. Newborn screening for X-linked adrenoleukodystrophy: evidence summary and advisory committeee recommendations. Genet Med 2017;19(1):121–6
Spinal Muscular Atrophy	Glascock J, Samspon J, Haidet-Phillips A. Treatment algorithm for infants diagnosed with spinal muscular atrophy through newborn screening. J Neuromuscul Dis 2018;5(2):145–58

1, carnitine uptake deficiency, carnitine transporter deficiency, or 3-methylcrotonyl-CoA carboxylase deficiency, may cause false-positive test results. Use of certain medications during the pregnancy may also affect screening for disorders such as congenital adrenal hyperplasia and congenital hypothyroidism (**Table 8**).

Limitations of newborn screening
For a variety of reasons, such as lack of a specific analyte or marker molecule to measure, absence of optimized treatment, or poorly described pathophysiology, other inborn errors of metabolism that may present in the neonatal period are not part of

Table 7
Factors that may affect newborn screening in a premature and sick infant

Conditions of the Newborn Affecting Newborn Screening Results	NICU Interventions Affecting Newborn Screening Results
• Immaturity—Poorly developed hypothalamic-pituitary axis, liver, and kidney • Hypoxia • Liver disease • Hyperbilirubinemia • Acute illness	• Red cell transfusion and extracorporeal membrane oxygenation (ECMO) • Medications: antibiotics (ampicillin, cefotaxime), steroids, dopamine, iodine (from antiseptics) • Total parenteral nutrition • Early specimen collection

Table 8	
Maternal disorders and medications that may affect newborn screening results	
Maternal Disorders	**Medications**
• Vitamin B12 deficiency	• Propylthiouracil (PTU)
• Glutaric aciduria type 1	• Radioactive iodine
• Primary carnitine deficiency	• Steroids
• Hyper/Hypothyroidism	
• Congenital adrenal hyperplasia	

the newborn testing. Mitochondrial disorders and congenital lactic acidosis syndromes, which may present with lactic acidosis, hypotonia, and seizures in the neonatal period, still cannot be screened. Practitioners should be aware of the disorders being screened for in their respective states and understand that a negative newborn screen does not rule-out all inborn errors of metabolism. Because this is a screening test, not a diagnostic test, both false-negatives and false-positives can occur. Therefore, all metabolic disorders should remain in the differential, even if a patient has had a normal newborn screen. Consultation with a Clinical Geneticist and/or Clinical/Medical Biochemical Geneticist is recommended for all patients in whom an inborn error of metabolism is suspected.

Ethical Issues

There are many ethical issues that must be considered in the newborn screening setting. Some of the more common ones are discussed in this section.

Parental education and consent

Unfortunately, many parents do not understand the newborn screening process for various reasons. Some parents do not know or even remember that newborn screening was performed. This is understandable, as the newborn screen is usually performed 24 to 48 hours after birth, when parents are exhausted and focused on taking care of their newborn. Education about newborn screening is not mandatory; therefore, only about half the states provide any formal education. In addition, this education can vary from having a hospital staff member discuss the testing to simply handing a parent a pamphlet.[6] Surveys of parents have suggested that education should ideally be done in the prenatal period, but this would require involvement before delivery.[7,8] Also, most newborn screening programs are "opt out," meaning testing is mandatory unless a parent specifically signs a form allowing them to opt out. Lack of information regarding the newborn screening process and purpose can lead to parents either opting in or opting out without truly understanding the risks and benefits.

Ambiguity of results

Some patients will have nondiagnostic follow-up test results. This may lead to weeks or months of additional testing to determine if a child is affected or not. This can cause significant stress to the child and family. Other times, infants are identified as having very mild disease or "biochemical only" disease (that is, abnormality by laboratory testing that would have never resulted in a clinical phenotype). This can lead to confusion over whether treatment is actually needed or not.[6]

Unintentional results

Sometimes, children with positive newborn screens are found to be genetic carriers of a disorder rather than affected. The identification of carriers without consent of the patient is discouraged by professional organizations, such as the American Academy of Pediatrics[9] and ACMG,[10] because this takes away their autonomy to decide whether they want to know their carrier status.

In addition, during the workup of metabolic disorders, parents sometimes undergo genetic testing, and this could potentially lead to the revelation of misattributed paternity.[11]

Obligation to other family members

Disclosing results that could have reproductive or health implications to family members other than the parents is not uncommon when a genetic disease is diagnosed. Although parents are encouraged to discuss results with other family members, there is currently no legal obligation to do so. The physician may offer to help other family members better understand the disorder and their own risks if requested by the parents.

Storage of dried blood spots

Many states store dried blood spots and use deidentified spots for research or other purposes. These dried blood spots can be a resource for researchers, especially those doing population-based genetic studies. There have been legal proceedings in some states related to privacy concerns that have led to the destruction of archived dried blood spots.[6] Some states require parents to sign a consent form to allow for long-term storage and permission to use these deidentified samples for research purposes.

Variable resources

There are certainly differences in newborn screening logistics related to access and resources. Follow-up specialized metabolic services may be many hours away for some patients. Insurance coverage for special formulas, medical foods, and rare medications can vary as well, making it difficult for some families to afford treatment. There may also be differences in the number of disorders screened for in different states.

Future of Newborn Screening

The introduction of tandem mass spectrometry revolutionized newborn screening over a decade ago. Since then, new technologies used in diagnosing rare genetic disorders have emerged and continue to evolve. The number of disorders included in the RUSP because of new treatment options also continues to increase. As a result, there are continuous efforts to expand the list of treatable disorders that can be detected from a dried blood spot.

Disorders being considered for newborn screening

The approval of nusinersen for the treatment of spinal muscular atrophy type 1 (SMA1) led to recent inclusion for SMA testing in the RUSP. At the time of writing this article, there are currently 4 states (Indiana, Minnesota, Missouri, and Utah) that have started screening their newborns for SMA. Other states offer optional SMA screening. Duchenne muscular dystrophy is being evaluated for inclusion in the RUSP. Other inborn errors of metabolism, such as GAMT deficiency, are also being studied for inclusion in the RUSP. More studies are needed to determine which disorders should be added.

Technology being evaluated for use in newborn screening

DNA-based technology is the most frequently proposed type of future testing but other developments in enzyme-based assays have been used increasingly, specifically in screening for lysosomal storage disorders. **Table 9** summarizes current technologies being studied as potential screening platforms. As always, it is essential to

Table 9
Current technologies being studied for newborn screening

Test	Methodology	Advantages	Disadvantages
Next-generation sequencing gene panels	Sequencing of a panel of genes specific for a specific disorder or symptom	Genes being tested are specific to patient's clinical presentation	Potential for VOUS Diagnosis may be missed if gene is not included in the panel Long TAT
Whole exome sequencing (WES)	Sequencing of all coding regions (exons) of the genome	Most exonic regions are covered	Higher risk for having VOUS Potential for false-negative result if pathogenic variant is in an intron Long TAT
Whole genome sequencing	Sequencing of both coding and noncoding regions of the genome (exons and introns)	Most exons and introns are covered	Highest risk for having VOUS Long TAT
Fluorimetric assay using digital microfluidics	Measures enzyme activity using fluorimetry	Simultaneous measurement of multiple enzymes on samples from multiple DBS in a single run Short run time	New equipment or workstations must be acquired
Metabolomic profiling	Measurement of all biomolecules/ metabolites in body fluids	Able to detect multiple biomarkers at the same time Has the potential to provide subclassifications of diseases	May be affected by external factors May still need DNA-based testing to confirm the diagnosis

Abbreviations: DBS, dried blood spot; TAT, turnaround time; VOUS, variant of uncertain significance.

keep in mind the fundamental characteristics of newborn screening: a highly sensitive test with reasonable costs, short turnaround time (TAT), and an effective treatment.

In the past few years, next-generation sequencing (NGS) panels, whole exome sequencing (WES), and whole genome sequencing (WGS) have been considered as NBS platforms. NGS can test for multiple disorders at the same time and those with milder disease forms, which may not be easily differentiated by metabolite screening and biochemical testing. Pilot studies are in process in some states, mostly funded through grants from the National Human Genome Research Institute and the National Institute of Health; some commercial companies are already offering such tests.[12] However, cost and prolonged TAT remain as the biggest barriers in adopting DNA-based tests for newborn screening at this time.[13]

Depending on the type of test used, there is also a risk of having false-negative results if particular segments of a gene or genome are sequenced. In addition, there are ethical issues, such as the loss of patient autonomy; the potential to identify adult-onset disorders; the detection of variants of uncertain clinical significance or detectable DNA changes that currently cannot be determined as benign or disease causing; and the identification of carriers.[14]

Aside from DNA tests, several assays have been developed to measure enzyme activity from dried blood spots. These assays have been used mostly in the screening for lysosomal storage disorders, such as Pompe disease, MPS-I, Fabry disease, Gaucher disease, and Krabbe disease. Platforms that use both TMS and fluorimetry are currently being used by multiple states.

Another method currently being studied as a tool for newborn screening is metabolomic profiling. The metabolome is the collection of biomolecules or metabolites that are produced by cells and present in body fluids. It is a reflection of genetic factors, illness, and external factors such as diet and environment. Certain diseases may be identified by this method by looking for the presence or absence of particular metabolites. At this time, more studies are still needed to validate its use as a newborn screening method.

Summary

The goal of newborn screening is to prevent morbidity and mortality through the early detection of treatable disorders. Many of these disorders may present in the neonatal period; therefore, neonatologists or pediatricians may be the first physicians to manage these patients. Although specialists will ultimately manage these patients, it is important for neonatologists and pediatricians to have a basic understanding of the newborn screening process as well as the basic evaluation and management of these disorders. In the future, more and more disorders will be added to newborn screening panels. We are experiencing exciting times in the genomic era. However, similar to all aspects of medicine, this expansion comes with many technical and ethical issues, some of which have been addressed in this article.

REFERENCES

1. American College of Medical Genetics Newborn Screening Expert Group. Newborn screening: toward a uniform screening panel and system–executive summary. Pediatrics 2006;117(5 Pt 2):S296–307.
2. US Preventive Services Task Force. Universal screening for hearing loss in newborns: US Preventive Services Task Force recommendation statement. Pediatrics 2008;122(1):143–8.
3. Oster ME, Kochilas L. Screening for critical congenital heart disease. Clin Perinatol 2016;43(1):73–80.
4. Qian J, Wang X, Liu J, et al. Applying targeted next generation sequencing to dried blood spot specimens from suspicious cases identified by tandem mass spectrometry-based newborn screening. J Pediatr Endocrinol Metab 2017; 30(9):979–88.
5. Cummings JJ. Guideline addresses challenges of newborn screening in preterm, ill infants. AAP News 2012.
6. Tarini BA, Goldenberg AJ. Ethical issues with newborn screening in the genomics era. Annu Rev Genomics Hum Genet 2012;13:381–93.
7. Etchegary H, Nicholls SG, Tessier L, et al. Consent for newborn screening: parents' and health-care professionals' experiences of consent in practice. Eur J Hum Genet 2016;24(11):1530–4.
8. Hasegawa LE, Fergus KA, Ojeda N, et al. Parental attitudes toward ethical and social issues surrounding the expansion of newborn screening using new technologies. Public Health Genomics 2011;14(4–5):298–306.

9. Committee on Bioethics. Ethical issues with genetic testing in pediatrics. Pediatrics 2001;107(6):1451–5.
10. Ross LF, Saal HM, David KL, et al, American Academy of Pediatrics, American College of Medical Genetics and Genomics. Technical report: ethical and policy issues in genetic testing and screening of children. Genet Med 2013;15(3): 234–45.
11. van der Burg S, Oerlemans A. Fostering caring relationships: suggestions to rethink liberal perspectives on the ethics of newborn screening. Bioethics 2018;32(3):171–83.
12. Friedman JM, Cornel MC, Goldenberg AJ, et al. Genomic newborn screening: public health policy considerations and recommendations. BMC Med Genomics 2017;10(1):9.
13. Almannai M, Marom R, Sutton VR. Newborn screening: a review of history, recent advancements, and future perspectives in the era of next generation sequencing. Curr Opin Pediatr 2016;28(6):694–9.
14. Reinstein E. Challenges of using next generation sequencing in newborn screening. Genet Res (Camb) 2015;97:e21.
15. Kölker S, Christensen E, Leonard JV, et al. Diagnosis and management of glutaric aciduria type I--revised recommendations. J Inherit Metab Dis 2011;34(3): 677–94.
16. Baumgartner MR, Hörster F, Dionisi-Vici C, et al. Proposed guidelines for the diagnosis and management of methylmalonic and propionic acidemia. Orphanet J Rare Dis 2014;9:130.
17. Vockley J, Ensenauer R. Isovaleric acidemia: new aspects of genetic and phenotypic heterogeneity. Am J Med Genet C Semin Med Genet 2006;142C(2):95–103.
18. New England consortium of metabolic programs: acute illness protocols. Available at: http://newenglandconsortium.org/for-professionals/acute-illness-protocols/. Accessed July 15, 2018.
19. Huemer M, Kožich V, Rinaldo P, et al. Newborn screening for homocystinurias and methylation disorders: systematic review and proposed guidelines. J Inherit Metab Dis 2015;38(6):1007–19.
20. Chinsky JM, Singh R, Ficicioglu C, et al. Diagnosis and treatment of tyrosinemia type I: a US and Canadian consensus group review and recommendations. Genet Med 2017;19(12):1–16.
21. Häberle J, Boddaert N, Burlina A, et al. Suggested guidelines for the diagnosis and management of urea cycle disorders. Orphanet J Rare Dis 2012;7:32.
22. Strauss KA, Puffenberger EG, Morton DH. Maple syrup urine disease. In: Adam MP, Ardinger HH, Pagon RA, et al, editors. GeneReviews®. Seattle (WA): University of Washington, Seattle; 2013. p. 1993–2018. Available at: https://www-ncbi-nlm-nih-gov.proxy.lib.wayne.edu/books/NBK1319/.
23. Spiekerkoetter U. Mitochondrial fatty acid oxidation disorders: clinical presentation of long-chain fatty acid oxidation defects before and after newborn screening. J Inherit Metab Dis 2010;33(5):527–32.
24. Wilcken B. Fatty acid oxidation disorders: outcome and long-term prognosis. J Inherit Metab Dis 2010;33(5):501–6.

Late Preterm Infants

Morbidities, Mortality, and Management Recommendations

Katie Huff, MD, Rebecca S. Rose, MD, William A. Engle, MD*

KEYWORDS

- Late preterm • Morbidity • Mortality • Monitoring • Management

KEY POINTS

- Late preterm infants are defined as those infants born between, and including, 34 weeks and 0 days and 36 weeks and 6 days.
- During the birth hospitalization, late preterm infants are at increased risk for morbidities such as respiratory distress, hypothermia, feeding difficulties, hyperbilirubinemia, and hypoglycemia.
- After discharge, late preterm infants are at increased risk for rehospitalization, mortality, and other morbidities, including neurologic, respiratory, developmental, and psychiatric/behavioral disorders.
- Monitoring for short-term and long-term morbidities is important in the late preterm population both during the birth hospitalization and into the future.

A significant increase in preterm births (those born <37 weeks of gestation) from 10.62% to 12.73% of all births occurred between 1990 and 2005.[1] Throughout this time, infants born later in the preterm period (variably referred to as near term, marginally preterm, mildly preterm, among other descriptors) continued to account for most, nearly three quarters, of these preterm births. To emphasize the importance of better optimizing the care of late preterm infants, along with supporting epidemiologic investigations into morbidity and mortality, the National Institute of Child Health and Human Development of the National Institutes of Health gathered a panel of experts to define this group. This panel defined infants born just before term as late preterm to emphasize their vulnerability and prematurity. Furthermore, late preterm was precisely defined as those born between, and including, the gestational ages of 34 weeks and 0 days (239 days) and 36 weeks and 6 days (259 days).[2]

Disclosure: The authors have no conflicts of interest to disclose.
Department of Neonatology, Indiana University School of Medicine, 699 Riley Hospital Drive, RR 208, Indianapolis, IN 46202, USA
* Corresponding author. Riley Research Room 208, 699 Riley Drive, Indianapolis, IN 46202.
E-mail address: wengle@iu.edu

Pediatr Clin N Am 66 (2019) 387–402
https://doi.org/10.1016/j.pcl.2018.12.008
0031-3955/19/© 2018 Elsevier Inc. All rights reserved.

pediatric.theclinics.com

This article describes epidemiologic trends in the rate of late preterm births and the associated risks for morbidities and mortality of being born late preterm. Furthermore, it discusses the importance of reducing the rate of late preterm births, monitoring and managing for short-term and long-term complications, and understanding factors that increase risk for morbidity and mortality in this subgroup of preterm infants.

Late preterm infants are a population with historically underappreciated increased risk for significant morbidity and mortality compared with term infants.[2,3] In 2017, the rate of late preterm births in the United States increased for the third year in a row, up 5% since 2014, to 7.17% (**Table 1**).[4,5] Late preterm births account for more than 70% of all preterm births, which equaled 279,382 births in 2016 alone (**Fig. 1**).[4] Although morbidities occur in only a fraction of these infants, given the large number of late preterm births annually, these infants contribute to a large burden of care and cost to the health care and education systems compared with term infants.[6]

The recent increased rate of late preterm birth is concerning given the already large number that occur annually and prior successes in reducing such births between 2006 and 2014. The exact cause of this trend is unclear. Possible causes include the ongoing changes in maternal demographics (including increasing maternal age) and maternal health (including increasing rates of obesity and opioid use) that contribute to preterm birth.[7–9] The increase in late preterm birth rate was observed across all maternal age groups, not just the older subgroups, so maternal age is less likely a new contributor.[4] Past cited causes, including increased number of multiple gestations, high rate of elective inductions, or cesarean sections, have decreased in recent years and are less likely to contribute to this recent increase.[4] Additional investigation is needed to clarify causation of this recent increase in late preterm birth rate and guide interventions to reverse this trend.

ACUTE MORBIDITIES DURING BIRTH HOSPITALIZATION

Late preterm infants are at risk for acute morbidities starting immediately after birth in the delivery room. Compared with term infants, late preterm infants more often require resuscitation (46% vs 28%; odds ratio [OR], 2.14; 95% confidence interval [CI], 1.88–2.44) including bag mask ventilation (14% vs 6%; OR, 2.61; 95% CI, 2.14–3.17).[10] These increased rates of delivery room intervention persist even when controlling for variables such as cesarean delivery. The level of resuscitation required decreases

Table 1
Percentage of annual births by gestational age 2014 to 2016

Year	Number	<28	28–31	32–33	34–36	37–38	39–40
2010	3,999,386	0.71	0.94	1.18	7.15	27.29	56.08
2011	3,953,590	0.70	0.93	1.18	6.99	26.09	57.51
2012	3,952,841	0.71	0.92	1.17	6.96	25.47	58.30
2013	3,932,181	0.70	0.92	1.17	6.83	24.81	58.85
2014	3,988,076	0.69	0.91	1.15	6.82	24.76	58.72
2015	3,978,487	0.68	0.91	1.17	6.87	24.99	58.47
2016	3,945,875	0.68	0.92	1.17	7.09	25.47	57.94
2017	3,853,472	—	—	—	7.17	—	—

Data from Martin JA, Hamilton BE, Osterman MJK, et al. Births: final data for 2016. US Department of Health and Human Services; 2018; and Hamilton BE, Martin JA, Osterman MJK, et al. Births: provisional data for 2017. Hyattsville (MD): National Center for Health Statistics; 2018.

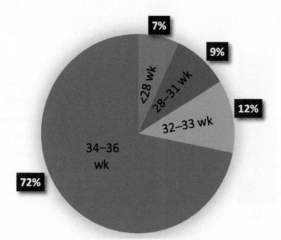

Fig. 1. Breakdown of preterm births for 2016. (*Data from* Martin JA, Hamilton BE, Osterman MJK, et al. Births: final data for 2016. Hyattsville (MD): U. S. Department of Health and Human Services; 2018.)

with increasing gestational age between 34 and 39 weeks of gestation.[11] After delivery, late preterm infants are at increased risk of neonatal intensive care unit (NICU) admission.[11,12] NICU admission criteria vary by institution but, even when comparing low-risk spontaneous late preterm delivery, late preterm infants continue to have an increased rate of NICU admission.[12] Reasons for NICU admission in this population include respiratory distress, hypothermia, feeding difficulties, hyperbilirubinemia, and hypoglycemia (**Fig. 2**).[12,13]

Late preterm infants more often have symptoms of respiratory distress than term infants.[13] With decreasing gestational age, there is an increase in respiratory distress syndrome, transient tachypnea of the newborn, pneumonia, apnea, and pneumothorax (**Fig. 3**).[11,14] These respiratory morbidities lead to an increased need for respiratory support, including oxygen therapy, noninvasive ventilation, invasive ventilation, and surfactant replacement.[11,14,15] Late preterm infants have structurally and functionally immature lungs with decreased surface area, decreased capacity for pulmonary fluid absorption at birth, and decreased surfactant

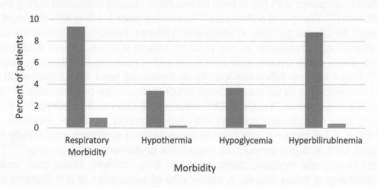

Fig. 2. Clinical morbidities noted during birth hospitalization from pooled data for late preterm and term patients. (*Data from* Refs.[11–13,77,78,90,91])

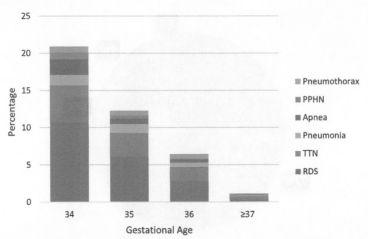

Fig. 3. Respiratory morbidities by gestational age. (*Data from* Teune MJ, Bakhuizen S, Gyamfi Bannerman C, et al. A systematic review of severe morbidity in infants born late preterm. Am J Obstet Gynecol 2011;205(4):374.e1-9.)

production.[16–21] Antenatal betamethasone therapy has been shown to decrease the rates of respiratory morbidities in the late preterm population.[22] Based on these observations, it is now recommended that women at risk of delivery between 34 0/7 weeks and 36 6/7 weeks of gestation receive a single course of corticosteroids.[23] Additional studies are needed to further understand the effect of this new recommendation on the rate of respiratory and other short-term and long-term morbidities in the late preterm population.[24]

About 10% of late preterm infants experience temperature instability early during the birth hospitalization.[13] Neonates in general rely on nonshivering thermogenesis to maintain body temperature.[25] Late preterm infants have lower amounts of brown adipose tissue and regulatory hormone concentrations compared with term infants, leading to a diminished ability to produce heat. Late preterm infants also have more heat loss than term infants because of lower amounts of white adipose tissue and higher surface area to mass ratio.[3,19,25,26]

Feeding problems increase with decreasing gestational age; about 32% of late preterm infants compared with 7% of term infants have feeding difficulties during the birth hospitalization.[13] Wang and colleagues[13] found that poor feeding was the most common reason for discharge delay in late preterm infants. Feeding difficulties are caused by the physiologic immaturity of late preterm infants with decreased suck efficacy, abnormal sleep wake cycles, and problems with breathing and feeding coordination.[27,28] These feeding difficulties lead to an increased need for supplemental feeds and an increased time to full oral feedings (median time to full oral feedings of 12 days at 34 weeks of gestation, 3 days at 35 weeks, and 2 days at 36 weeks).[28,29] Feeding immaturity also complicates success with breastfeeding. However, because of the normal delay in full maternal milk supply, breastfeeding problems may initially be unrecognized until a larger amount of breastmilk is delivered by suckling.[3,30,31] It is important to educate mothers, particularly first-time mothers, about such problems before discharging these infants. A higher rate of separation of late preterm infants from their mothers because of medical complications is also associated with a higher rate of difficulties with breastfeeding compared with term infants (eg, decreased maternal milk supply, increased time to oral feedings).[29,32]

Feeding problems can increase the risk of physiologic morbidities such as hypogly-cemia and hyperbilirubinemia in late preterm infants. Late preterm infants have lower glucose stores and glucose production compared with more mature infants because of hepatic enzymatic immaturity.[3,33-35] Hepatic immaturity also contributes to more prolonged and clinically significant hyperbilirubinemia because of the lower concen-trations of uridine diphosphate-glucoronosyltransferase, a key enzyme in the meta-bolism of hemoglobin.[36]

As previously noted, late preterm infants are neurologically immature. At 34 weeks gestational age, a neonate's brain weighs 65% that of a term neonate.[37] Even at term postmenstrual gestational age, late preterm infants continue to have increased cere-bral spinal fluid spaces, and decreased myelination, brain size, and biparietal diameter.[38] Such neurologic immaturity increases vulnerability to brain injury and long-term impairments in late preterm infants.[37]

During the birth hospitalization, late preterm infants have a longer length of stay compared with more mature infants, with length of stay increasing with decreasing gestational age. During the initial birth hospitalization, infants born at 34 weeks' gesta-tion stay on average 12.6 days compared with 6.1 days at 35 weeks birth gestational age and 3.8 days at 36 weeks birth gestational age (**Fig. 4**).[39] The most common fac-tors contributing to increased length of stay in late preterm infants are feeding diffi-culties (75.9%), respiratory distress (30.8%), and jaundice (16.3%).[13] In addition to gestational age, hospital practice variation regarding neonatal intensive care, interme-diate nursery care, or well newborn nursery admission also affects the length of stay.[40] Such practice variation may lead to differences in outcomes after hospital discharge, given readmission rates vary in late preterm infants based on NICU admission and duration of birth hospitalization.[41]

Late preterm infants have an increased rate of mortality compared with term infants. In 2013, per 1000 live births, the infant mortality for gestational ages 34 to 36 weeks was 7.23 compared with 3.01 for 37 to 38 weeks and 1.85 for 39 to 40 weeks of gesta-tion.[42] Notably, mortality in late preterm infants varies with the reason for delivery.[43] Those infants born because of isolated spontaneous preterm labor have a neonatal mortality of 1.9 per 1000 live births. In comparison, late preterm infants born with no specific indication, a medical indication, or an obstetric indication have neonatal mor-talities of 3.3, 3.8, and 8.6 per 1000 live births, respectively. Such different neonatal

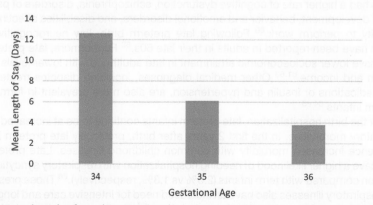

Fig. 4. Mean length of stay by gestational age in weeks. (*Data from* Pulver LS, Denney JM, Silver RM, et al. Morbidity and discharge timing of late preterm newborns. Clin Pediatr (Phila) 2010;49(11):1061–7.)

mortalities emphasize the importance of causality of late preterm birth and associated intrauterine adversity for outcomes.

MORBIDITY IN LATE PRETERM INFANTS FOLLOWING THE BIRTH HOSPITALIZATION

Among infants of all gestational ages, readmission rates are highest among late preterm infants (<34 weeks, 3%; 34–36 weeks, 4.4%; >37 weeks, 2.0%).[44] A higher rate of readmission in late preterm infants correlates with a short duration of birth hospitalization (<4 days).[41] Other risk factors for readmission include any labor or delivery complication, primigravid mother, breastfeeding, and Asian/Pacific Islander ethnicity.[45] Common reasons for readmission include jaundice, feeding difficulties, respiratory distress/apnea, and infection.[41,44,46,47] Jaundice is also a frequent presenting complaint for emergency department visits among neonates, with late preterm infants, especially those born at 36 weeks of gestation, presenting more often than infants of other gestational ages.[48]

Later in life, long-term morbidities encountered by late preterm infants include neurodevelopmental, respiratory, and medical illnesses. Mortality during young adulthood is also higher in late preterm infants than in term infants, with rates of 0.65 per 1000 person years versus 0.46 per 1000 person years, respectively (hazard ratio, 1.31; 95% CI, 1.13–1.50).[49] Late preterm infants have increased rates of developmental delay and cerebral palsy compared with term infants.[50–52] For example, rates of developmental delay/cognitive dysfunction and cerebral palsy at 34 weeks of gestation are 12 per 1000 children and 9 per 1000 children, respectively; at 38 to 41 weeks of gestation, comparable rates are 9 per 1000 and 3 per 1000 children, respectively.[50,52] Partly because of higher rates of neurodevelopmental impairments, more late preterm infants are enrolled in early intervention programs compared with term infants (23.5% vs 11.9%, respectively).[53]

Late preterm infants are also more likely to have behavioral problems, school difficulties, and autism.[51,54–56] Behavioral problems are more common in those diagnosed with developmental delays.[54] However, an increased risk of attention-deficit/hyperactivity disorder has not been consistently found.[57,58] A higher rate of psychiatric hospitalization among adolescents born late preterm has been reported.[59,60] Neurodevelopmental disabilities and impairments are also found in adults born late preterm.[60,61] In a Norwegian cohort of adults aged 20 to 36 years, former late preterm infants had a higher rate of cognitive dysfunction, schizophrenia, disorders of psychological development, behavior and emotional disorders, and disabilities affecting their capacity to perform work.[60] Following late preterm birth, low neurocognitive test scores have been reported in adults in their late 60s.[62] Furthermore, late preterm infants have lower socioeconomic attainment in late adulthood with lower levels of education and income.[61,63] Other medical diagnoses, including diabetes treated with oral medications or insulin and hypertension, are also more prevalent in former late preterm infants.[64,65]

After the birth hospitalization, late preterm infants continue to be at increased risk of respiratory morbidities. In the first 2 years after birth, previously late preterm infants experience increased morbidity with common childhood illnesses. Late preterm infants have a higher likelihood of needing hospitalization with respiratory syncytial virus infection compared with term infants (2.5% vs 1.3%, respectively).[66] Those presenting with respiratory illnesses also have an increased need for intensive care and longer durations of hospital stay than more mature infants.[67] At 18 months of age there is an increased rate of persistent asthma (adjusted OR [aOR], 1.68; 95% CI, 1.01–2.80), need for inhaled corticosteroids (aOR, 1.66; 95% CI, 1.20–2.29), and number of urgent visits for respiratory disorders (incident rate ratio, 1.45; 95% CI, 1.25–1.68).[68] During late childhood and adolescence, poor pulmonary function tests are found in late preterm compared with term infants.[69,70] To control for environmental confounders, especially smoke exposure, contributing to respiratory morbidity, Todisco and colleagues[70] compared late preterm infants with their term siblings and found increased residual volume and residual volume to total lung capacity ratio. Therefore, even when accounting for postnatal exposures, respiratory outcome differences persist, suggesting that intrinsic pulmonary abnormalities are present during childhood and beyond in former late preterm infants.

RISK FACTORS FOR MORBIDITY AND MORTALITY IN LATE PRETERM INFANTS

Given the increased rate of morbidity and mortality of late preterm infants, close monitoring for social, neurodevelopmental, and medical disabilities beyond the neonatal period is warranted. However, most late preterm infants survive, grow, and develop without identifiable medical or social difficulties. This lack of morbidities and mortality may reflect an absence of complications or evaluation at an age when problems have not yet presented.[71–76] Thus, an important question is: what factors are associated with development of complications of late prematurity? The answer is likely multifactorial and may include combinations of influences that include physical and physiologic immaturity, genetic endowment, fetal environmental exposures and stressors, congenital anomalies, infections, medical disorders, and complications associated with any of the preceding factors, along with the postnatal environment.[71,77,78]

In the United States, congenital anomalies are the leading cause of infant mortality (129 per 1000 live births) and second leading cause of neonatal mortality after prematurity-associated complications (92.1 per 1000 live births).[79] In a Swedish cohort of 14,030 late preterm infants, 41% of late preterm neonatal deaths (1.14 per 1000 live births) were attributed to congenital anomalies.[77] Comparing the most commonly noted indications for late preterm delivery, major congenital anomaly is associated with the highest rate of neonatal (107.9 per 1000 live births) and infant (140.7 per 1000 live births) mortality.[43]

The cause of late preterm birth may be associated with an adverse intrauterine environment and is an important determinant of fetal outcomes, including neonatal and infant mortality; acute birth hospitalization conditions; and long-term neurodevelopmental, medical, and social health.[43,77] In addition to congenital anomalies, other causes of late preterm delivery, categorized as obstetric, medical, no recorded indication, and isolated spontaneous labor, are associated with infant mortalities of 13.3, 7.0, 6.8, and 4.8 per 1000 live births, respectively.[43] Maternal factors affecting late preterm delivery and neonatal and infant outcomes include maternal race, marital status, age, smoking status, health (including diabetes and hypertensive disorders), diet, income, and educational levels.[42,71,76–78,80,81] Pregnancy, labor, and delivery complications, including multiple gestation, intrauterine growth restriction, antepartum hemorrhage, abruption, preterm prelabor rupture of membranes, and chorioamnionitis, also occur at higher rates in late preterm pregnancies.[77,78,81,82] Such complications contribute to premature birth and likely morbidity and mortality of late preterm infants.

Physiologic and structural immaturity are important fetal and neonatal contributions to the risks of morbidity and mortality in late preterm infants.[3,30,51,74] The rates of neonatal intensive care admission and acute birth hospital morbidities increase with decreasing gestational age, consistent with a major impact of immaturity on such outcomes.[11,13,77] Immaturity also adversely affects neurodevelopmental outcomes with decreasing gestational age in neonates without other genetic, metabolic, or neurologic disorders.[51,72] Across the gestational age spectrum from 32 to 41 weeks, the risk for neurodevelopmental delay compared with a term cohort is much higher in the younger gestational age groups. This risk of developmental delay for the moderately preterm (32 0/7 to 33 6/7 weeks), late preterm (34 0/7 to 36 6/7 weeks), and early term (37 0/7 to 38 6/7 weeks) infants is 3-fold (aOR, 3.01; 95% CI, 1.59–5.71), 2.6-fold (aOR, 2.58; 95% CI, 1.66–4.01), and 1.6-fold (aOR, 1.56; 95% CI, 1.19–2.06), respectively, compared with those born at 39 0/7 to 41 6/7 weeks gestational age.[72] In a cohort of 22,552 healthy late preterm infants (ie, discharged from birth hospitalization within 3 days of birth), 4.24% of late preterm and 2.96% of full-term infants were diagnosed with developmental delay or disability (adjusted RR, 1.36; 95% CI, 1.29–1.43).[51] In this same cohort, referral for prekindergarten services, exceptional student education, retention in kindergarten, and suspension in kindergarten were all significantly increased in the late preterm group.

In contrast with the association of immaturity with poor neurodevelopmental outcomes in nonanomalous late preterm versus term infants, conflicting evidence has been reported for an association with specific outcomes during early childhood, such as intellectual disability (intelligence quotient <70), overall developmental score, problem solving, attention and behavior disorders, and learning disabilities.[57,71,73–75,83] Such contrasting results may be associated with absence of true difference in outcomes, variations in sensitivity of study methods to differentiate outcomes at some ages, methodologic issues, and population sample size limitations. Despite some contradictory evidence, the preponderance of information, including differences observed through adulthood, support an important contribution of immaturity on neurodevelopmental, educational, social, medical, and behavioral outcomes of infants born late preterm.[3,30,51,60–63,74]

In addition to immaturity, other fetal/neonatal factors, including sex and birth weight, specifically infants small for gestational age, are associated with late preterm delivery in addition to other outcomes, including mortality.[42,77,82] Late preterm infants who are also small for gestational age have been shown to have an increased risk for poor neurocognitive intelligence test scores in young adulthood (full-scale intelligence quotient score, −11.84; 95% CI, −18.33 to −5.36 compared with term appropriate for gestational age infants) and cerebral palsy in childhood (pooled OR, 3.47; 95% CI, 1.29–9.31), indicating the lasting impact of intrauterine growth restriction on this population.[71,84]

The morbidity and mortality risks found in late preterm infants compared with term infants are numerous. Adverse outcomes throughout the lifespan of infants born late preterm are the result of an interplay between immaturity and a host of unique pathobiological and social determinants that also contribute to poor outcomes in infants born at other gestational ages.

COSTS ATTRIBUTABLE TO LATE PRETERM BIRTHS

The costs, including emotional and financial, for families and society attributable to consequences of late preterm birth are extensive.[85–87] Although the percentage of late preterm infants without congenital anomalies that have long-term impairments is low compared with extreme and moderate preterm infants, the large absolute number of late preterm births (in 2016, 279, 382 late preterm vs 108,836 extreme and moderate preterm infants) contributes to the large number of children in need of special care and support services.[4] For example, using population-based data from Finland, where 0.55% of late preterm and 0.85% of combined extremely and moderately

Table 2
Sample management and monitoring guideline for late preterm infants during the birth hospitalization

Delivery Room[30,88,89,92]	• Monitor for signs of respiratory distress • NRP Guidelines followed if resuscitation is needed • Thermoregulation measures: hat and skin to skin or radiant warmer • Vital signs (heart rate, respiratory rate, and temperature) measured within the first hour of birth
NICU Admission Decision[30]	• Significant resuscitation in the delivery room (ie, positive pressure ventilation, chest compressions, medications) or clinical concerns, observe patient with continuous vital sign monitoring for at least 6 h • Institution-specific guideline for gestational age and weight parameters for NICU admission considered when determining admission placement
Thermoregulation[30,88,89]	• Temperature measurement every hour for the first 6 h and then minimum of every 6 h until discharge • If temperature is < 36.0°C, swaddle infant and cover head with a hat. In 30 min, if temperature remains <36.0°C, place infant under radiant warmer. If still <36.0°C despite radiant warmer, admit infant to higher level of care, if in Well Baby Nursery, for further evaluation and management.
Respiratory Distress[30,89]	• During the first 2 h after delivery infants may have abnormal respiratory rates (rate 25–100 breaths per minute). Normalization is expected after this transitional period (respiratory rate 40–60 breaths per minute). • Monitor for signs of respiratory distress throughout the birth hospitalization. • If signs of respiratory distress arise, institute cardiorespiratory monitoring with consideration to move infant to higher level of care. • Apnea with pause in breathing >20 s also requires closer cardiorespiratory monitoring and transfer to higher level of care.
Feeding[3,30,88,89]	• All aspects of feedings monitored including latch, frequency, volume, and duration. • Daily weights monitored. • Optimize feeding by having a health care professional observe at least one feeding each shift. If the infant is breastfeeding, this may be performed by a lactation consultant. • If feeding difficulty noted, early consultation with speech therapy or occupational therapy. • If excessive weight loss (more than 3% per day of age or more than 7% of birth weight total) consider further evaluation for dehydration and possible supplementation. • If the infant is unable to maintain adequate oral intake other forms of feeding, such as gavage feedings are recommended.
Hypoglycemia[93]	• *Birth to 4 h of age*: Encourage feeding within 1 h of birth and measure glucose 30 min after feeding. If glucose is < 25 mg/dL refeeding is recommended. If glucose still <25 mg/dL 1 hour after feeding IV glucose is recommended. If glucose is 25–40 mg/dL refeeding or IV glucose is recommended. • *From 4 h to 24 h of age*: Glucose measurement is recommended before each feeding. If < 35 mg/dL feed, and recheck in 1 h. If still <35 mg/dL IV glucose is recommended. If glucose 35–45 mg/dL encourage feeding or consider IV glucose. • If symptomatic hypoglycemia, give IV glucose.

(continued on next page)

Table 2 (continued)	
Hyperbilirubinemia[94,95]	• Assess risk factors for hyperbilirubinemia, including ABO incompatibility and presence of maternal antibody for each infant. • If maternal blood type is Rh negative or O Rh positive, determine infant blood type. • Monitor clinical signs of jaundice regularly. • Within the first 24 h, obtain transcutaneous or serum total bilirubin. • For infants >35 wk of age, treat hyperbilirubinemia with phototherapy per the AAP guidelines. • For infants <35 wk, initiate phototherapy at a lower threshold. Because of inadequate evidence regarding the treatment threshold in this group, each institution should establish their own guidelines.

Abbreviation: NRP, neonatal resuscitation program.

preterm infants have intellectual disability, late preterm births would contribute 1537 children with intellectual disability compared with 926 extremely and moderately preterm births in 2016 alone.[83]

MONITORING AND MANAGEMENT OF LATE PRETERM INFANTS

Given the significant morbidities encountered by late preterm infants, this population warrants increased observation and close monitoring during birth hospitalization, soon after discharge, and throughout life. Understanding the morbidities and the time frame during which they may occur can guide health care professionals to care for this at-risk population. Monitoring for these morbidities and ensuring adequate care of late preterm infants will help to decrease rates of negative outcomes.

During the birth hospitalization, as previously mentioned, late preterm infants are at risk for respiratory distress, hypothermia, hypoglycemia, hyperbilirubinemia, and feeding difficulties.[12,13] **Table 2** provides a sample guideline for monitoring and managing these morbidities. Clinicians who care for late preterm infants during their birth hospitalization should consider setting guidelines to care for these infants, because

Table 3
Discharge criteria recommendations for late preterm infants

• In general, a minimum of 48 h of age unless necessary competencies established beforehand • 12–24 h of stable vital signs (heart rate, respiratory rate, temperature) • Physical examination without abnormalities for which ongoing hospital management is necessary • Adequate feeding for at least 24 h with at least 2 feedings observed by health care professionals • If weight loss more than 3% per day, or 7% total, at time of discharge, consider dehydration evaluation and/or supplementation before release	• Passage of at least 1 stool • Bilirubin level (transcutaneous or serum) documented and does not require intervention • All state-mandated screening evaluations performed (newborn metabolic, hearing, congenital heart screens) • Car seat study passed if applicable • Family and social situation assessed and appropriate for discharge • Outpatient follow-up scheduled within 24–48 h of discharge

Data from Refs.[3,30,88,89]

variation in practice effects the length of stay, care received, and potentially outcomes after discharge (eg, readmission rates).[40] Before discharge, it is recommended that specific goals be met (**Table 3**). Other considerations before discharge include the parents' ability to provide care for the infant at the bedside. This ability of parents to care for their infants during the birth hospitalization has been linked to outcomes and future maternal infant interactions after discharge.[87]

After birth hospitalization, it is recommended that late preterm infants be followed closely by their primary care physicians. Initial follow-up is recommended within 24 to 48 hours to evaluate the infant for feeding issues, jaundice, and other concerns.[30,88,89] Frequency of follow-up can be increased if issues arise, until the infant is clearly thriving and developing.[89] It is important for previously late preterm infants to have an established primary care physician.[89] These infants should receive all recommended screens throughout childhood, with care taken to diagnose disabilities or medical disorders as early as possible. If a problem is identified, such as a developmental delay, referral for the appropriate intervention or therapies should be made as early as possible. Parents should be informed of the increased risk of long-term morbidities associated with prematurity, to emphasize the importance of continued timely follow-up of late preterm infants.

SUMMARY

Late preterm infants are at increased risk of significant morbidity and mortality. During birth hospitalization, these morbidities include respiratory distress, hypothermia, feeding difficulties, hypoglycemia, and hyperbilirubinemia.[12,13] After discharge, these infants are at increased risk of rehospitalization because of feeding difficulties and jaundice, especially with shorter birth hospitalization.[41,43,44,46,47] Risks for morbidity and mortality continue throughout life for late preterm infants. This persistence emphasizes the need for well-defined long-term follow-up.

REFERENCES

1. Martin JA, Hamilton BE, Ventura SJ, et al. Births: final data for 2010. Natl Vital Stat Rep 2012;61(1):1–72.
2. Raju TN, Higgins RD, Stark AR, et al. Optimizing care and outcome for late-preterm (near-term) infants: a summary of the workshop sponsored by the National Institute of Child Health and Human Development. Pediatrics 2006; 118(3):1207–14.
3. Engle WA, Tomashek KM, Wallman C. "Late-preterm" infants: a population at risk. Pediatrics 2007;120(6):1390–401.
4. Martin JA, Hamilton BE, Osterman MJK, et al. Births: final data for 2016. Hyattsville (MD): US Department of Health and Human Services; 2018.
5. Hamilton BE, Martin JA, Osterman MJK, et al. Births: provisional data for 2017. Hyattsville (MD): National Center for Health Statistics; 2018.
6. McLaurin KK, Hall CB, Jackson EA, et al. Persistence of morbidity and cost differences between late-preterm and term infants during the first year of life. Pediatrics 2009;123(2):653–9.
7. Deputy NP, Dub B, Sharma AJ. Prevalence and trends in prepregnancy normal weight - 48 states, New York City, and District of Columbia, 2011-2015. MMWR Morb Mortal Wkly Rep 2018;66(5152):1402–7.
8. Martin JA, Hamilton BE, Osterman MJK. Births in the United States, 2016. Hyattsville (MD): National Center for Health Statistics; 2017.

9. Norgaard M, Nielsson MS, Heide-Jorgensen U. Birth and neonatal outcomes following opioid use in pregnancy: a Danish population-based study. Subst Abuse 2015;9(Suppl 2):5–11.

10. de Almeida MF, Guinsburg R, da Costa JO, et al. Resuscitative procedures at birth in late preterm infants. J Perinatol 2007;27(12):761–5.

11. Hibbard JU, Wilkins I, Sun L, et al. Respiratory morbidity in late preterm births. JAMA 2010;304(4):419–25.

12. Melamed N, Klinger G, Tenenbaum-Gavish K, et al. Short-term neonatal outcome in low-risk, spontaneous, singleton, late preterm deliveries. Obstet Gynecol 2009; 114(2 Pt 1):253–60.

13. Wang ML, Dorer DJ, Fleming MP, et al. Clinical outcomes of near-term infants. Pediatrics 2004;114(2):372–6.

14. Teune MJ, Bakhuizen S, Gyamfi Bannerman C, et al. A systematic review of severe morbidity in infants born late preterm. Am J Obstet Gynecol 2011;205(4): 374.e1-9.

15. Gouyon JB, Vintejoux A, Sagot P, et al. Neonatal outcome associated with singleton birth at 34-41 weeks of gestation. Int J Epidemiol 2010;39(3):769–76.

16. Bland RD. Loss of liquid from the lung lumen in labor: more than a simple "squeeze". Am J Physiol Lung Cell Mol Physiol 2001;280(4):L602–5.

17. Kallapur SG, Jobe AH. Lung development and maturation. In: Martin RJ, Fanaroff AA, Walsh MC, editors. Fanaroff and Martin's neonatal perinatal medicine. Philadelphia: Elsevier Saunders; 2015. p. 1042–59.

18. Pike KC, Lucas JS. Respiratory consequences of late preterm birth. Paediatr Respir Rev 2015;16(3):182–8.

19. Ramachandrappa A, Jain L. The late preterm infant. In: Martin R, Fanaroff A, Walsh M, editors. Fanaroff and Martin's neonatal-perinatal medicine. Philadelphia: Elsevier Saunders; 2015. p. 577–91.

20. Rozycki HJ, Hendricks-Munoz KD. Structure and development of alveolar epithelial cells. In: Polin RA, Abman SH, Rowitch DH, et al, editors. Fetal and neonatal physiology, vol. 1, 5th edition. Philadelphia: Elsevier; 2017. p. 809–13.

21. Smith DE, Otulakowski G, Yeger H, et al. Epithelial Na(+) channel (ENaC) expression in the developing normal and abnormal human perinatal lung. Am J Respir Crit Care Med 2000;161(4 Pt 1):1322–31.

22. Gyamfi-Bannerman C, Thom EA, Blackwell SC, et al. Antenatal betamethasone for women at risk for late preterm delivery. N Engl J Med 2016;374(14):1311–20.

23. Committee on Obstetric Practice. Committee opinion no. 713: antenatal corticosteroid therapy for fetal maturation. Obstet Gynecol 2017;130(2):e102–9.

24. Kaempf JW, Suresh G. Antenatal corticosteroids for the late preterm infant and agnotology. J Perinatol 2017;37(12):1265–7.

25. Sahni R. Temperature control in newborn infants. In: Polin RA, Abman SH, Rowitch DH, et al, editors. Fetal and neonatal physiology, vol. 1, 5th edition. Philadelphia: Elsevier; 2017. p. 459–82.

26. Symonds ME, Mostyn A, Pearce S, et al. Endocrine and nutritional regulation of fetal adipose tissue development. J Endocrinol 2003;179(3):293–9.

27. Margolis KG, Picoraro JA. Development of gastrointestinal motility. In: Polin RA, Abman SH, Rowitch DH, et al, editors. Fetal and neonatal physiology, vol. 1, 5th edition. Philadelphia: Elsevier; 2017. p. 881–8.

28. Mizuno K, Ueda A. The maturation and coordination of sucking, swallowing, and respiration in preterm infants. J Pediatr 2003;142(1):36–40.

29. Jackson BN, Kelly BN, McCann CM, et al. Predictors of the time to attain full oral feeding in late preterm infants. Acta Paediatr 2016;105(1):e1–6.

30. Engle WA. Morbidity and mortality in late preterm and early term newborns: a continuum. Clin Perinatol 2011;38(3):493–516.
31. McManaman JL. Physiology of lactation. In: Polin RA, Abman SH, Rowitch DH, et al, editors. Fetal and neonatal physiology, vol. 1, 5th edition. Philadelphia: Elsevier; 2017. p. 281–7.
32. Briere CE, Lucas R, McGrath JM, et al. Establishing breastfeeding with the late preterm infant in the NICU. J Obstet Gynecol Neonatal Nurs 2015;44(1):102–13 [quiz: E101–2].
33. Garg M, Devaskar SU. Glucose metabolism in the late preterm infant. Clin Perinatol 2006;33(4):853–70.
34. Hume R, Burchell A. Abnormal expression of glucose-6-phosphatase in preterm infants. Arch Dis Child 1993;68(2):202–4.
35. Stanley CA, Rozance PJ, Thornton PS, et al. Re-evaluating "transitional neonatal hypoglycemia": mechanism and implications for management. J Pediatr 2015; 166(6):1520–5.e1.
36. Kawade N, Onishi S. The prenatal and postnatal development of UDP-glucuronyltransferase activity towards bilirubin and the effect of premature birth on this activity in the human liver. Biochem J 1981;196(1):257–60.
37. Kinney HC. The near-term (late preterm) human brain and risk for periventricular leukomalacia: a review. Semin Perinatol 2006;30(2):81–8.
38. Walsh JM, Doyle LW, Anderson PJ, et al. Moderate and late preterm birth: effect on brain size and maturation at term-equivalent age. Radiology 2014;273(1): 232–40.
39. Pulver LS, Denney JM, Silver RM, et al. Morbidity and discharge timing of late preterm newborns. Clin Pediatr 2010;49(11):1061–7.
40. Aliaga S, Boggess K, Ivester TS, et al. Influence of neonatal practice variation on outcomes of late preterm birth. Am J Perinatol 2014;31(8):659–66.
41. Escobar GJ, Joffe S, Gardner MN, et al. Rehospitalization in the first two weeks after discharge from the neonatal intensive care unit. Pediatrics 1999;104(1):e2.
42. Mathews TJ, MacDorman MF, Thoma ME. Infant mortality statistics from the 2013 period linked birth/infant death data set. Natl Vital Stat Rep 2015;64(9):1–30.
43. Reddy UM, Ko CW, Raju TN, et al. Delivery indications at late-preterm gestations and infant mortality rates in the United States. Pediatrics 2009;124(1):234–40.
44. Escobar GJ, Greene JD, Hulac P, et al. Rehospitalisation after birth hospitalisation: patterns among infants of all gestations. Arch Dis Child 2005;90(2):125–31.
45. Shapiro-Mendoza CK, Tomashek KM, Kotelchuck M, et al. Risk factors for neonatal morbidity and mortality among "healthy," late preterm newborns. Semin Perinatol 2006;30(2):54–60.
46. Tomashek KM, Shapiro-Mendoza CK, Weiss J, et al. Early discharge among late preterm and term newborns and risk of neonatal morbidity. Semin Perinatol 2006; 30(2):61–8.
47. Young PC, Korgenski K, Buchi KF. Early readmission of newborns in a large health care system. Pediatrics 2013;131(5):e1538–44.
48. Jain S, Cheng J. Emergency department visits and rehospitalizations in late preterm infants. Clin Perinatol 2006;33(4):935–45 [abstract: xi].
49. Crump C, Winkleby MA, Sundquist J, et al. Risk of asthma in young adults who were born preterm: a Swedish national cohort study. Pediatrics 2011;127(4): e913–20.
50. Hirvonen M, Ojala R, Korhonen P, et al. Cerebral palsy among children born moderately and late preterm. Pediatrics 2014;134(6):e1584–93.

51. Morse SB, Zheng H, Tang Y, et al. Early school-age outcomes of late preterm infants. Pediatrics 2009;123(4):e622–9.

52. Petrini JR, Dias T, McCormick MC, et al. Increased risk of adverse neurological development for late preterm infants. J Pediatr 2009;154(2):169–76.

53. Shapiro-Mendoza C, Kotelchuck M, Barfield W, et al. Enrollment in early intervention programs among infants born late preterm, early term, and term. Pediatrics 2013;132(1):e61–9.

54. Potijk MR, de Winter AF, Bos AF, et al. Co-occurrence of developmental and behavioural problems in moderate to late preterm-born children. Arch Dis Child 2016;101(3):217–22.

55. Talge NM, Holzman C, Wang J, et al. Late-preterm birth and its association with cognitive and socioemotional outcomes at 6 years of age. Pediatrics 2010;126(6): 1124–31.

56. Chan E, Quigley MA. School performance at age 7 years in late preterm and early term birth: a cohort study. Arch Dis Child Fetal Neonatal Ed 2014;99(6):F451–7.

57. Harris MN, Voigt RG, Barbaresi WJ, et al. ADHD and learning disabilities in former late preterm infants: a population-based birth cohort. Pediatrics 2013;132(3): e630–6.

58. Linnet KM, Wisborg K, Agerbo E, et al. Gestational age, birth weight, and the risk of hyperkinetic disorder. Arch Dis Child 2006;91(8):655–60.

59. Lindstrom K, Lindblad F, Hjern A. Psychiatric morbidity in adolescents and young adults born preterm: a Swedish national cohort study. Pediatrics 2009;123(1): e47–53.

60. Moster D, Lie RT, Markestad T. Long-term medical and social consequences of preterm birth. N Engl J Med 2008;359(3):262–73.

61. Lindstrom K, Winbladh B, Haglund B, et al. Preterm infants as young adults: a Swedish national cohort study. Pediatrics 2007;120(1):70–7.

62. Heinonen K, Eriksson JG, Lahti J, et al. Late preterm birth and neurocognitive performance in late adulthood: a birth cohort study. Pediatrics 2015;135(4): e818–25.

63. Heinonen K, Eriksson JG, Kajantie E, et al. Late-preterm birth and lifetime socioeconomic attainments: the Helsinki Birth Cohort Study. Pediatrics 2013;132(4): 647–55.

64. Crump C, Winkleby MA, Sundquist K, et al. Risk of diabetes among young adults born preterm in Sweden. Diabetes Care 2011;34(5):1109–13.

65. Gunay F, Alpay H, Gokce I, et al. Is late-preterm birth a risk factor for hypertension in childhood? Eur J Pediatr 2014;173(6):751–6.

66. Helfrich AM, Nylund CM, Eberly MD, et al. Healthy late-preterm infants born 33-36+6 weeks gestational age have higher risk for respiratory syncytial virus hospitalization. Early Hum Dev 2015;91(9):541–6.

67. Gunville CF, Sontag MK, Stratton KA, et al. Scope and impact of early and late preterm infants admitted to the PICU with respiratory illness. J Pediatr 2010; 157(2):209–14.e1.

68. Goyal NK, Fiks AG, Lorch SA. Association of late-preterm birth with asthma in young children: practice-based study. Pediatrics 2011;128(4):e830–8.

69. Kotecha SJ, Watkins WJ, Paranjothy S, et al. Effect of late preterm birth on longitudinal lung spirometry in school age children and adolescents. Thorax 2012; 67(1):54–61.

70. Todisco T, de Benedictis FM, Iannacci L, et al. Mild prematurity and respiratory functions. Eur J Pediatr 1993;152(1):55–8.

71. Heinonen K, Lahti J, Sammallahti S, et al. Neurocognitive outcome in young adults born late-preterm. Dev Med Child Neurol 2018;60(3):267–74.

72. Schonhaut L, Armijo I, Perez M. Gestational age and developmental risk in moderately and late preterm and early term infants. Pediatrics 2015;135(4): e835–41.

73. Gurka MJ, LoCasale-Crouch J, Blackman JA. Long-term cognition, achievement, socioemotional, and behavioral development of healthy late-preterm infants. Arch Pediatr Adolesc Med 2010;164(6):525–32.

74. Hornman J, de Winter AF, Kerstjens JM, et al. Stability of developmental problems after school entry of moderately-late preterm and early preterm-born children. J Pediatr 2017;187:73–9.

75. Shah P, Kaciroti N, Richards B, et al. Developmental outcomes of late preterm infants from infancy to kindergarten. Pediatrics 2016;138(2) [pii:e20153496].

76. Woythaler M, McCormick MC, Mao WY, et al. Late preterm infants and neurodevelopmental outcomes at kindergarten. Pediatrics 2015;136(3):424–31.

77. Bonnevier A, Brodszki J, Bjorklund LJ, et al. Underlying maternal and pregnancy-related conditions account for a substantial proportion of neonatal morbidity in late preterm infants. Acta Paediatr 2018;107:1521–8.

78. Dimitriou G, Fouzas S, Georgakis V, et al. Determinants of morbidity in late preterm infants. Early Hum Dev 2010;86(9):587–91.

79. Ely DM, Hoyert DL. Differences between rural and urban areas in mortality rates for the leading causes of infant death: United States, 2013-2015. NCHS Data Brief 2018;(300):1–8.

80. Smith LK, Draper ES, Evans TA, et al. Associations between late and moderately preterm birth and smoking, alcohol, drug use and diet: a population-based case-cohort study. Arch Dis Child Fetal Neonatal Ed 2015;100(6):F486–91.

81. Manuck TA, Rice MM, Bailit JL, et al. Preterm neonatal morbidity and mortality by gestational age: a contemporary cohort. Am J Obstet Gynecol 2016;215(1): 103.e1–14.

82. Mathiasen R, Hansen BM, Andersen AM, et al. Gestational age and basic school achievements: a national follow-up study in Denmark. Pediatrics 2010;126(6): e1553–61.

83. Hirvonen M, Ojala R, Korhonen P, et al. Intellectual disability in children aged less than seven years born moderately and late preterm compared with very preterm and term-born children - a nationwide birth cohort study. J Intellect Disabil Res 2017;61(11):1034–54.

84. Zhao M, Dai H, Deng Y, et al. SGA as a risk factor for cerebral palsy in moderate to late preterm infants: a system review and meta-analysis. Sci Rep 2016;6: 38853.

85. Haataja P, Korhonen P, Ojala R, et al. Hospital admissions for lower respiratory tract infections in children born moderately/late preterm. Pediatr Pulmonol 2018;53(2):209–17.

86. Isayama T, Lewis-Mikhael AM, O'Reilly D, et al. Health services use by late preterm and term infants from infancy to adulthood: a meta-analysis. Pediatrics 2017;140(1) [pii:e20170266].

87. Premji SS, Pana G, Currie G, et al. Mother's level of confidence in caring for her late preterm infant: a mixed methods study. J Clin Nurs 2018;27(5–6):e1120–33.

88. Kilpatrick S, Papile L, Macones G. Guidelines for perinatal care. 8th edition. Elk Grove Village, IL and Washington, DC: American Academy of Pediatrics and American College of Obstetricians and Gynecologists; 2017.

89. Phillips RM, Goldstein M, Hougland K, et al. Multidisciplinary guidelines for the care of late preterm infants. J Perinatol 2013;33(Suppl 2):S5–22.

90. Boyle EM, Johnson S, Manktelow B, et al. Neonatal outcomes and delivery of care for infants born late preterm or moderately preterm: a prospective population-based study. Arch Dis Child Fetal Neonatal Ed 2015;100(6):F479–85.

91. Sarici SU, Serdar MA, Korkmaz A, et al. Incidence, course, and prediction of hyperbilirubinemia in near-term and term newborns. Pediatrics 2004;113(4):775–80.

92. Weiner G, Zaickin J. Textbook of neonatal resuscitation. 7th edition. Elk Grove Village (IL): American Academy of Pediatrics; 2016.

93. Adamkin DH. Postnatal glucose homeostasis in late-preterm and term infants. Pediatrics 2011;127(3):575–9.

94. American Academy of Pediatrics Subcommittee on Hyperbilirubinemia. Management of hyperbilirubinemia in the newborn infant 35 or more weeks of gestation. Pediatrics 2004;114(1):297–316.

95. Maisels MJ, Watchko JF, Bhutani VK, et al. An approach to the management of hyperbilirubinemia in the preterm infant less than 35 weeks of gestation. J Perinatol 2012;32(9):660–4.

Intrauterine Growth Restriction
Postnatal Monitoring and Outcomes

Kalpashri Kesavan, MD[a],*, Sherin U. Devaskar, MD[b]

KEYWORDS

- Intrauterine growth restriction (IUGR) • Small for gestational age (SGA)
- Fetal programming • Metabolic programming • Growth hormone

KEY POINTS

- IUGR is one of the major causes of perinatal-neonatal morbidity and mortality.
- IUGR and SGA infants experience several immediate postnatal complications such as hypothermia, hypoglycemia, polycythemia, jaundice, and feeding difficulties.
- The adverse uterine environment and/or genetic factors that lead to growth restriction predisposes IUGR infants to long-term health issues.
- Optimal catch-up growth is vital for normal neurologic development in IUGR infants.
- Growth hormone is recommended for treatment of persistent short stature in SGA infants.

INTRODUCTION

Intrauterine growth restriction (IUGR) continues to be a challenging problem for clinicians despite advances in both obstetric and neonatal care. IUGR is defined as a rate of fetal growth that is less than normal for the expected growth potential of a specific infant, based on the race and gender of the fetus. The terms IUGR and small for gestational age (SGA) have been used interchangeably in the literature, albeit there is a difference. IUGR is a clinical definition that indicates that a neonate is born with clinical features of malnutrition and in utero growth compromise irrespective of their birth weight percentile, having deviated from the intrauterine growth curves. Therefore, an infant with normal anthropometric measurements can still be designated as IUGR if the infant demonstrates signs of in utero growth deceleration compromise (eg, Doppler flow abnormalities) and evidence of malnutrition at birth. In contrast, SGA is a term used for neonates

Disclosure Statement: Authors report no conflicts of interest.
[a] Division of Neonatology & Developmental Biology, Department of Pediatrics, David Geffen School of Medicine at UCLA, UCLA Mattel Children's Hospital, 10833 Le Conte Avenue, B2-413 MDCC, Los Angeles, CA 90095, USA; [b] Department of Pediatrics, David Geffen School of Medicine at UCLA, UCLA Mattel Children's Hospital, 10833 Le Conte Avenue, 22-412 MDCC, Los Angeles, CA 90095, USA
* Corresponding author.
E-mail address: kkesavan@mednet.ucla.edu

Pediatr Clin N Am 66 (2019) 403–423
https://doi.org/10.1016/j.pcl.2018.12.009
0031-3955/19/© 2018 Elsevier Inc. All rights reserved.

whose birth weight is less than the 10th percentile for that specific gestational age, or at least 2 SD below a given population norm. An SGA infant can also be described as IUGR, although the latter signifies intrauterine compromise while the former may merely reflect the infant's genetic potential. Most studies pertaining to IUGR and/or SGA do not clearly make these distinctions between the terms. For example, a neonate who is SGA may not have evidence of fetal growth restriction and yet referred to interchangeably as IUGR,[1] causing significant confusion. For the purpose of this Review, we will use IUGR as a proxy for either IUGR or SGA as referred to in the literature, but if any entity is specific to SGA infants only, we will make that distinction.

IUGR is one of the leading causes of perinatal-neonatal morbidity and mortality, and contributes to long-term chronic diseases. Perinatal problems posed by IUGR include perinatal asphyxia, difficult cardiopulmonary transition after birth, meconium aspiration, and persistent pulmonary hypertension. In addition, IUGR infants are at higher risk of immediate postnatal complications, such as hypothermia, hypoglycemia, polycythemia, jaundice, feeding difficulties, necrotizing enterocolitis, and late-onset sepsis.[2] Furthermore, changes in the fetal nutritional environment, prenatal programming, and postnatal catch-up growth in IUGR infants lead to long-term adverse consequences such as neurodevelopmental impairment, increased risk of cardiovascular disease, and metabolic syndrome that span over a lifetime.[3–5]

IUGR is an important public health concern, especially in under-resourced countries. The incidence of SGA in well-resourced countries such as the United States is ~10% and one-third of these cases represent IUGR. On the other hand, rates of IUGR in under-resourced countries are estimated to be 6 times higher than in well-resourced countries. Approximately 30 million infants per year suffer from IUGR in the non-Western world, with Asia accounting for 75% of all affected infants, and Africa and Latin America contributing toward 20% and 5% of IUGR cases, respectively.[6]

The etiology, pathophysiology, diagnosis, maternal management, and fetal and neonatal therapies, as well as long-term ramifications of IUGR, continue to confront perinatal health care providers and pediatric care providers who follow these vulnerable infants. In this Review, we address the immediate postnatal issues and monitoring of infants affected by IUGR, as well as tracking of long-term adverse outcomes, to help guide clinicians who follow these infants to adulthood in transitional, adolescence, and young adult programs.

ETIOLOGIES AND MECHANISMS OF INTRAUTERINE GROWTH RESTRICTION

The etiology and "type" of IUGR dictate the diagnostic testing that needs to be undertaken, guide the immediate postnatal management, and aid in predicting long-term sequelae that will ensure clinicians take preventive measures and provide anticipatory guidance. The etiology of IUGR is broadly classified into maternal, placental, and fetal causes, and are summarized in **Table 1**. In addition to these factors, several maternal, fetal, and placental gene polymorphisms encoding various proteins and hormones have been implicated in IUGR (**Table 2**). Finally, the interplay of various hormones is fundamental to normal fetal growth by modifying metabolism and gene expression in fetal tissues. Any disruption in these "endocrine factors" will result in IUGR (**Table 3**).

POSTNATAL DIAGNOSIS
Clinical Examination

A thorough examination of neonates with IUGR can demonstrate clinical features reflecting varying degrees of nutrient deficiency **Fig. 1**; extreme cases can be akin to malnutrition/starvation. Neurologic maturity using the Ballard scoring system is

Table 1
Maternal, placental and fetal causes of IUGR

Category	Causes	Specifics
Maternal	Demographics[7–10]	Extremes of age
		Race
		Lower socioeconomic status
		Poor nutritional status
		Low pre-pregnancy weight
		Poor pregnancy weight gain
	Environmental[11–15]	High altitude (because of reduced blood volume and lower oxygen carrying capacity that lead to poor placental blood flow)
		Maternal alcohol intake and maternal drug use
		Smoking (including passive smoking) (owing to increased carbon monoxide in maternal blood leading to secondary fetal tissue hypoxemia; also due to direct vasoconstrictive effects of nicotine)
		Air pollution
	Maternal health/ disease status[16–19]	Chronic hypertension
		Pre-eclampsia
		Diabetes
		Renal insufficiency
		Autoimmune diseases (eg, lupus)
		Pulmonary diseases (eg, asthma, chronic obstructive pulmonary disease, cystic fibrosis)
		Cardiac diseases (eg, cyanotic congenital heart disease, heart failure)
		Hematologic disorders (eg, severe anemia)
		Gastrointestinal disease (eg, Crohn's disease, ulcerative colitis)
		Infections (eg, malaria, TORCH, tuberculosis, urinary tract infections, bacterial vaginosis)
	Obstetric and gynecologic conditions[20,21]	Short inter-pregnancy interval
		Artificial reproductive techniques
		Prior history of delivering an SGA infant
		Maternal history of SGA as infant
		Uterine fibroids that limit uterine capacity
Fetal	[a]Genetic[22–25]	Chromosomal abnormalities (trisomy 13, 18, or 21; deletions of chromosome X, 4, 5, 13 or 18; ring chromosomes)
		Uniparental disomy of chromosome 6, 14, or 18
		Single gene disorders (Cornelia de Lange syndrome, Fanconi's anemia, some skeletal dysplasias)
	[b]Congenital malformations[26–28] (1% to 2%)	Tracheo-esophageal fistula
		Congenital heart disease
		Congenital diaphragmatic hernia
		Abdominal wall defects (gastroschisis or omphalocele)
		Neural tube defects (eg, anencephaly)
		Anorectal malformations
	[c]Congenital infections (5%)[17,29–31]	Bacterial, viral and parasitic (eg, malaria) infections:
		• Western nations: toxoplasmosis, cytomegalovirus
		• Africa and South-East Asia: rubella, syphilis, human immunodeficiency virus, malaria

(continued on next page)

Table 1
(continued)

Category	Causes	Specifics
	Metabolic[32–35]	Agenesis of the pancreas, congenital lipodystrophy, galactosemia, gangliosidoses, hypophosphatasia, leprechaunism, I-cell disease, fetal phenylketonuria, and transient neonatal diabetes mellitus
	Other[36]	Multiple gestation
		• Due to "uterine overcrowding," dissimilar placental sizes, an increased risk of in velamentous cord insertion, twin-to-twin transfusion, or a primary uterine/placental pathology)
		• More common in monochorionic than dichorionic twins.
		• Higher risk with higher order multiples
[d]Placental	Low placental weight[37,38]	Placental weight is directly proportional to the functional mass of the placenta, leading to a reduction in the area of exchange of nutrition between the pregnant woman and the fetus
	Abnormal utero-placental vasculature[37,39]	Associated with a decrease in the number and surface area of villi, as well as inadequate trophoblastic invasion and narrow spiral arteries with increased vascular resistance
	[e]Vascular anomalies and disruptions[40,41]	Velamentous cord insertion
		True knots in umbilical cord
		Placental infarcts
		Placental abruption
	Placental infections[42]	Leads to dysregulation of angiogenic factors necessary for remodeling of placental vasculature to match fetal growth, thereby leading to placental insufficiency
	Confined placental mosaicism[43]	Associated with greater decidual vasculopathy, infarction, or intervillous thrombus formation
	Chronic villitis of unknown etiology[44]	Associated with focal areas of inflammation with mononuclear cells and areas of fibrinoid necrosis in chorionic villi
	Overexpression of placental endoglin gene[45]	Results in vascular dysfunction leading to chronic fetal hypoxia
		Induces vascular endothelium growth factor A leading to increased angiogenesis to attempt to restore fetal placental circulation

[a] Note: genetic causes of growth restriction typically impact growth earlier in pregnancy than non-genetic causes.

[b] It is unclear whether the malformations lead to IUGR or if IUGR is merely associated with malformations in the fetus; an increase in the number of structural defects increases the frequency of IUGR.[28]

[c] Infections can activate inflammatory processes such as cytokine release, oxidative stress, and cellular apoptosis that disrupt placental and fetal growth; viral infections cause intra-amniotic inflammation, which is associated with preterm birth.

[d] A mismatch between placental supply and fetal demand is the leading cause of IUGR.

[e] Vascular anomalies and disruptions can lead to decreased nutrient transfer.

Table 2
Genes associated with IUGR

Type of Gene	Functions	Genes
Placental	Development and maintenance of blood and lymphatic systems	Homeobox genes
	Proteolysis	Cullin genes
	Trophoblast function	STOX1 gene, NEAT gene
	Vasculogenesis and angiogenesis	Placental growth factor, PIGF
	Apoptosis	Apoptosis Bcl-2 gene, Bax gene
	Optimizing glucose and insulin metabolism	Insulin-like growth factors (IGF) 1 and 2
	Placental size	Epidermal growth factor
Fetal	Cell growth, cell-cell communication, cell structure, energy metabolism	Protein S100B
	Cell growth and differentiation	N-terminal parathyroid hormone-related protein
	Uteroplacental vasodilation	
	Uterine muscle relaxation	
	Placental transport	
	Regulation of glucose supply	IGF1
	Cell proliferation	
	Skeletal development	SHOX
	Cell division	IGF-1R
	IGF binding	
Maternal	Normal fetal growth and healthy placenta	Endothelin-1
		Leptin
		Vistafin T
		Thrombophilia genes

Data from Sharma D, Sharma P, Shastri S. Genetic, metabolic and endocrine aspect of intrauterine growth restriction: an update. J Matern Fetal Neonatal Med 2017;30(19):2263–75.

unaffected in IUGR infants. However, the physical maturity scores are not reliable because of features of intrauterine nutritional (including oxygen) deprivation. Examples of these findings are:

- Cracking/peeling of the skin and a mature crease pattern on the soles of feet; these are not indicative of maturity, but rather, occur in response to exposure to amniotic fluid without the protective effect of the vernix caseosa.
- Under-developed ear cartilage and diminished breast buds, which are due to decreased blood flow, low estradiol concentrations, and low subcutaneous fat.
- Immature appearance of the female genitalia, which is due to reduced fat deposition in the labia majora.

In infants with IUGR beginning early in gestation, it is important to be vigilant about dysmorphic features as a result of genetic disorders or sequelae of congenital infections. The additional common stigmata of the TORCHS group of infections include: microcephaly, petechiae, blueberry muffin lesions, hepatosplenomegaly, cataracts, and cardiac defects.

Anthropometric Indices

Ponderal Index

To determine the degree of malnutrition, the Ponderal Index[53] can be used:

$$\text{Ponderal Index} = \frac{\text{Weight(grams)} \times 100}{\text{Length}^3(\text{cm})}$$

Table 3
Endocrine factors implicated in IUGR

Hormone	Function	Disruption
Insulin	Mitogenic effect, controls cell number Promotes glucose uptake and consumption Limits protein breakdown	Insulin deficiency causes reduction in fetal growth due to decrease in uptake of nutrients by fetal tissues Pancreatic agenesis leads to fetal hyperglycemia → secondary decrease in maternal-fetal glucose concentration gradient → decrease glucose transport to fetus → IUGR[46,47]
Insulin-like growth factor-I (IGF-I)	Mitogenic properties, somatic cell growth and proliferation (including oligodendrocytes and neuronal growth, dendritic arborization and axon terminal fields) Transport of glucose and amino acids across placenta	Decreased expression of IGF-I markedly decreases fetal growth[48]
IGF-II, IGF-binding protein (IGFBP)-2, IGF BP-3 and vasoactive intestinal peptide (VIP)	Cellular growth Whole body growth Neuronal growth	Decrease in fetal size[49,50]
Thyroid hormone[51]		Developmental abnormalities in certain tissues Decreases O_2 consumption and oxidation of glucose Decreases fetal energy supply Lowers circulating and tissue concentrations of IGF-I
Pregnancy-associated plasma protein-A (PAPP-A)	Increases activity of local IGFs by cleaving IGFBP-4 an inhibitor of IGF action	IUGR[52]

Data from Refs.[46–52]

Although a Ponderal Index less than the 10th percentile reflects malnutrition, a Ponderal Index less than the third percentile indicates severe wasting. Based on anthropometric indices, IUGR can be classified as asymmetric (type I) or symmetric (type II); comparisons of these types are described in **Table 4**.

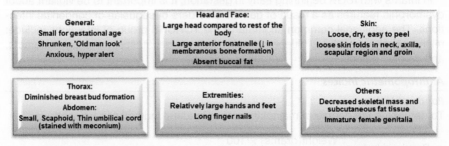

Fig. 1. Clinical features of IUGR infants. Head-to-toe description of IUGR infants in the early neonatal period demonstrating varying degrees of intrauterine malnutrition.

Table 4
Comparison of asymmetric and symmetric IUGR

	Type I: Asymmetric IUGR	Type II: Symmetric IUGR
Anthropometry	Head sparing	All growth parameters affected
Common cause(s)	Uteroplacental insufficiency	Genetic disorders Congenital anomalies Infections
Incidence	70% to 80% of IUGR	20% to 30% of IUGR
Ponderal Index	Normal >2	Low <2
Prognosis	Good (lower mortality and morbidity)	Poor (high mortality and morbidity)

Mid-arm circumference/head circumference ratio
Mid-arm circumference of the newborn is strongly associated with birth weight and is a very good indicator of low and insufficient birth weight.[54]

Clinical assessment of nutrition score
The clinical assessment of nutrition (CAN) score is a simple, systematic method of identifying fetal malnutrition and compromise. The score is composed of visible signs of fetal malnutrition, and estimates the loss of subcutaneous tissue and muscle mass in 8 regions of the body, including the cheeks, neck, chin, arms, legs, buttocks, chest, and abdomen. The texture of the infant's hair constitutes the ninth parameter (**Fig. 2**), which is generally thinner, smoother, and straight with areas of depigmentation. The CAN score is considered superior to anthropometry, the Ponderal Index, weight for age, mid-arm circumference/head circumference ratio, and BMI in determining the nutritional status of the newborn.[55]

APPROACH TO POSTNATAL MANAGEMENT OF GROWTH-RESTRICTED NEONATES

The management of an infant with IUGR begins with understanding the likely timing of the insult (ie, early vs late), the type of IUGR (ie, symmetric vs asymmetric), and the possible underlying etiology/mechanisms of growth restriction (ie, maternal vs fetal vs placenta). However, the clinician must first anticipate and treat the immediate perinatal morbidities, some of which need urgent/emergent intervention. Next, initiation of appropriate diagnostic testing may be helpful to elucidate the cause of the growth failure to better manage the immediate and long-term consequences. Finally, it is important for clinicians to attempt to prevent and/or prepare for the long-term sequelae of IUGR. This begins with establishing early optimal growth followed by surveillance of growth percentiles, cardiovascular health, neurodevelopmental testing, and metabolic/endocrine parameters that have lasting effects into adulthood. **Table 5** summarizes the immediate and long-term complications associated with IUGR.

Hair	Neck	Chest	CAN Score is based on 9 parameters shown in the table on the left: Each parameter can get a 1. Maximum score of 4 (no malnutrition) 2. Minimum score of 1 (evidence of malnutrition) Score<25: malnourished
Cheeks	Arms	Abdomen	
Chin	Legs	Buttocks	

Fig. 2. Clinical assessment of nutrition score. Systematic method of identifying intrauterine compromise and undernourishment based on the appearance of 9 different body parts.

Table 5 Immediate and long-term complications of IUGR	
Immediate Complications	**Long-Term Complications**
Perinatal/neonatal mortality	Poor physical growth
Perinatal asphyxia	Neurodevelopmental outcomes
Pulmonary complications	Metabolic syndrome
• Persistent pulmonary hypertension of the newborn	• Insulin resistance/type II diabetes
	• Obesity
• Pulmonary hemorrhage	• Hypertension
• Meconium aspiration	• Dyslipidemia
Gastrointestinal disturbances	Endocrinology issues
• Feeding intolerance	• Growth hormone/insulin growth factor abnormalities
• Necrotizing enterocolitis	
• Hepatocellular dysfunction	• Hypothalamus-pituitary axis abnormalities
Thermoregulatory disturbances	• Reproductive issues
Metabolic disturbances	Renal insufficiency
• Glucose issues (hypo/hyperglycemia)	Respiratory morbidity
• Hypocalcemia	Abnormal bone development
Hematologic disturbances	Vision and hearing impairment
• Polycythemia	
• Thrombocytopenia	
• Neutropenia/Leukopenia	
Immunodeficiency	
Renal dysfunction	

POSTNATAL COMPLICATIONS
Management of Immediate Complications

IUGR fetuses and infants have a higher risk of *perinatal and neonatal mortality* compared with AGA fetuses/infants of the same gestational age.[56,57] The most common causes of mortality are severe placental insufficiency and chronic hypoxia, congenital malformations, congenital infections, placental abruption, cord accidents, cord prolapse, placental infarcts, and severe perinatal depression. Thus, it is important to closely monitor the fetal wellbeing of growth-restricted fetuses and plan to deliver at a tertiary care center.

IUGR infants have a greater risk of *perinatal asphyxia*.[58] This can be attributable to fetal hypoxia superimposed on chronic fetal hypoxia from placental insufficiency or associated with a sentinel event such as placental abruption or a cord accident. This risk emphasizes the importance of delivery at a tertiary care center.

Regardless of birth gestational age, growth-restricted fetuses are at greater risk of developing *persistent pulmonary hypertension of the newborn*.[59] This is due to remodeling of the pulmonary vasculature in the setting of chronic hypoxia with thick tunica media up to the level of the acinar arteries. Pulmonary hypertension can also occur due to other co-morbidities such as prolonged intrauterine hypoxia, perinatal depression, polycythemia, or sepsis. Growth-restricted neonates also have a higher incidence of meconium aspiration[60] as a result of chronic hypoxia from placental insufficiency or a sentinel event leading to distress and acute hypoxia.

Feeding intolerance and *necrotizing enterocolitis* are more common in IUGR neonates due to decreased intestinal perfusion in utero as a result of preferential distribution of blood to vital organs (heart, brain, and adrenals), known as "the diving reflex," in the setting of chronic hypoxia.[61] Prolonged in utero hypoxia-ischemia can impact the metabolic capacity of hepatocytes, which can affect protein metabolism as well as bile salt transport. This can lead to intolerance of proteins and increased incidence of total parenteral nutrition cholestasis in IUGR infants compared with AGA infants.[62,63] These effects can last for several weeks post-delivery. Ideally, IUGR infants should receive breast milk and some infants may benefit from probiotics and lactoferrin.

Hypothermia is common in IUGR neonates owing to the infant's relatively large body surface area and decreased body and subcutaneous fat.[2] In addition, growth-restricted infants may have impaired thermoregulation, catecholamine depletion, or concurrent hypoxia and/or hypoglycemia that interferes with fueling heat production. It is important to maintain a thermo-neutral environment for IUGR infants (eg, plastic wrap, warming mattress, radiant warmer or servo-controlled isolette, and early skin-to-skin contact) after delivery.

Hypoglycemia is common in IUGR newborns in the initial days after birth as a result of delay in postnatal metabolic adaptation.[64,65] Infants often have insufficient glycogen stores, inadequate glycogenesis, decreased gluconeogenesis, suboptimal concentrations of counter-regulatory hormones (eg, catecholamines and glucagon), and increased insulin sensitivity. Co-morbidities such as perinatal depression, polycythemia, and hypothermia can exacerbate the risks of hypoglycemia. IUGR infants are at risk for prolonged neonatal hyperinsulinism,[66] which highlights the need to maintain a higher plasma glucose target; the Pediatric Endocrine Society recommends a plasma glucose target of greater than 50 mg/dL prior to 48 hours of age and increases the target to greater than 60 mg/dL beyond 48 hours of age in growth-restricted infants.[67]

Growth-restricted infants are also at risk of *hyperglycemia* due to immaturity of the pancreas leading to decreased insulin production or secretion, insulin resistance, excessive exogenous glucose delivery, or increased catecholamine and glucagon levels following perinatal depression.[68] *Hypocalcemia* is found in IUGR infants who are preterm or have perinatal asphyxia.[69–71] This is most frequently noted in the first 3 days after birth. Causes of hypocalcemia include:

- Decrease in intrauterine calcium transfer, if associated with prematurity
- Rapid skeletal accretion of calcium and relative resistance of the intestinal tract and bone to calcitriol
- Parathyroid gland dysfunction from hypoxic-ischemic injury
- Increased calcitonin production, increased endogenous phosphate load and renal insufficiency owing to perinatal asphyxia

Polycythemia occurs in IUGR infants as a result of increased erythropoietin levels from chronic hypoxia. Placental insufficiency and chronic hypoxia can lead to *thrombocytopenia*, *neutropenia*, and/or *leukopenia*. Infants affected by IUGR are at *increased risk of infections* as a result of immunologic compromise, congenital infection, and low T and B cells in peripheral blood.[72,73] IUGR infants also have *renal dysfunction* because of reduced nutrient delivery and decreased renal blood flow during fetal development resulting in fewer nephrons/glomeruli and reduced renal volume.[74] Renal tubular injury can occur as a result of chronic intrauterine hypoxia and perinatal asphyxia.[74]

Management of Long-Term Consequences

An unfavorable uterine environment that leads to IUGR not only results in significant concerns during the perinatal period, but has potentially long-lasting implications for the rest of the child's life. IUGR infants can have suboptimal growth, neurodevelopmental impairments, metabolic and endocrine alterations, and increased cardiovascular morbidity that occur as a result of prenatal/developmental programming.

Children affected by IUGR and especially those born SGA may continue to have *growth issues* through infancy, childhood, and adulthood. Infants with symmetric IUGR experience poor postnatal growth and tend to remain small throughout life. Asymmetric IUGR infants have better growth outcomes as they generally demonstrate catch-up postnatal growth. Levels of growth hormone (GH), insulin-like growth factor (IGF)-I, and IGF-binding protein-3, the Ponderal Index, and other scores described above, are not predictive of subsequent growth.[75] Most IUGR infants experience catch-up growth in the first 2 years of age, with the majority of growth occurring within the first 6 months after birth.[76,77] The more premature the infant and/or more severe the growth restriction, the lower likelihood that the child will attain a normal height.[78] An estimated 10% of infants born SGA due to IUGR remain short in late childhood.

As a result of these growth risks, pediatric providers should measure growth parameters of IUGR infants every 3 months for the first year of age and every 6 months thereafter. Absence of demonstrated catch-up growth in the first 6 months or those that remain short at 2 years of age require considerations of other conditions contributing toward poor postnatal growth. Catch-up growth is defined as weight or length gain greater than 0.67 SD score, which represents the width of each percentile band in standard growth charts, indicating clinically significant centile crossing.[79] If the infant was born preterm, catch-up growth can take longer (up to 4 years or more) to achieve height in the normal range.[80]

Efficacy of GH therapy for short stature have been reported in children born less than 10th percentile at birth (ie, SGA). Growth hormone is approved by the US Food and Drug Administration and the European Medicines Agency for short stature in SGA infants. It should be noted that the etiology for short stature in SGA babies is variable, and therefore the response and ultimate height achieved is also variable. A consensus statement by the International Societies of Pediatric Endocrinology and the GH Research Society proposed that children born SGA with height below −2.5 standard deviation score at the age of 2 years or with height below −2 SD score at the age of 4 years are eligible for GH treatment.[81] The US Food and Drug Administration has approved the use of GH at a dose of up to 0.48 mg/kg/wk for long-term treatment of growth failure in children born SGA who fail to manifest catch-up growth by the age of 2 years. The primary care provider should refer a child who is eligible for GH treatment to pediatric endocrinology. Growth hormone treatment also favorably affects body composition, blood pressure, and lipid metabolism.[82]

IUGR infants are at high risk for *neurodevelopmental abnormalities* including motor delay and cognitive impairments (**Fig. 3**).[83] One-third of adults who were born SGA with evidence of IUGR at term had a low IQ.[84] A suboptimal intrauterine environment increases the stress on the developing fetus, which leads to increased glucocorticoid levels that may contribute to detrimental effects on the developing brain.[85] Animal studies demonstrate a decrease in volume and number of neurons in the hippocampus and cerebellum.[86] Damage to the basal ganglia can lead to difficulties in executive functions,[87] whereas damage to frontal/parietal cortices and white matter tracts connecting these areas lead to problems with higher level cognition.[88] Altered brain growth, particularly in the frontal lobe, leads to neuropsychological difficulties and reduction in IQ.[89] Cognitive impairment is independently associated with low birth weight, reduced birth length, and small head circumference. Poor catch-up growth, especially in length and head circumference, is associated with worse outcomes.[90] IUGR infants can present later with poor school achievement and lower scholastic performance. They also perform poorly on tests of muscle strength and have lower work capacity. Growth hormone treatment induces head growth and can improve IQ in these infants.[91]

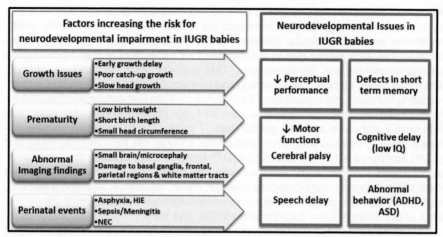

Fig. 3. Neurodevelopmental implications of IUGR. Risk factors that predispose to poor neurodevelopmental outcomes in IUGR infants; IUGR infants are at high risk for neurodevelopmental abnormalities, including motor delay and cognitive impairments. (*Data from* Baschat AA. Neurodevelopment following fetal growth restriction and its relationship with antepartum parameters of placental dysfunction. Ultrasound Obstet Gynecol 2011;37(5):501–14.)

The fetal programming that occurs as a result of an adverse intrauterine environment along with postnatal catch-up growth can have long-lasting *metabolic consequences* (also known as the nutritional mismatch concept) (**Fig. 4**). To survive, the growth-restricted fetus adapts by:

1. Redistributing blood flow and nutrients to vital organs, sparing blood flow to the brain at the expense of other organs; and
2. Changing the production of placental and fetal hormones that affect fetal growth (insulin, IGFs, and hormones in the hypothalamic-pituitary-adrenal [HPA] axis).[92]

This developmental programming can cause epigenetic modifications that occur during a critical period of growth and maturation, thus resulting in permanent effects.[93]

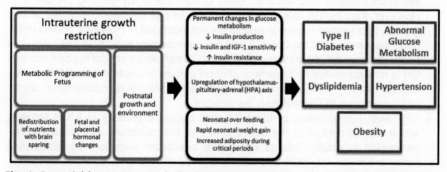

Fig. 4. Potential long-term metabolic derangements associated with IUGR. Adverse intrauterine environment results in fetal programming, which, along with postnatal catch-up growth, has long-lasting metabolic consequences including, insulin resistance, dyslipidemia, and cardiovascular disease.

Along with these prenatal changes, the addition of excessive postnatal nutrition and a subsequent sedentary life style increases the risk for metabolic syndrome, insulin resistance, and cardiovascular disease.[94] IUGR infants can have voracious appetites because they lack satiety due to derangement (or imbalance) of their hypothalamic orexigenic/anorexigenic neuropeptides. This appetite leads to catch-up growth, which one needs for brain development, and perhaps bone development, but is detrimental to the heart and metabolism. As reported by Soto and colleagues[95] in SGA infants, insulin resistance can appear as early as 1 year of age and is closely associated with rapid weight gain and BMI greater than 17 kg/m^2. Insulin-mediated glucose uptake is lower in these infants, who demonstrate a higher risk for metabolic syndrome (2.3%) compared with AGA infants (0.4%).[96] Preterm IUGR children have increased risk of arterial stiffness, aortic wall thickness, metabolic dysfunction that predisposes them to hypertension, cardiovascular disease, insulin resistance, and type II diabetes mellitus.[5,97] Children and adults with a history of IUGR can have abnormal concentrations of circulating insulin, catecholamines, GH, and IGFs.[98]

Visceral adipose tissue is relatively increased in IUGR fetuses, even though body fat mass overall is reduced.[99] Their abdominal adipose tissue is hypersensitive to catecholamine and insulin resistance.[100] With rapid catch-up growth, the central fat mass increases, yet at times registers a normal BMI. Changes in leptin quantity, responsiveness, and function prenatally and after birth also affect adiposity and body composition.[101,102]

Because of the risks of metabolic syndrome, pediatric care providers should consider the following preventive and treatment strategies in IUGR infants with:

- Anthropometric measurements every 3 months for the first year and then every 6 months thereafter
- Annual blood pressure measurements
- Close observation of growth patterns toward predicting metabolic syndrome/cardiovascular disease
- Close monitoring of BMI, fasting glucose, and lipids
- Early introduction of lifestyle modifications

Several studies demonstrate evidence for long-term *endocrinologic disturbances* in IUGR infants (**Fig. 5**). It is important to note that in the studies described below, authors have reported data in SGA infants and did not distinguish between IUGR and SGA:

- *Growth hormone-IGF axis*: In SGA children, there are alterations in diurnal GH secretion patterns and reduced levels of IGF-1 and IGF-binding protein 3.[103] However, the GH-IGF axis in early postnatal life has not been predictive of later growth, thus routine hormone assays are not indicated.[75] However, later in childhood, assessment of the GH-IGF axis will be important in an SGA child who has persistent poor height growth with signs of GH deficiency and/or hypopituitarism. GH is now approved for treatment of short stature in children born SGA, as discussed earlier.[81] Because the etiology for short stature is multifactorial, an infant's response to GH will likely be variable.
- *HPA axis*: Upregulation of the HPA axis occurs prenatally in IUGR fetuses, which can contribute to the development of the metabolic syndrome and hypertension in adults. Infants born after significant exposure to intrauterine stress are frequently SGA and have a blunted HPA axis response to stressors. Animal models of prenatal stress and maternal malnutrition produce low-birth-weight offspring with HPA hyperactivity and lifelong hypertension and glucose intolerance.[104]

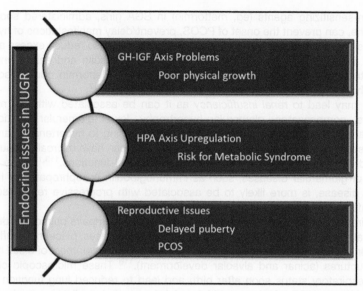

Fig. 5. Long-term endocrine problems associated with IUGR. IUGR causes programming of key endocrine pathways, namely the GH-IGF axis leading to short stature and the HPA axis contributing to metabolic derangements, as well as the reproductive axes in both boys and girls affecting fertility.

- *Puberty, polycystic ovarian syndrome (PCOS), and reproductive issues*: Menarche can occur 5 to 10 months earlier than normal in SGA girls, and this can potentially lead to reduced adult stature.[105] In both boys and girls who had IUGR, pubertal growth is modestly decreased. The variation in pubertal timing and progression also depends on ethnicity, background population trends, and nutrition. Rapid catch-up growth, increased adiposity and over-weight in girls has been associated with earlier onset of puberty.[106] This may be related to circulating leptin concentrations that have effects on gonadotropin releasing hormone secretion, the concentrations of which are dependent on optimal fat mass accumulation. Analysis of hypothalamic DNA also demonstrates significant changes in the methylation patterns associated with the onset of puberty in girls.[107] Onset of puberty is slightly delayed in growth-restricted boys although early puberty can be found in boys with remarkable pre-pubertal weight gain. Adolescent girls who were SGA at birth may have reduced ovulation rates, increased secretion of adrenal and ovarian androgens, excess abdominal fat, and hyperinsulinemia.[108] Insulin resistance, dyslipidemia, and hyperandrogenism can lead to PCOS in adolescence. Boys who were born SGA may have smaller testicular volume and lower serum inhibin B and testosterone concentrations.[109] Growth-restricted boys could have abnormal sperm counts as a result of lower birth weight. Maternal smoking, which is associated with IUGR, has a significant impact on reducing sperm counts in the offspring.[110] Low birth weight/SGA are also associated with hypospadias, cryptorchidism, and testicular cancer.[111] Reproductive abnormalities associated with IUGR depend on the timing of fetal growth restraint. Early fetal growth suppression is associated with germ cell tumors (seminoma), hypospadias, and subfertility. Later fetal growth suppression leads to cryptorchidism, testicular cancer, premature adrenarche, PCOS, and low fertility.

Insulin-sensitizing agents (eg, metformin) in SGA girls, administered soon after menarche, can prevent the onset of PCOS, prevent/delay manifestations of hyperandrogenism, and increase ovulation rates. Metformin can also reduce excess abdominal fat, increase lean body mass, decrease fasting insulin and serum androgen concentrations, and improve the serum lipid profile. Metformin could also delay menarche and prolong the growth period in SGA girls.[108,112]

IUGR may lead to *renal insufficiency* as it can be associated with low nephron numbers, compensatory glomerular hypertrophy, lower glomerular filtration rate (GFR), and higher albumin: creatinine ratio, predisposing to hypertension, and later renal disease.[97] Young adults with a history of IUGR can have microalbuminuria and reduced GFR, but typically have grossly normal renal functions.[113,114] The clinical course of glomerular diseases, such as immunoglobulin A nephropathy or minimal change disease, is more likely to be associated with progressive renal disease in IUGR infants.[115]

Impaired fetal nutrition and oxygen availability in utero impairs pulmonary development that affects long-term *lung function*. In most IUGR cases, placental insufficiency occurs in the late second trimester, which parallels the development of distal respiratory structures (acinar and alveolar development).[116] These microscopic changes affect respiratory status soon after birth and lead to reduced lung function lasting into adulthood. IUGR infants are at higher risk for respiratory distress syndrome and bronchopulmonary dysplasia.[117] Impaired fetal growth and rapid postnatal growth/obesity can increase the risk for childhood asthma.[118]

Nutritional deficits in utero and leptin dynamics can lead to *impaired bone metabolism* and predispose toward osteoporosis due to reduced bone mineral content and bone density.[119,120] Lower birth length and poor linear growth between 7 and 11 years of life is associated with more osteoporosis in adulthood, as demonstrated by increased hip fractures in the growth-restricted group compared with the ones that had optimal height gain.[121]

IUGR can lead to *impaired visual function* as a result of retinal damage.[122] IUGR increases the risk for *sensorineural hearing loss* due to abnormalities in the cochlea, auditory neurons, auditory ganglion cells and brainstem-evoked potentials.[123,124]

SUMMARY

IUGR infants suffer significant morbidity with immediate and long-term health consequences. These infants are at high risk throughout their life and should be carefully monitored at different stages to ensure timely interventions toward prevention and management of various disorders affecting most organ systems. In the immediate postnatal period and infancy, a balance has to be struck between achieving catch-up growth necessary for promoting normal brain and bone development, against the subsequent development of cardiovascular and metabolic disorders if the catch-up growth is excessive. A caution toward moderation in diet is necessary while meeting the needs of neurodevelopment. It is important to note that GH is one of the few therapies that can be administered to SGA children with persistent growth failure after evaluation by a pediatric endocrinologist. This therapy, while targeting improved stature, favorably affects body composition, blood pressure and lipid metabolism.

REFERENCES

1. Battaglia FC, Lubchenco LO. A practical classification of newborn infants by weight and gestational age. J Pediatr 1967;71(2):159–63.
2. Rosenberg A. The IUGR newborn. Semin Perinatol 2008;32(3):219–24.

3. Longo S, Bollani L, Decembrino L, et al. Short-term and long-term sequelae in intrauterine growth retardation (IUGR). J Matern Fetal Neonatal Med 2013; 26(3):222–5.

4. von Beckerath AK, Kollmann M, Rotky-Fast C, et al. Perinatal complications and long-term neurodevelopmental outcome of infants with intrauterine growth restriction. Am J Obstet Gynecol 2013;208(2):130.e1-6.

5. Zanardo V, Visentin S, Trevisanuto D, et al. Fetal aortic wall thickness: a marker of hypertension in IUGR children? Hypertens Res 2013;36(5):440–3.

6. de Onis M, Blossner M, Villar J. Levels and patterns of intrauterine growth retardation in developing countries. Eur J Clin Nutr 1998;52(Suppl 1):S5–15.

7. Cetin I, Mando C, Calabrese S. Maternal predictors of intrauterine growth restriction. Curr Opin Clin Nutr Metab Care 2013;16(3):310–9.

8. Cavazos-Rehg PA, Krauss MJ, Spitznagel EL, et al. Maternal age and risk of labor and delivery complications. Matern Child Health J 2015;19(6):1202–11.

9. Blumenshine P, Egerter S, Barclay CJ, et al. Socioeconomic disparities in adverse birth outcomes: a systematic review. Am J Prev Med 2010;39(3):263–72.

10. Parraguez VH, Mamani S, Cofre E, et al. Disturbances in maternal steroidogenesis and appearance of intrauterine growth retardation at high-altitude environments are established from early pregnancy. effects of treatment with antioxidant vitamins. PLoS One 2015;10(11):e0140902.

11. Pruett D, Waterman EH, Caughey AB. Fetal alcohol exposure: consequences, diagnosis, and treatment. Obstet Gynecol Surv 2013;68(1):62–9.

12. Rayburn WF. Maternal and fetal effects from substance use. Clin Perinatol 2007; 34(4):559–71, vi.

13. Norsa'adah B, Salinah O. The effect of second-hand smoke exposure during pregnancy on the newborn weight in Malaysia. Malays J Med Sci 2014;21(2): 44–53.

14. Milnerowicz-Nabzdyk E, Bizon A. Effect of cigarette smoking on vascular flows in pregnancies complicated by intrauterine growth restriction. Reprod Toxicol 2014;50:27–35.

15. Miyake Y, Tanaka K, Arakawa M. Active and passive maternal smoking during pregnancy and birth outcomes: the Kyushu Okinawa Maternal and Child Health Study. BMC Pregnancy Childbirth 2013;13:157.

16. Hendrix N, Berghella V. Non-placental causes of intrauterine growth restriction. Semin Perinatol 2008;32(3):161–5.

17. Adams Waldorf KM, McAdams RM. Influence of infection during pregnancy on fetal development. Reproduction 2013;146(5):R151–62.

18. Howarth C, Gazis A, James D. Associations of type 1 diabetes mellitus, maternal vascular disease and complications of pregnancy. Diabet Med 2007; 24(11):1229–34.

19. Cyganek A, Pietrzak B, Kociszewska-Najman B, et al. Intrauterine growth restriction in pregnant renal and liver transplant recipients: risk factors assessment. Transplant Proc 2014;46(8):2794–7.

20. Zhu BP, Rolfs RT, Nangle BE, et al. Effect of the interval between pregnancies on perinatal outcomes. N Engl J Med 1999;340(8):589–94.

21. Turkgeldi E, Yagmur H, Seyhan A, et al. Short and long term outcomes of children conceived with assisted reproductive technology. Eur J Obstet Gynecol Reprod Biol 2016;207:129–36.

22. Maulik D. Fetal growth restriction: the etiology. Clin Obstet Gynecol 2006;49(2): 228–35.

23. Soong YK, Wang TH, Lee YS, et al. Genome-wide detection of uniparental disomy in a fetus with intrauterine growth restriction using genotyping microarrays. Taiwan J Obstet Gynecol 2009;48(2):152–8.

24. Dicke JM, Crane JP. Sonographic recognition of major malformations and aberrant fetal growth in trisomic fetuses. J Ultrasound Med 1991;10(8):433–8.

25. Snijders RJ, Sherrod C, Gosden CM, et al. Fetal growth retardation: associated malformations and chromosomal abnormalities. Am J Obstet Gynecol 1993; 168(2):547–55.

26. Wallenstein MB, Harper LM, Odibo AO, et al. Fetal congenital heart disease and intrauterine growth restriction: a retrospective cohort study. J Matern Fetal Neonatal Med 2012;25(6):662–5.

27. Balayla J, Abenhaim HA. Incidence, predictors and outcomes of congenital diaphragmatic hernia: a population-based study of 32 million births in the United States. J Matern Fetal Neonatal Med 2014;27(14):1438–44.

28. Khoury MJ, Erickson JD, Cordero JF, et al. Congenital malformations and intrauterine growth retardation: a population study. Pediatrics 1988;82(1):83–90.

29. Khan NA, Kazzi SN. Yield and costs of screening growth-retarded infants for torch infections. Am J Perinatol 2000;17(3):131–5.

30. Walker PG, ter Kuile FO, Garske T, et al. Estimated risk of placental infection and low birthweight attributable to *Plasmodium falciparum* malaria in Africa in 2010: a modelling study. Lancet Glob Health 2014;2(8):e460–7.

31. Rogerson SJ, Grau GE, Hunt NH. The microcirculation in severe malaria. Microcirculation 2004;11(7):559–76.

32. Priyadarshi A, Verge CF, Vandervliet L, et al. Transient neonatal diabetes mellitus followed by recurrent asymptomatic hypoglycaemia: a case report. BMC Pediatr 2015;15:200.

33. Brassier A, Ottolenghi C, Boddaert N, et al. Prenatal symptoms and diagnosis of inherited metabolic diseases]. Arch Pediatr 2012;19(9):959–69.

34. Jacquinet A, Verloes A, Callewaert B, et al. Neonatal progeroid variant of Marfan syndrome with congenital lipodystrophy results from mutations at the 3' end of FBN1 gene. Eur J Med Genet 2014;57(5):230–4.

35. Planchenault D, Martin-Coignard D, Rugemintwaza D, et al. Donohue syndrome or leprechaunism. Arch Pediatr 2014;21(2):206–10 [in French].

36. Townsend R, Khalil A. Fetal growth restriction in twins. Best Pract Res Clin Obstet Gynaecol 2018;49:79–88.

37. Salavati N, Sovio U, Mayo RP, et al. The relationship between human placental morphometry and ultrasonic measurements of utero-placental blood flow and fetal growth. Placenta 2016;38:41–8.

38. Heinonen S, Taipale P, Saarikoski S. Weights of placentae from small-for-gestational age infants revisited. Placenta 2001;22(5):399–404.

39. Zygmunt M, Herr F, Munstedt K, et al. Angiogenesis and vasculogenesis in pregnancy. Eur J Obstet Gynecol Reprod Biol 2003;110(Suppl 1):S10–8.

40. Madazli R, Somunkiran A, Calay Z, et al. Histomorphology of the placenta and the placental bed of growth restricted foetuses and correlation with the Doppler velocimetries of the uterine and umbilical arteries. Placenta 2003;24(5):510–6.

41. Shilling C, Walsh C, Downey P, et al. Umbilical artery thrombosis is a rare but clinically important finding: a series of 7 cases with clinical outcomes. Pediatr Dev Pathol 2014;17(2):89–93.

42. Conroy AL, Silver KL, Zhong K, et al. Complement activation and the resulting placental vascular insufficiency drives fetal growth restriction associated with placental malaria. Cell Host Microbe 2013;13(2):215–26.

43. Wilkins-Haug L, Quade B, Morton CC. Confined placental mosaicism as a risk factor among newborns with fetal growth restriction. Prenat Diagn 2006;26(5): 428–32.

44. Boog G. Chronic villitis of unknown etiology. Eur J Obstet Gynecol Reprod Biol 2008;136(1):9–15.

45. Szentpeteri I, Rab A, Kornya L, et al. Placental gene expression patterns of endoglin (CD105) in intrauterine growth restriction. J Matern Fetal Neonatal Med 2014;27(4):350–4.

46. Carver TD, Anderson SM, Aldoretta PA, et al. Glucose suppression of insulin secretion in chronically hyperglycemic fetal sheep. Pediatr Res 1995;38(5): 754–62.

47. Hay WW Jr. Recent observations on the regulation of fetal metabolism by glucose. J Physiol 2006;572(Pt 1):17–24.

48. Martin-Estal I, de la Garza RG, Castilla-Cortazar I. Intrauterine growth retardation (iugr) as a novel condition of insulin-like growth factor-1 (IGF-1) deficiency. Rev Physiol Biochem Pharmacol 2016;170:1–35.

49. Leger J, Oury JF, Noel M, et al. Growth factors and intrauterine growth retardation. I. Serum growth hormone, insulin-like growth factor (IGF)-I, IGF-II, and IGF binding protein 3 levels in normally grown and growth-retarded human fetuses during the second half of gestation. Pediatr Res 1996;40(1):94–100.

50. Gressens P, Paindaveine B, Hill JM, et al. Vasoactive intestinal peptide shortens both G1 and S phases of neural cell cycle in whole postimplantation cultured mouse embryos. Eur J Neurosci 1998;10(5):1734–42.

51. Saki F, Dabbaghmanesh MH, Ghaemi SZ, et al. Thyroid function in pregnancy and its influences on maternal and fetal outcomes. Int J Endocrinol Metab 2014;12(4):e19378.

52. Poon LC, Zaragoza E, Akolekar R, et al. Maternal serum placental growth factor (PlGF) in small for gestational age pregnancy at 11(+0) to 13(+6) weeks of gestation. Prenat Diagn 2008;28(12):1110–5.

53. Landmann E, Reiss I, Misselwitz B, et al. Ponderal index for discrimination between symmetric and asymmetric growth restriction: percentiles for neonates from 30 weeks to 43 weeks of gestation. J Matern Fetal Neonatal Med 2006; 19(3):157–60.

54. Georgieff MK, Sasanow SR, Chockalingam UM, et al. A comparison of the mid-arm circumference/head circumference ratio and ponderal index for the evaluation of newborn infants after abnormal intrauterine growth. Acta Paediatr Scand 1988;77(2):214–9.

55. Soundarya M, Basavaprabhu A, Raghuveera K, et al. Comparative assessment of fetal malnutrition by anthropometry and CAN score. Iran J Pediatr 2012;22(1): 70–6.

56. Pilliod RA, Cheng YW, Snowden JM, et al. The risk of intrauterine fetal death in the small-for-gestational-age fetus. Am J Obstet Gynecol 2012;207(4):318.e1-6.

57. Madden JV, Flatley CJ, Kumar S. Term small-for-gestational-age infants from low-risk women are at significantly greater risk of adverse neonatal outcomes. Am J Obstet Gynecol 2018;218(5):525.e1-9.

58. Flamant C, Gascoin G. Short-term outcome and small for gestational age newborn management. J Gynecol Obstet Biol Reprod 2013;42(8):985–95.

59. Steurer MA, Jelliffe-Pawlowski LL, Baer RJ, et al. Persistent pulmonary hypertension of the newborn in late preterm and term infants in California. Pediatrics 2017;139(1) [pii:e20161165].

60. Pariente G, Peles C, Perri ZH, et al. Meconium-stained amniotic fluid–risk factors and immediate perinatal outcomes among SGA infants. J Matern Fetal Neonatal Med 2015;28(9):1064–7.

61. Bozzetti V, Tagliabue PE, Visser GH, et al. Feeding issues in IUGR preterm infants. Early Hum Dev 2013;89(Suppl 2):S21–3.

62. Baserga MC, Sola A. Intrauterine growth restriction impacts tolerance to total parenteral nutrition in extremely low birth weight infants. J Perinatol 2004; 24(8):476–81.

63. Boehm G, Senger H, Braun W, et al. Metabolic differences between AGA- and SGA-infants of very low birthweight. I. Relationship to intrauterine growth retardation. Acta Paediatr Scand 1988;77(1):19–23.

64. Hosagasi NH, Aydin M, Zenciroglu A, et al. Incidence of hypoglycemia in newborns at risk and an audit of the 2011 American Academy of Pediatrics guideline for hypoglycemia. Pediatr Neonatol 2018;59(4):368–74.

65. Hawdon JM, Weddell A, Aynsley-Green A, et al. Hormonal and metabolic response to hypoglycaemia in small for gestational age infants. Arch Dis Child 1993;68(3 Spec No):269–73.

66. Hoe FM, Thornton PS, Wanner LA, et al. Clinical features and insulin regulation in infants with a syndrome of prolonged neonatal hyperinsulinism. J Pediatr 2006; 148(2):207–12.

67. Thornton PS, Stanley CA, De Leon DD, et al. Recommendations from the Pediatric Endocrine Society for Evaluation and Management of Persistent Hypoglycemia in Neonates, Infants, and Children. J Pediatr 2015;167(2):238–45.

68. Mitanchez D. Ontogenesis of glucose regulation in neonate and consequences in neonatal management. Arch Pediatr 2008;15(1):64–74.

69. Jain A, Agarwal R, Sankar MJ, et al. Hypocalcemia in the newborn. Indian J Pediatr 2010;77(10):1123–8.

70. Hyman SJ, Novoa Y, Holzman I. Perinatal endocrinology: common endocrine disorders in the sick and premature newborn. Pediatr Clin North Am 2011; 58(5):1083–98, ix.

71. Hsu SC, Levine MA. Perinatal calcium metabolism: physiology and pathophysiology. Semin Neonatol 2004;9(1):23–36.

72. Mukhopadhyay D, Weaver L, Tobin R, et al. Intrauterine growth restriction and prematurity influence regulatory T cell development in newborns. J Pediatr Surg 2014;49(5):727–32.

73. Neumann CG, Stiehm ER, Zahradnick J, et al. Immune function in intrauterine growth retardation. Nutr Res 1998;18(2):201–24.

74. Bagby SP. Maternal nutrition, low nephron number, and hypertension in later life: pathways of nutritional programming. J Nutr 2007;137(4):1066–72.

75. Leger J, Noel M, Limal JM, et al. Growth factors and intrauterine growth retardation. II. Serum growth hormone, insulin-like growth factor (IGF) I, and IGF-binding protein 3 levels in children with intrauterine growth retardation compared with normal control subjects: prospective study from birth to two years of age. Study Group of IUGR. Pediatr Res 1996;40(1):101–7.

76. Karlberg J, Albertsson-Wikland K. Growth in full-term small-for-gestational-age infants: from birth to final height. Pediatr Res 1995;38(5):733–9.

77. Albertsson-Wikland K, Boguszewski M, Karlberg J. Children born small-for-gestational age: postnatal growth and hormonal status. Horm Res 1998; 49(Suppl 2):7–13.

78. Wit JM, Finken MJ, Rijken M, et al. Preterm growth restraint: a paradigm that unifies intrauterine growth retardation and preterm extrauterine growth

retardation and has implications for the small-for-gestational-age indication in growth hormone therapy. Pediatrics 2006;117(4):e793–5.

79. Boersma B, Wit JM. Catch-up growth. Endocr Rev 1997;18(5):646–61.

80. Gibson AT, Carney S, Cavazzoni E, et al. Neonatal and post-natal growth. Horm Res 2000;53(Suppl 1):42–9.

81. Clayton PE, Cianfarani S, Czernichow P, et al. Management of the child born small for gestational age through to adulthood: a consensus statement of the International Societies of Pediatric Endocrinology and the Growth Hormone Research Society. J Clin Endocrinol Metab 2007;92(3):804–10.

82. Sas T, Mulder P, Hokken-Koelega A. Body composition, blood pressure, and lipid metabolism before and during long-term growth hormone (GH) treatment in children with short stature born small for gestational age either with or without GH deficiency. J Clin Endocrinol Metab 2000;85(10):3786–92.

83. Baschat AA. Neurodevelopment following fetal growth restriction and its relationship with antepartum parameters of placental dysfunction. Ultrasound Obstet Gynecol 2011;37(5):501–14.

84. Lohaugen GC, Ostgard HF, Andreassen S, et al. Small for gestational age and intrauterine growth restriction decreases cognitive function in young adults. J Pediatr 2013;163(2):447–53.

85. Seckl JR, Meaney MJ. Glucocorticoid programming. Ann N Y Acad Sci 2004; 1032:63–84.

86. Mallard C, Loeliger M, Copolov D, et al. Reduced number of neurons in the hippocampus and the cerebellum in the postnatal guinea-pig following intrauterine growth-restriction. Neuroscience 2000;100(2):327–33.

87. Tideman E, Marsal K, Ley D. Cognitive function in young adults following intrauterine growth restriction with abnormal fetal aortic blood flow. Ultrasound Obstet Gynecol 2007;29(6):614–8.

88. Barbey AK, Colom R, Solomon J, et al. An integrative architecture for general intelligence and executive function revealed by lesion mapping. Brain 2012; 135(Pt 4):1154–64.

89. Geva R, Eshel R, Leitner Y, et al. Neuropsychological outcome of children with intrauterine growth restriction: a 9-year prospective study. Pediatrics 2006; 118(1):91–100.

90. Lundgren EM, Cnattingius S, Jonsson B, et al. Intellectual and psychological performance in males born small for gestational age with and without catch-up growth. Pediatr Res 2001;50(1):91–6.

91. van Pareren YK, Duivenvoorden HJ, Slijper FS, et al. Intelligence and psychosocial functioning during long-term growth hormone therapy in children born small for gestational age. J Clin Endocrinol Metab 2004;89(11):5295–302.

92. Fukuoka H. DOHaD (developmental origins of health and disease) and birth cohort research. J Nutr Sci Vitaminol 2015;61(Suppl):S2–4.

93. Huang RC, Prescott SL, Godfrey KM, et al. Assessment of cardiometabolic risk in children in population studies: underpinning developmental origins of health and disease mother-offspring cohort studies. J Nutr Sci 2015;4:e12.

94. Barker DJ. The origins of the developmental origins theory. J Intern Med 2007; 261(5):412–7.

95. Soto N, Bazaes RA, Pena V, et al. Insulin sensitivity and secretion are related to catch-up growth in small-for-gestational-age infants at age 1 year: results from a prospective cohort. J Clin Endocrinol Metab 2003;88(8):3645–50.

96. Jaquet D, Deghmoun S, Chevenne D, et al. Dynamic change in adiposity from fetal to postnatal life is involved in the metabolic syndrome associated with reduced fetal growth. Diabetologia 2005;48(5):849–55.

97. Chan PY, Morris JM, Leslie GI, et al. The long-term effects of prematurity and intrauterine growth restriction on cardiovascular, renal, and metabolic function. Int J Pediatr 2010;2010:280402.

98. Phillips DI. Fetal growth and programming of the hypothalamic-pituitary-adrenal axis. Clin Exp Pharmacol Physiol 2001;28(11):967–70.

99. Ibanez L, Lopez-Bermejo A, Suarez L, et al. Visceral adiposity without overweight in children born small for gestational age. J Clin Endocrinol Metab 2008;93(6):2079–83.

100. Boiko J, Jaquet D, Chevenne D, et al. In situ lipolytic regulation in subjects born small for gestational age. Int J Obes (Lond) 2005;29(6):565–70.

101. McMillen IC, Muhlhausler BS, Duffield JA, et al. Prenatal programming of postnatal obesity: fetal nutrition and the regulation of leptin synthesis and secretion before birth. Proc Nutr Soc 2004;63(3):405–12.

102. Martinez-Cordero C, Amador-Licona N, Guizar-Mendoza JM, et al. Body fat at birth and cord blood levels of insulin, adiponectin, leptin, and insulin-like growth factor-I in small-for-gestational-age infants. Arch Med Res 2006;37(4):490–4.

103. de Waal WJ, Hokken-Koelega AC, Stijnen T, et al. Endogenous and stimulated GH secretion, urinary GH excretion, and plasma IGF-I and IGF-II levels in prepubertal children with short stature after intrauterine growth retardation. The Dutch Working Group on Growth Hormone. Clin Endocrinol 1994;41(5):621–30.

104. Langley-Evans SC, Gardner DS, Jackson AA. Maternal protein restriction influences the programming of the rat hypothalamic-pituitary-adrenal axis. J Nutr 1996;126(6):1578–85.

105. Bhargava SK, Ramji S, Srivastava U, et al. Growth and sexual maturation of low birth weight children: a 14 year follow up. Indian Pediatr 1995;32(9):963–70.

106. Neville KA, Walker JL. Precocious pubarche is associated with SGA, prematurity, weight gain, and obesity. Arch Dis Child 2005;90(3):258–61.

107. Roth CL, Sathyanarayana S. Mechanisms affecting neuroendocrine and epigenetic regulation of body weight and onset of puberty: potential implications in the child born small for gestational age (SGA). Rev Endocr Metab Disord 2012;13(2):129–40.

108. Ibanez L, Potau N, Ferrer A, et al. Reduced ovulation rate in adolescent girls born small for gestational age. J Clin Endocrinol Metab 2002;87(7):3391–3.

109. Cicognani A, Alessandroni R, Pasini A, et al. Low birth weight for gestational age and subsequent male gonadal function. J Pediatr 2002;141(3):376–9.

110. Jensen TK, Jorgensen N, Punab M, et al. Association of in utero exposure to maternal smoking with reduced semen quality and testis size in adulthood: a cross-sectional study of 1,770 young men from the general population in five European countries. Am J Epidemiol 2004;159(1):49–58.

111. Main KM, Jensen RB, Asklund C, et al. Low birth weight and male reproductive function. Horm Res 2006;65(Suppl 3):116–22.

112. Chernausek SD. Update: consequences of abnormal fetal growth. J Clin Endocrinol Metab 2012;97(3):689–95.

113. Abitbol CL, Rodriguez MM. The long-term renal and cardiovascular consequences of prematurity. Nat Rev Nephrol 2012;8(5):265–74.

114. Bacchetta J, Harambat J, Dubourg L, et al. Both extrauterine and intrauterine growth restriction impair renal function in children born very preterm. Kidney Int 2009;76(4):445–52.

115. Teeninga N, Schreuder MF, Bokenkamp A, et al. Influence of low birth weight on minimal change nephrotic syndrome in children, including a meta-analysis. Nephrol Dial Transplant 2008;23(5):1615–20.
116. Pike K, Jane Pillow J, Lucas JS. Long term respiratory consequences of intrauterine growth restriction. Semin Fetal Neonatal Med 2012;17(2):92–8.
117. Sharma P, McKay K, Rosenkrantz TS, et al. Comparisons of mortality and pre-discharge respiratory outcomes in small-for-gestational-age and appropriate-for-gestational-age premature infants. BMC Pediatr 2004;4:9.
118. Kallen B, Finnstrom O, Nygren KG, et al. Association between preterm birth and intrauterine growth retardation and child asthma. Eur Respir J 2013;41(3):671–6.
119. Javaid MK, Godfrey KM, Taylor P, et al. Umbilical cord leptin predicts neonatal bone mass. Calcif Tissue Int 2005;76(5):341–7.
120. Tobias JH, Cooper C. PTH/PTHrP activity and the programming of skeletal development in utero. J Bone Miner Res 2004;19(2):177–82.
121. Cooper C, Eriksson JG, Forsen T, et al. Maternal height, childhood growth and risk of hip fracture in later life: a longitudinal study. Osteoporos Int 2001;12(8):623–9.
122. Loeliger M, Briscoe T, Lambert G, et al. Chronic placental insufficiency affects retinal development in the guinea pig. Invest Ophthalmol Vis Sci 2004;45(7):2361–7.
123. Pettigrew AG, Edwards DA, Henderson-Smart DJ. The influence of intra-uterine growth retardation on brainstem development of preterm infants. Dev Med Child Neurol 1985;27(4):467–72.
124. Barrenas ML, Bratthall A, Dahlgren J. The association between short stature and sensorineural hearing loss. Hear Res 2005;205(1–2):123–30.

Hearing Loss in Pediatrics
What the Medical Home Needs to Know

Jane E. Stewart, MD[a],*, Jennifer E. Bentley, AuD[b]

KEYWORDS

- Audiology • Hearing loss • Risk-factors

KEY POINTS

- The "1-3-6" approach to diagnose and manage hearing loss: Screening before 1 month, diagnosis before 3 months, habilitation/treatment before 6 months.
- Hearing loss can develop at any time during childhood with even mild, unilateral, and fluctuating loss having a major impact of developmental outcomes.
- The evaluation for deafness-associated medical and genetic conditions provides important information that can impact parental choice of communication and outcome for the affected child and other family members.
- Early access to language therapy and developing a rich language environment is important in shaping language development.
- Advances in technology (eg, hearing aids and cochlear implants) have improved outcomes of infants with hearing loss.

INTRODUCTION

Congenital hearing loss occurs in approximately 1 to 3 per 1000 newborns[1,2]; preterm infants are especially at risk, with hearing loss reported in approximately 30 per 1000 live preterm births.[3,4] Early detection of hearing loss is vital. Children whose hearing loss is identified after 6 months of age show delays in language development compared with peers identified before 6 months.[5]

As part of the 2000 and 2007 position statements, the Joint Committee on Infant Hearing (JCIH) recommended that all newborns should be screened for hearing loss before 1 month of age.[6,7] Infants who do not pass their newborn hearing screen should have a diagnostic evaluation as soon as possible and before 3 months of age. Those diagnosed with hearing loss should obtain intervention promptly and before 6 months of age. Currently, 47 of 50 states have legislation or regulations requiring newborns to

[a] Department of Neonatology, Beth Israel Deaconess Medical Center, Harvard Medical University, Boston Children's Hospital, Rose 3, 330 Brookline Avenue, Boston, MA 02215, USA; [b] Department of Neonatology, Beth Israel Deaconess Medical Center, Rose 3, 330 Brookline Avenue, Boston, MA 02215, USA
* Corresponding author.
E-mail address: jstewart@bidmc.harvard.edu

Pediatr Clin N Am 66 (2019) 425–436
https://doi.org/10.1016/j.pcl.2018.12.010
0031-3955/19/© 2019 Elsevier Inc. All rights reserved.
pediatric.theclinics.com

have their hearing screened before discharge from the birthing center. According to data collected by the Centers for Disease Control and Prevention,[8] 98% of infants were screened for hearing loss in 2016. Of those who did not pass the newborn screening, only 47% had a completed diagnostic hearing evaluation before 3 months of age and only 45% of infants diagnosed with hearing loss were enrolled in Early Intervention (EI) before 6 months of age.

COMMON MISSTEPS IN THE EARLY HEARING DETECTION AND INTERVENTION PROCESS

Outcomes for children who are deaf or hard of hearing (D/HH) are dependent on the timing of intervention and affected children are vulnerable to oversights within the process. Oversights can occur at various stages of a child's development. Awareness by the medical home can ensure optimal language acquisition.

- *Giving false reassurances:* Statistics show that most infants who do not pass their newborn hearing screening will have normal hearing on their diagnostic test, but there is no definitive way to determine from the newborn screen which infants will have true hearing loss. Giving families false reassurance that the diagnostic test will be normal may lead to a lack of appreciation of the importance of follow-up and result in delay or complete lack of follow-up.
- *Lack of or delay in additional testing:* The most common reason for delay in audiology follow-up is poor accessibility to services, but maternal sociodemographic features, lack of insurance, and lack of family education about screenings are also factors.
- *Failure to complete an evaluation for medical disorders associated with hearing loss:* It is important to assess for disorders associated with hearing loss (eg, visual, cardiac, and renal disorders) to ensure optimal medical management and assist decision-making on mode of communication.[9] If facilities test for congenital cytomegalovirus as a risk for hearing loss, sample collection is time-sensitive in determining eligibility for antiviral treatment.
- *Failure to initiate appropriate, individualized and targeted EI from specialized providers:* Language development is dependent on early input to the infant's developing language acquisition center during the critical window. Establishment of EI services is complex and decisions about the best plan for providing an enriched language environment require parent education.[10] Prompt initiation of amplification, auditory input, and language input (spoken and visual) is associated with improved long-term language and cognitive outcomes. Providers of EI services for infants who are D/HH must have specialized training.
- *Lack of support and education of parents in a timely, understandable and culturally sensitive manner:* Parents may not be aware of the vast number of resources available to help them through this journey. Support groups, specialized intervention services, and sign language programs are available. The universal newborn hearing program in each state is able to provide the medical home and parents with a wealth of information in a language that they can understand. Programs often use parents of a D/HH child and deaf mentors to supplement information provided by medical professionals. It is important to listen to and respect the family culture and understand that the goals of parents may be different. For example, the traditional medical model of considering D/HH individuals as having a defect or disability that can be "fixed" is not a view accepted by many in the Deaf Community. This understanding is critical in supporting families in their decision-making and facilitating the appropriate resources.

- *Lack of prompt pick-up of auditory/language concerns in first year of life:* Infants who are unable to attain auditory or speech and language developmental milestones should be scheduled for a hearing evaluation even if they initially passed their newborn screen. Hearing loss can develop at any age. "A pass on a newborn hearing screen is not a vaccine against hearing loss" (Personal Communication, Brian James Fligor, AuD, ScD, former Director of Audiology, Boston Children's Hospital, 2013).

REVIEW OF AUDIOLOGY BASICS
Screening Tests

Two methods are recommended for screening an infant's hearing at birth. A threshold of $\geq$35 dB is the standard cutoff for an abnormal screen (termed "refer"), prompting further testing. Both tests may be influenced by debris or fluid in the external or middle ears.

- Screening Otoacoustic Emissions (OAE): This test is based on the detection of low level sounds emitted by the cochlea in response to acoustic stimulation. These sounds are measured in the external ear and represent the function of the auditory pathway up to the cochlear outer hair cells.
- Automated Auditory Brainstem Response (AABR): In this test, electroencephalographic waves generated in response to click stimuli presented in the external ear are recorded via electrodes placed on an infant's scalp. This test evaluates the function of the auditory pathway including the auditory nerve.

Birthing centers may use 1 or both methods for screening newborns, depending on their states' Department of Public Health policy. The JCIH recommends that infants who are admitted to the neonatal intensive care unit (NICU) for longer than 5 days should be screened with the AABR to help determine status of neural hearing.[6]

Medical home facilities may also have hearing screening equipment. It is important that all screening equipment is calibrated annually and that personnel are properly trained in test administration and interpretation of results.

Diagnostic Tests

Diagnostic evaluations should be completed only by an audiologist and may include the use of a combination of objective and subjective test methods, depending on the age of a child and their ability to participate. Some of the more common tests are listed as follows.

- Diagnostic Auditory Brainstem Response: Ideal for infants younger than 3 months, but can be used with sedation for infants age 6 months and older. The diagnostic ABR will assess the function of the auditory system to clicks as well as low and high frequency tone bursts. This will help to define auditory thresholds and provide a starting point for amplification should a hearing loss be identified.
- Tympanometry: Assesses middle ear function using air pressure and tones. Abnormal results on tympanometry are typically a result of fluid in the middle ear, otitis media, perforation of the ear drum or sequela of infection.
- Diagnostic Otoacoustic Emissions: Measures cochlear hair cell function over a wider range of frequencies (as compared with screening OAEs) and can include click or tonal stimuli.
- Behavioral Hearing Assessment: Ideal for children who are developmentally older than 6 months of age. This testing requires subjective responses to both tones and speech stimuli and is conducted in a sound proof environment.

Definition of Hearing Loss

Hearing is assessed through air and bone conduction stimulation and defined by degree, configuration and type. Describing hearing based on these 3 categories allows for the comparison between known acoustic features of speech and a child's hearing sensitivity. This results in an estimation of a patient's audibility. Based on this information, providers can determine the potential therapeutic options. Hearing is typically plotted on a graph called an audiogram (**Fig. 1**).

- Degree: Measured in decibels (dB) with threshold defined as the ability to detect a sound approximately 50% of the time. Severity of hearing loss is graded between slight (16–25 dB) and profound (91+ dB). Hearing levels can be fixed or fluctuating, any degree of hearing loss outside normal can have a significant impact on speech/language development and developmental outcomes.
- Configuration: Hearing thresholds are measured bilaterally over a range of frequencies (pitches) so that information from low (base) tones and high (treble) tones are obtained. Configuration of hearing provides a description of the frequency range where hearing loss occurs. Low-frequency hearing occurs below 750 Hz, mid-frequency hearing is from 750 to 2000 Hz, and high-frequency hearing involves frequencies over 2000 Hz. The configuration also highlights differences between the ears. Although most people recognize the need for intervention created by bilateral hearing loss, many are unaware that unilateral hearing loss has been linked to significant educational difficulties.

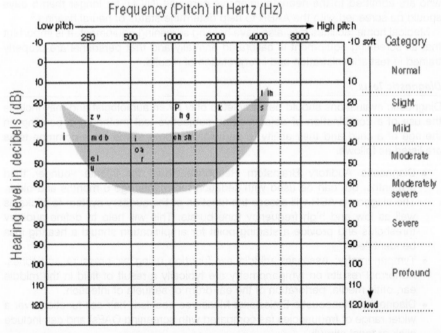

Fig. 1. Blank audiogram where hearing thresholds would be displayed and the range of conversational speech (shaded area). (*From* American Speech Language Hearing Association. Hearing loss- beyond early childhood. Available at: https://www.asha.org/Practice-Portal/Clinical-Topics/Hearing-Loss. Accessed July 31, 2018.)

- Type: Depends on the part of the auditory system impaired. Type can be divided into 5 major categories.
  - Conductive Hearing Loss (CHL):
    - Occurs secondary to problems in the outer or middle ear and is mostly the result of a blockage in sound transmission.
    - Audiogram shows a significant difference between the elevated thresholds for air conducted sound and normal thresholds for bone conducted sound.
    - Most common causes of conductive loss in the infant population are fluid in the middle ear or middle ear effusion. Less common causes are microtia or canal stenosis that may occur in infants with or without other craniofacial malformations.
  - Sensorineural Hearing Loss (SNHL):
    - Occurs secondary to problems in the inner ear and is the result of damage to the cochlear hair cells or auditory nerve.
    - Audiogram shows elevated but symmetric thresholds for both air and bone conducted sound.
  - Mixed Hearing Loss (MHL):
    - Results from both damage to the inner ear and a blockage in the outer or middle ear.
    - Audiogram shows elevated thresholds for both air and bone conducted sound, but with a significant difference between air and bone thresholds.
  - Auditory Neuropathy/Auditory Dyssynchrony (AN/AD):
    - Results from the disruption of the signal between a normal functioning inner ear cochlea and the auditory nerve.
    - Audiogram shows various degree and configuration of results.
    - Rare type of hearing loss with unclear etiology but occurring more often in infants with a history of extreme prematurity, hypoxia, severe hyperbilirubinemia, and immune disorders.
  - Central Hearing Loss:
    - Result of abnormal auditory processing at higher levels of the central nervous system.
    - Audiogram shows various degree and configuration of results.

Etiology

A thorough family history and review for risk factors should be performed. **Fig. 2** provides a graphical breakdown of causes of hearing loss.[11]

- Genetic risk factors: Congenital sensorineural hearing loss is inherited in approximately half of the cases, with most children born to parents with normal hearing and demonstrating a recessive nonsyndromic hearing loss. The most common cause of genetic nonsyndromic hearing loss is a mutation in the gene that encodes the protein connexin 26 (Cx26) (DFNB1).[12] There are more than 125 different loci that result in hearing loss ranging from mild to profound. Almost one-third of infants with genetic hearing loss have other medical issues associated with a syndrome. More than 700 syndromes are known to be associated with some degree of hearing loss.[13]
- Nongenetic/Environmental risk factors: Injury to the developing auditory system in the prenatal, intrapartum or perinatal period accounts for the other 50% of cases of childhood hearing loss. Injury may be the result of infection, hypoxia, ischemia, metabolic disease, hyperbilirubinemia, or ototoxic medications. Cytomegalovirus (CMV) congenital infection is the most common cause of

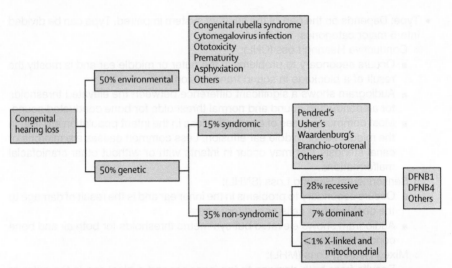

Fig. 2. Environmental and genetic contributions to total congenital SNHL. (*From* Smith RJH, Bale JF Jr, White KR. Sensorineural hearing loss in children. Lancet 2005;365(9462):882; with permission.)

nonhereditary sensorineural hearing loss. Although only 10% of newborns born with CMV infection will show any signs at birth, 1 in 3 will develop hearing loss. Of those infants who have no clinical signs, approximately 10% will still develop hearing loss and it is often progressive. In infants who have signs of infection at birth (thrombocytopenia, microcephaly) 30% to 50% are diagnosed with hearing loss. Hearing loss with CMV is typically congenital but delayed onset also occurs.[14] Routine screening for CMV is becoming more common, with some states (UT, CT) recently enacting laws mandating testing for infants who do not pass their hearing screen. If indicated due to hearing screen refer, or demonstration of clinical signs, CMV testing of urine or saliva should be performed within the first 21 days to distinguish between congenital or acquired infection.

Although 1 to 3 per 1000 infants are born with congenital hearing loss, it is estimated that another 1 to 2 per 1000 children will develop hearing loss by age 16.[15] The current recommendation of the JCIH is for all infants to have ongoing, developmentally appropriate audiological surveillance and those with one or more risk factors to be referred for at least 1 diagnostic audiology assessment by 24 to 30 months. Some risk factors are highly associated with later-onset or progressive hearing loss and warrant earlier and more frequent follow-up.

Because of a higher incidence of hearing loss, the JCIH recommends routine monitoring of infants with risk indicators listed as follows and summarized in **Fig. 3**.[6]

1. Caregiver concern[a] regarding hearing, speech, language, or developmental delay.
2. Family history of permanent childhood hearing loss.
3. Neonatal intensive care of more than 5 days or any of the following regardless of length of stay: ECMO[a], assisted ventilation, exposure to ototoxic medications (gentamicin and tobramycin) or loop diuretics (furosemide) and hyperbilirubinemia that requires exchange transfusion (some centers use a level of ≥20 mg/dL as a general guideline for risk).

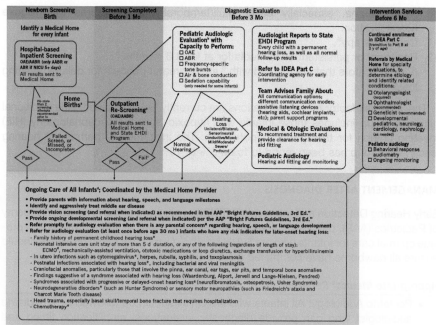

Fig. 3. Early Hearing Detection and Intervention (EHDI) Guidelines for Pediatric Medical Home Providers. IDEA, individuals with disabilities education act. Notes: [a] In screening programs that do not provide Outpatient Screening, infants will be referred directly from Inpatient Screening to Pediatric Audiologic Evaluation. Likewise, infants at higher risk for hearing loss (or loss to follow-up) also may be referred directly to Pediatric Audiology. [b] Part C of IDEA may provide diagnostic audiologic evaluation services as part of Child Find activities. [c] Even infants who fail screening in only one ear should be referred for further testing of both ears. [d] Includes infants whose parents refused initial or follow-up hearing screening. [e] Denotes risk indicators of greater concern. Earlier and/or more frequent referral should be considered. (*Adapted from* Joint Committee on Infant Hearing. Year 2007 position statement: principles and guidelines for early hearing detection and intervention programs. Pediatrics 2007;120(4):921; with permission.)

4. In utero infections such as CMV[a], herpes, rubella, syphilis, and toxoplasmosis.
5. Craniofacial anomalies, including those that involve the pinna, ear canal, ear tags, ear pits, and temporal bone anomalies.
6. Physical findings, such as a white forelock (Waardenberg syndrome), coloboma (CHARGE association), hypopigmentation of skin and hair (oculocutaneous albinism) that are associated with a syndrome known to include a sensorineural or permanent conductive hearing loss.
7. Syndromes associated with progressive or late-onset hearing loss, such as neurofibromatosis, osteopetrosis, and Usher syndrome. Other frequently identified syndromes include Waardenburg, Alport, Pendred (enlarged vestibular aqueduct/hypothyroidism), and Jervell and Lange-Neilson.
8. Neurodegenerative disorders[a], such as Hunter syndrome, or sensory motor neuropathies, such as Friedreich's ataxia and Charcot-Marie-Tooth syndrome.
9. Culture-positive postnatal infections associated with sensorineural hearing loss[a], including bacterial and viral (especially herpes viruses and varicella) meningitis.

10. Head trauma, especially basal skull/temporal bone fractures that require hospitalization.
11. Chemotherapy[a].
12. Recurrent or persistent otitis media for at least 3 months.[6]
(Risk indicators that are marked with [a] are of greater concern for delayed hearing loss).

The JCIH risk factor recommendations are currently being updated. One additional high-risk group includes those infants with hypoxic-ischemic encephalopathy (HIE) meeting criteria for therapeutic hypothermia. The incidence of permanent hearing loss in this group has been reported to be 6% to 10%.

MANAGEMENT AFTER DIAGNOSIS

Early Hearing Detection and Intervention (EHDI), a program of the American Academy of Pediatrics (AAP), provides guidelines for pediatric medical home providers to provide optimal care for infants who are D/HH.[6,10,16,17] All medical home providers should ensure all newborns have completed the 1-3-6 timeline as appropriate.

Appropriate Medical Referrals

- Pediatric Audiology: All infants who are D/HH should be followed by a pediatric audiologist who can provide diagnostic evaluations, amplification fitting and ongoing care.
- Otolaryngology: An otolaryngologist provides information and participates in the assessment of eligibility for amplification, assistive devices, and surgical intervention, including reconstruction, bone-anchored hearing aids, and cochlear implantation.
- Ophthalmology: A complete evaluation by a pediatric ophthalmologist is recommended because children who are D/HH use their vision to augment their communication in multiple ways and also because of the risk of associated visual problems including progressive later onset blindness with associated syndromes such as Usher Syndrome and Stickler Syndrome.
- Genetics: An evaluation by a geneticist is important to determine a possible genetic etiology that would allow for a better understanding of audiological prognosis and prompt a targeted evaluation for associated medical diagnoses.
- Infectious diseases: If an infant is diagnosed with congenital CMV, prompt treatment with antiviral agents such as valganciclovir may halt the progression of or improve hearing loss and neurodevelopmental outcome.[18] Likewise, special follow-up should be arranged for infants infected with congenital rubella, syphilis, and Zika virus.
- Consultations with Developmental Pediatrics, Neurology, Cardiology (risk of prolonged QT syndrome), and Nephrology (branchio-oto-renal syndrome) are also recommended when specific problems are suspected.

Referral to Early Intervention

The key role of EI is to provide an enriched language environment as early as possible to the infant's developing brain and promote optimal early language learning during this sensitive period of development.[19] Early diagnosis and intervention, and avoiding language deprivation are crucial to the development of speech, language, cognitive, and psychosocial abilities.

Guidelines for the implementation of early intervention services

- Ideally, the first contact by an EI coordinator with a family of an infant newly diagnosed as D/HH should occur within a few days after diagnosis.[10]
- EI service coordinators for infants who are D/HH should have specialized knowledge and skills that allow them to: assist the family in gaining access to services, facilitating the infant and family in receiving information about their rights, procedural safeguards, and services available in their state, coordinate assessments, facilitate the development of an Individual Family Service Plan (IFSP) and coordinate and monitor the delivery of services with an EI provider.
- EI providers for D/HH children and their families should be highly qualified with specific core knowledge and skills necessary to optimize their overall development and well-being. Medical home should verify that services are meeting appropriate standards.

Essential parent information: this includes

- Support in understanding the diagnosis and results of their child's hearing diagnostic evaluation.
- Information on communication development from infancy through childhood.
- Communication choices and language exposure: this refers to all listening, spoken and visual or signed language or combination thereof (eg, auditory-verbal therapy, auditory-oral, cued speech, sign language, total communication). For example, some families planning on cochlear implants may opt to use multiple modes initiating the use of sign language during the child's first year before being old enough for cochlear implant.
- Choices in amplification (see later in this article).
- Educational resources and choices.

For families who choose visual/sign language as part of their communication with their infant, access to an EI provider who is a fluent or native American Sign Language speaker is critical. There are different models in different states, including Deaf Mentor programs.

Cultural and linguistic diversity must be considered from the start to ensure that families of children who are D/HH receive comparable quality and quantity of information. It is critical to know details about the parents hearing status (90% of D/HH children are born to hearing parents) and each parent's primary language (eg, English, oral, sign language) to understand the baseline home environment.

Children who are D/HH should be monitored closely developmentally with regular standardized assessments of their language and overall development every 6 months for the first 3 years of age to allow tracking of their progress and to prompt augmentation of their services in identified areas of need.

Improving Auditory Input

Families that choose to pursue amplification will require multiple appointments with the audiologist to select devices, learn how to manage them, and for routine maintenance to ensure appropriate outcomes. Device options are based on degree, type, and configuration of hearing loss as well as age of patient and amplification goals.

- Hearing Aids: Sound is amplified through the device and transmitted into the ear with frequencies altered to emphasize areas of decreased hearing. Infants with sensorineural hearing loss are typically fitted with behind the ear devices with custom ear molds due to ongoing growth of ear concha.

- Implants:
  - ○ Bone-anchored hearing aids: Sound is amplified through a small abutment that vibrates to transmit sound through skull to reach cochlea. These are typically recommended for children older than 5 years with permanent conductive hearing loss. A nonimplantable option is available for children younger than 5 years.
  - ○ Cochlear implants: Sound is amplified through an external processor and sent electronically through the skin to an electrode array surgically implanted in the cochlea. Current US Food and Drug Administration regulations require children to be at least 1 year of age and have a bilateral profound sensorineural hearing loss to be eligible for implantation. The degree of hearing loss requirement changes as the child gets older.
- Assistive Listening Devices: Personal or universal devices can be obtained for classrooms, homes, and public venues to help override poor acoustics through frequency modulation, infrared, and inductive loop systems. Alerting/safety devices can also be used in the home without personal amplification.

OUTCOMES

The implementation of universal newborn hearing screening has led to a marked decrease in the average age of diagnosis from approximately 2 to 3 years to 2 to 3 months with many infants being diagnosed within a few weeks after birth.[8,20] However, we continue to identify areas in need of improvement; specifically, fewer than half of infants who did not pass their hearing screen having a final audiologic diagnosis by 3 months of age or fewer than half of infants diagnosed with hearing loss enrolled in EI by 6 months of age. There has been concomitant improvement in long-term language development, with children who met the 1-3-6 EHDI guidelines having better vocabulary outcomes than those who were diagnosed later (mean Verbal Quotient [VQ] 82 compared with 71); however, affected children still had mean vocabulary scores that were below average (mean VQ 82 compared with 100).[17] With earlier diagnosis and implementation of EI, language communication and general developmental outcomes have clearly improved; however, further research into the best way to provide intervention is still needed.

Prognosis of pediatric hearing loss depends on multiple variables including degree of loss, timing of identification and treatment as well as the presence of additional disabilities (eg, visual impairment, cognitive impairment).[21,22]

Children with hearing loss that was detected early and whose intervention was initiated in the first 3 to 9 months had consistently better outcomes in terms of expressive and receptive language skills and speech production and reading skills.[23,24] Multiple longitudinal studies are ongoing to evaluate the relationship of the quality of EI services and variables associated with improved outcomes. Likewise, the use of multiple modalities to learn language is also being studied.

Factors such as early age at exposure to sign language, age at fitting of hearing aids, age of cochlear implant are also being studied and most likely have a positive influence on outcomes.

Children who receive cochlear implants early in life (younger than than age 2 years) can develop age-appropriate spoken language development. This is of course dependent on associated high-quality intensive intervention service. Even with optimal timing, children with implants may demonstrate language deficits when compared with peers with normal hearing in areas such as speech production, perception, and vocabulary.[25–28]

In summary, children who are D/HH will achieve their best outcomes with appropriate specialized multidisciplinary EI services for the child and family. Providing a

Medical Home that facilitates this long-term support, monitoring, and adjustment as needed is a critical component of this child's medical care.

REFERENCES

1. Vohr B. Overview: infants and children with hearing loss – part 1. Ment Retard Dev Disabil Res Rev 2003;9:62–4.
2. Davis A, Wood S. The epidemiology of childhood hearing impairment: factors relevant to planning of services. Br J Audiol 1992;26:77–90.
3. Robertson CMT, Howarth TM, Bork DLR, et al. Permanent bilateral sensory and neural hearing loss of children after neonatal intensive care because of extreme prematurity: a thirty-year study. Pediatrics 2009;123:e797–807.
4. Hille ETM, Van Straaten HLM, Verkerk PH. Prevalence and independent risk factors for hearing loss in NICU infants. The Dutch NICU Neonatal Hearing Screening Working Group. Acta Paediatr 2007;96:1155–8.
5. Yoshinagao-Itano C, Sedey AL, Coulter DK, et al. Language of early and later identified children with hearing loss. Pediatrics 1998;102(5):1161–71.
6. Joint Committee on Infant Hearing. Year 2007 position statement: principles and guidelines for early hearing detection and intervention programs. Pediatrics 2007;120(4):898–921.
7. Joint Committee on Infant Hearing. Year 2000 position statement: principles and guidelines for early hearing detection and intervention programs. Pediatrics 2000;106(4):798–819.
8. CDC EHDI hearing screening & follow-up survey (HSFS). Available at: www.cdc.gov/ncbddd/hearingloss/ehdi-data.html. Accessed July 31, 2018.
9. American Academy of Pediatrics Task Force for Improving Newborn Hearing Screening. Diagnosis and intervention. Early hearing detection and intervention (EHDI) guidelines for pediatric medical home providers 2010. Available at: www.medicalhomeinfo.org. Accessed August 7, 2018.
10. Yoshinaga-Itano C. Principles and guidelines for early intervention after confirmation that a child is deaf or hard of hearing. J Deaf Stud Deaf Educ 2014;19:143–75.
11. Smith RJH, Bale JF Jr, White KR. Sensorineural hearing loss in children. Lancet 2005;365(9462):879–90.
12. Egilmez OK, Kalcioglu MT. Genetics of nonsyndromic congenital hearing loss. Scientifica (Cairo) 2016;2016:7576064.
13. Koffler T, Ushakov K, Avraham KB. Genetics of hearing loss – syndromic. Otolaryngol Clin North Am 2015;48(6):1047–61.
14. Goderis J, Leenheer ED, Smets K, et al. Hearing loss and congenital CMV infection: a systematic review. Pediatrics 2014;134:972–82.
15. Fortnum HM, Summerfield AQ, Marshall DH, et al. Prevalence of permanent childhood hearing impairment in the United Kingdom and implications for universal neonatal hearing screening: questionnaire-based ascertainment study. BMJ 2001;323:536–40.
16. Russ SA, Hanna D, DesGeorges J, et al. Improving follow-up to newborn hearing screening: a learning-collaborative. Pediatrics 2010;126:S59–69.
17. Yoshinag-Itano C, Sedey AL, Wiggin M, et al. Early hearing detection and vocabulary of children with hearing loss. Pediatrics 2017;140(2) [pii:e20162964].
18. Kimberlin DW, Jester PM, Sanchez PJ, et al. Valganciclovir for symptomatic congenital cytomegalovirus disease. N Engl J Med 2015;372:933–43.

19. Werker CJ, Hensch TK. Critical periods in speech perception: new directions. Annu Rev Psychol 2015;66:173–96.
20. Sininger YS, Martinez A, Eisenberg L, et al. Newborn hearing screening speeds diagnosis and access to intervention by 20-25 months. J Am Acad Audiol 2009; 20:49–57.
21. Hall WC. What you don't know can hurt you: the risk of language deprivation by impairing sign language development in deaf children. Matern Child Health J 2017;21(5):961–5.
22. Moeller MP, Tomblin JB. An introduction to the outcomes of children with hearing loss study. Ear Hear 2015;36(Suppl 1):4S–13S.
23. Stika CJ, Eisnberg LS, Johnson KC, et al. Developmental outcomes of early-identified children who are hard of hearing at 12-18 months of age. Early Hum Dev 2015;91(1):47–55.
24. Vohr B, Jodoin-Krauzyk J, Tucker R, et al. Early language outcomes of early-identified infants with permanent hearing loss at 12 to 16 months of age. Pediatrics 2008;122(3):535–44.
25. Lund E. Vocabulary knowledge of children with cochlear implants: a meta-analysis. J Deaf Stud Deaf Educ 2016;21(2):107–21.
26. Davidson LS, Geers AE, Blamey PJ, et al. Factors contributing to speech perception scores in long-term pediatric CI users. Ear Hear 2011;32(1 Suppl):19S–26S.
27. Ruben RJ. Language development in the pediatric cochlear implant patient. Laryngoscope Investig Otolaryngol 2018;3:209–13.
28. Duchesne L, Sutton A, Bergeron F. Language achievement in children who received cochlear implants between 1 and 2 years of age: group trends and individual patterns. J Deaf Stud Deaf Educ 2009;14(4):465–85.

Diagnosis and Management of Infantile Hemangiomas in the Neonate

Nicole Harter, MD, Anthony J. Mancini, MD*

KEYWORDS

- Infantile hemangioma • Neonate • Propranolol • Timolol • PHACE

KEY POINTS

- Infantile hemangiomas (IH) are the most common benign tumor of infancy.
- IH have a characteristic and predictable growth pattern, which assists in planning timing of referral and intervention(s).
- The majority of IH are uncomplicated and require no intervention; however, treatment is indicated for life- or function-threatening IH, IH with potential for permanent disfigurement, and ulcerated or bleeding IH.
- The distribution and extent of IH can provide insight into potential IH-associated syndromes and/or complications.
- The discovery of the efficacy of oral propranolol in the treatment of hemangiomas has revolutionized the standard of care in treatment of IH.

INTRODUCTION

Infantile hemangiomas (IH) are the most common tumors in children, with an estimated incidence of 4% to 5%, with higher prevalence noted in Whites, girls, and preterm/low-birth-weight infants.[1–3] **Box 1** lists risk factors for IH, which are a type of vascular tumor, distinct from vascular malformations (**Table 1**). IH display a characteristic growth (and eventual involution) pattern after birth, whereas vascular malformations are developmental anomalies that are fully formed at birth, and remain relatively static without a similar natural history.[3]

Disclosure Statement: A.J. Mancini has served as a consultant to Pierre Fabre USA.
a Division of Dermatology, Ann & Robert H. Lurie Children's Hospital of Chicago, Northwestern University Feinberg School of Medicine, 225 East Chicago Avenue, Box 107, Chicago, IL 60611-2605, USA
* Corresponding author.
E-mail address: amancini@northwestern.edu

Box 1
Risk factors for infantile hemangiomas

Prematurity

Low birth weight

Multiple gestation pregnancy

Pre-eclampsia

Gestational hypertension

Placental abnormalities
• Placenta previa

Advanced maternal age

Female sex

Caucasian race

Invasive antepartum procedures (ie, chorionic villus sampling)

Assisted reproductive technologies (ie, in vitro fertilization)

Data from Refs.[1,15,55,56]

PATHOGENESIS

IH are composed of stem cells, immature endothelial cells, pericytes, and mesenchymal cells.[2,4] Despite significant investigation into this area, the pathogenesis of IH is not clearly defined, and there are several proposed mechanisms:

- *Tissue hypoxia:* hypoxic events may contribute to the development of IH via stimulation of hypoxia-inducible factor-1 alpha (HIF-1α), which upregulates pro-angiogenic mediators that are known to be increased in IH. This association is supported by the observation that some of the risk factors for the development of IH (see **Box 1**) are also often associated with hypoxic states.[1,2]
- *Vasculogenesis and angiogenesis:* IH stem cells may differentiate into endothelial cells in the setting of hypoxia, with subsequent stimulation of angiogenesis. Bone marrow-derived endothelial progenitor cells may also be stimulated by tissue ischemia, resulting in local vasculogenesis or angiogenesis.[2,5]

Table 1
Contemporary classification of vascular birthmarks (simplified)

Vascular Tumors	Vascular Malformations
Benign	Capillary malformation
• Infantile hemangioma	Lymphatic malformation
• Congenital hemangioma	Venous malformation
• Tufted angioma	Combined malformation
Locally aggressive or borderline	Arteriovenous malformation/fistula
• Kaposiform hemangioendothelioma	
Malignant	
• Angiosarcoma	

Data from Wassef M, Blei F, Adams D, et al. Vascular anomalies classification: recommendations from the International Society for the Study of Vascular Anomalies. Pediatrics 2015;136(1):e203–14.

- *Placental embolization:* an alternate theory of origin arises from the knowledge that certain vascular markers of IH, including glucose transporter-1, are found only in human placental vessels. Placental cells may embolize during gestation or delivery, resulting in the development of IH at distant tissue sites in the neonate.[2,5]

There is likely a complex interplay between host and environmental factors. Endothelial progenitor cells or placental angioblasts may be triggered to migrate and proliferate by a hypoxic event, with this ischemic stimulus resulting in a cascade of growth factor and cytokine release, resulting in vasculogenesis and angiogenesis.[5] Decline in growth factor stimulation, together with upregulation of enzymatic degradation and increased apoptotic activity, likely contributes to involution of IH with transition from vascular to fibrofatty tissue.[6,7]

CLASSIFICATION OF INFANTILE HEMANGIOMAS

IH can be classified based on their clinical depth or their configuration. The former classification includes:

- *Superficial* IH: bright red, thin, often cobblestoned or pebbly, vascular papules or plaques, previously termed "strawberry hemangiomas" (**Fig. 1**)
- *Deep* IH: blue-violaceous or skin-colored, compressible, subcutaneous papules or nodules, previously termed "cavernous hemangiomas" (**Fig. 2**)
- *Combined* IH: both superficial and deep components, frequently seen as a superficial IH overlying a deeper IH component (**Fig. 3**)

The anatomic configuration of IH is also important, and helps to define the following classifications:

- *Focal* IH: a solitary, isolated IH, usually a papule, plaque, or nodule (**Fig. 4**)
- *Segmental* IH: IH that involve a larger or entire region of the body (i.e. hand, lower leg, hemi-face) in a sharply demarcated territory (**Fig. 5**)
- *Indeterminate* IH: IH that do not uniformly fall into either category, or do not fully or uniformly proliferate (**Fig. 6**)
- *Multifocal* IH: multiple discrete focal IH that do not occupy a particular region or territory (**Fig. 7**).[1,8–10]

A less common type of hemangioma is a congenital hemangioma, which is fully formed at birth, and includes the rapidly involuting congenital hemangioma (RICH)

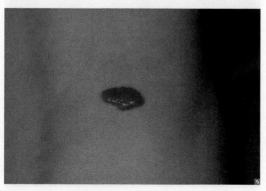

Fig. 1. Superficial hemangioma. This bright red, thin vascular plaque is characteristic of a superficial infantile hemangioma.

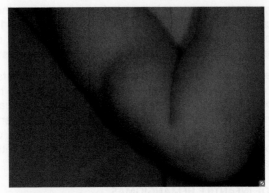

Fig. 2. Deep hemangioma. A faintly blue, compressible subcutaneous nodule on the upper arm.

and the non-involuting congenital hemangioma (NICH). RICH and NICH are characterized by their behavior after birth, with a RICH quickly decreasing in size and color, and usually demonstrating complete involution by 14 months, whereas a NICH remains static throughout the child's lifetime. Histologically, congenital hemangiomas are characterized by lack of GLUT-1 staining, which is uniformly positive in IH. Examination and natural history can usually help differentiate IH from congenital hemangiomas, with NICH presenting as a round pink to purple nodule with overlying coarse telangiectasias and a peripheral blanched rim (**Fig. 8**). RICH can present in a similar fashion to

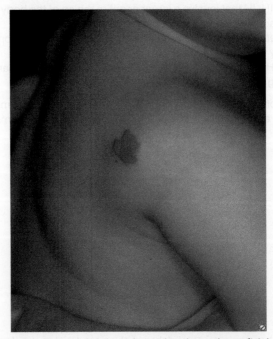

Fig. 3. Combined hemangioma. A bright red vascular plaque (superficial component) overlying a blue-hued compressible nodule (deep component) on the right posterior shoulder.

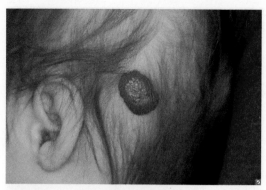

Fig. 4. Localized hemangioma. A single, discrete, bright red vascular plaque of the left post-auricular scalp.

NICH, or may present as a red to violaceous firm tumor, which can mimic other benign and malignant vascular tumors (**Fig. 9**).[11]

NATURAL HISTORY OF INFANTILE HEMANGIOMAS

As part of their definition, IH follow a specific pattern of growth and involution. They are most often not present at birth, and are noted in the first few weeks to months of age, although deep IH may take even longer to become clinically apparent. Precursor findings may include a faint red patch, vasoconstricted area of pallor, bruise-like findings, or telangiectasia (**Fig. 10**).[1,6,11–13] IH enter a period of rapid proliferation in the first few months of age, with maximal growth occurring between 5 and 7 weeks. The early proliferative phase is completed by around 5 months of age, a time when most (up to 80%) IH have completed growth, although deep IH may proliferate longer than more superficial lesions. After proliferation ends, IH may enter a stabilization or plateau phase, with eventual spontaneous involution, usually beginning around the first birthday. Involution is characterized by flattening, softening, and fading of color, which continues through approximately 4 to 5 years of age, although this may be delayed for deeper lesions (**Fig. 11**).[1,5,6,11–13] Knowledge of the normal growth pattern of IH helps providers in planning the appropriate timing of intervention and/or referral.

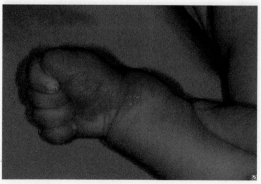

Fig. 5. Segmental hemangioma. A large, superficial bright red vascular plaque with irregular borders on the wrist, thenar palm, and thumb.

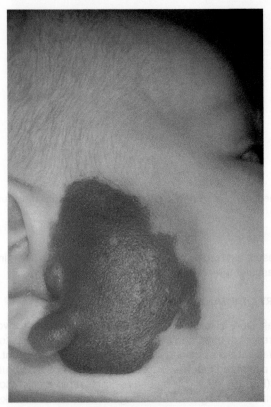

Fig. 6. Indeterminate hemangioma. Right pre-auricular cheek with a bright red vascular plaque with deeper component and irregular borders.

POTENTIAL COMPLICATIONS OF INFANTILE HEMANGIOMAS
Cutaneous and Extracutaneous Sequelae

The vast majority of IH are uncomplicated and do not require intervention. However, in 10% to 15% of cases, IH may be life-threatening, cause functional impairment, pose a

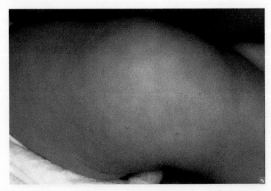

Fig. 7. Multifocal hemangiomas. Multiple, discrete, bright red, 1- to 2-mm papules; when numbering 5 or more, these lesions warrant further evaluation with abdominal ultrasound.

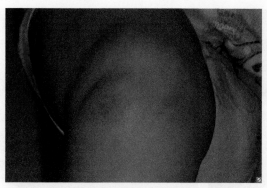

Fig. 8. Non-involuting congenital hemangioma (NICH). A thin blue-hued nodule with peripheral pallor and coarse surface telangiectasia.

risk for long-term disfigurement, or be predisposed to ulceration.[6,14] Factors that increase the risk for development of complications include segmental, indeterminate, large, and facial IH.[14–16] Preterm birth increases the risk for ulceration, whereas facial location makes the need for any intervention more likely.[15] Early management includes frequent re-evaluation in the first few weeks after birth, with the goal of initiating intervention as soon as clinically indicated.[5]

Up to 55% to 70% of IH have been reported to leave cutaneous sequelae following involution. The most common significant sequelae of IH and the clinical characteristics that are most likely to leave substantial residua are discussed in **Table 2** and shown in **Fig. 12**. Consideration of these features can assist with appropriate counseling of families and determination of the need or desirability for intervention.[5,17] Other potentially significant sequelae resulting in systemic or functional (extracutaneous) compromise are reviewed in **Table 3**.

Psychosocial Consequences

Even if IH are not life- or function-threatening during the proliferative phase, if the expected residua may lead to significant psychosocial compromise, treatment should be considered.[17] Long-term morbidity of IH has been linked to facial location, segmental or indeterminate subtypes, and history of complication or intervention.[15] Chamlin and

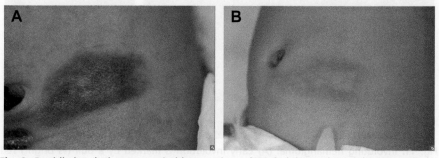

Fig. 9. Rapidly involuting congenital hemangioma (RICH). (*A*) A red to violaceous vascular plaque was present at birth in this infant. (*B*) At 3 months of age, the lesion has already largely resolved.

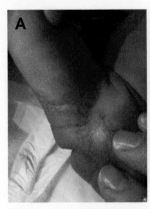
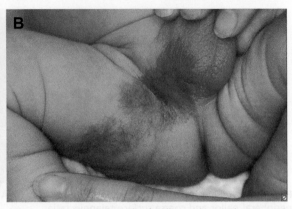

Fig. 10. Hemangioma precursor. (*A*) A vasoconstricted patch of pallor with prominent coarse telangiectasias was present at birth and involved the right scrotum, inguinal fold, and thigh of this neonate. (*B*) At 2 weeks of age, follow-up revealed a bright red vascular plaque more typical of superficial infantile hemangioma.

colleagues[18] noted a correlation between the location of IH on the head and neck and greater impact on quality of life. In another study, parents of children with disfiguring facial IH were found to exhibit reactions of disbelief, fear, and mourning, especially during the active growth phase of the IH, and reported that the reactions of strangers resulted in feelings of social stigmatization. These effects seem to also have an impact on parent-child interactions, which underscores the potential impact on quality of life.[19]

HEMANGIOMA SYNDROMES AND ASSOCIATIONS

Although the vast majority of IH are solitary, uncomplicated, and do not require treatment, there are several potential IH associations and syndromes that are important to consider. These are summarized in **Table 4**.

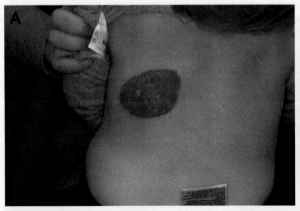
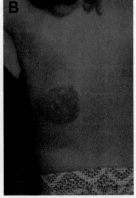

Fig. 11. Involuting hemangioma. (*A*) Early involution is marked by a dull (vs bright) red appearance and early appearance of more flesh-colored regions throughout. (*B*) With continued involution, the color is even lighter with flattening of the tumor and more areas appearing as flesh-colored.

Table 2
Characteristics of IH that increase the risk of significant cutaneous sequelae

Characteristics	Potential Sequelae
Combined type IH	Anetodermic (outpouching) skin Redundant skin (see **Fig. 12**)
IH with sharp elevation in border IH with cobblestoned surface	Anetodermic (outpouching) skin Redundant skin (see **Fig. 12**)
Ulceration	Scar

Data from Darrow DH, Greene AK, Mancini AJ, et al. Section on Dermatology, Section on Otolaryngology–Head and Neck Surgery, and Section on Plastic Surgery. Diagnosis and management of infantile hemangioma. Pediatrics 2015;136(4):e1060–104; and Baselga E, Roe E, Coulie J, et al. Risk factors for degree and type of sequelae after involution of untreated hemangiomas of infancy. JAMA Dermatol 2016;152(11):1239–43.

TREATMENT CONSIDERATIONS

Table 5 summarizes IH features that may suggest the need for therapy. Specific aspects of various treatment approaches are discussed below. Clinical practice guidelines for management of infantile hemangiomas have recently been published.[20]

Active Non-intervention

The majority of IH do not require treatment, although there are multiple factors that influence the decision to treat IH. Age of the patient, size and location of the

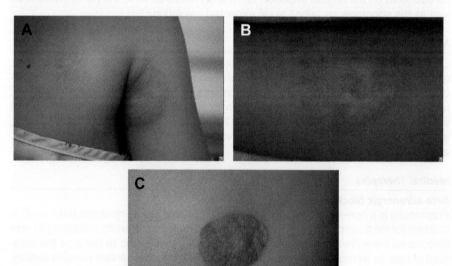

Fig. 12. Hemangioma residua. (*A*) Atrophy with faint telangiectasias at the site of an involuted hemangioma on the left upper arm; notice the telangiectasias on the left upper chest, where there was another hemangioma. (*B*) Telangiectasias on the lower leg at the site of an involuted hemangioma; note the central scarring, which resulted from prior ulceration within the lesion. (*C*) Fibrofatty tissue. A soft plaque with skin redundancy and telangiectasias at the site of an involuted combined hemangioma; surgical excision is the primary treatment for this type of hemangioma residua.

Table 3
Other potential complications of IH

Complication	Risk Factor(s)/Comment
Visual or feeding impairment	Periocular IH Perioral IH
Permanent deformity	Involvement of nasal tip (ie, Cyrano deformity) Involvement of auricular cartilage Large IH
Airway IH with risk of obstruction	Beard-distribution IH
High-output congestive heart failure	Large cutaneous or hepatic IH
Transient hypothyroidism	Large hepatic IH Parotid IH
Psychosocial compromise	Facial location Segmental subtype More likely with history of complication or need for intervention

Data from Refs.[11,14,15,57–65]

hemangioma, potential for future psychosocial impact, and parent/family preference are all factors considered.[5] Active non-intervention is an acceptable and often recommended treatment option in the setting of a low-risk, small, solitary IH. Parents should be educated on the natural evolution of IH, and reassured as to the benign nature, as well as the spontaneous (albeit slow) expected involution.[21–23]

Management of Ulceration

Ulceration is the most common complication of IH, seen in 10% to 30% of patients, usually early in the course, before 4 months of age.[11,14,24] Anatomic location may predispose to ulceration, with greater risk in intertriginous areas including the lower lip, neck, axillae, and anogenital regions. Large, superficial, segmental, and mixed IH are also predisposed to ulceration (**Fig. 17**).[14,24] Treatment, as outlined in **Table 6**, is indicated as ulceration is painful and creates the risks of bleeding, superinfection, and permanent scarring.[14]

Medical Therapies

Beta-adrenergic blocking agents

Propranolol is a non-selective beta-adrenergic receptor blocker that has been used in children for the treatment of cardiac conditions for decades. Its utility in treating IH was discovered serendipitously in 2008 and it subsequently evolved to become the standard of care for IH requiring therapy.[25] Although the exact mechanism remains elusive, the effects of propranolol on IH are believed to include vasoconstriction, endothelial cell apoptosis, and inhibition of angiogenesis.[26,27] In 2014, propranolol became the first treatment approved by the United States Food and Drug Administration (FDA) for the treatment of IH. Contraindications to propranolol therapy are listed in **Box 2**.

Propranolol is highly effective, with reports of up to 98% of IH responding favorably to treatment.[14] Positive effects include lightening in color and softening of texture. Treatment duration is determined by a variety of factors including age, hemangioma location, hemangioma subtype, and age at initiation of therapy. Propranolol is often tapered gradually, in an effort to allow for assessment of rebound growth, as well as the theoretic prevention of rebound sinus tachycardia.[5,27]

Table 4
Hemangioma syndromes and associations

Condition/Association	Clinical IH Features	Potential Associations	Recommended Evaluations	Treatment Considerations
Neonatal hemangiomatosis				
Benign neonatal hemangiomatosis	Multiple (<5) cutaneous IH	Usually none, unless individual IH lesions causing functional or other concern	Clinical examination and follow-up; liver ultrasonography if increasing lesions (≥5), hepatomegaly, abdominal distension	Treatment for cutaneous IH as indicated for functional impairment, potential deformity, or ulceration
Diffuse neonatal hemangiomatosis (Fig. 13)	Multiple (≥5) cutaneous IH	Hepatic IH, 3 subtypes: • Focal • Multifocal • Diffuse Risk of hypothyroidism (especially with diffuse form), high-output congestive heart failure	Liver ultrasonography, TSH, free T4, reverse T3 Echocardiography if concern for CHF	Pharmacologic therapy (propranolol, others); thyroid hormone replacement; treatment for CHF, if needed; occasionally embolization, surgery, transplantation
Hemangioma syndromes				
PHACES	Large (>5 cm) segmental IH, most often facial/scalp location	Posterior fossa malformations, most commonly Dandy-Walker Cerebrovascular/carotid artery and aortic arch anomalies Posterior or anterior eye segment abnormalities Sternal cleft, supraumbilical median abdominal raphe Hearing loss	MRI and MRA of the head and neck Echocardiography Ophthalmologic evaluation Other studies as clinically indicated	If oral propranolol being considered and significant intracranial vascular anomalies, consult neurologist/consider lower dosing and slower dose escalation given potentially increased risk of ischemic CVA

(continued on next page)

Table 4
(continued)

Condition/Association	Clinical IH Features	Potential Associations	Recommended Evaluations	Treatment Considerations
PELVIS/LUMBAR (Fig. 14)	Segmental IH over lower lumbosacral spine, perineum, genital regions	Tethering of spinal cord, spinal dysraphism, neurologic abnormalities Genitourinary and renal anomalies Anorectal malformations	Varies; consider ultrasonography (abdomen/pelvis, spine in children <3 mo of age), MRI/MRA (abdomen/pelvis, spine in children >3 mo of age) Other studies as clinically indicated	Treatment of IH as clinically indicated; referral to relevant specialists if other abnormalities noted on imaging
Other hemangioma associations				
Beard-distribution IH (Fig. 15)	Segmental IH of lower face: pre-auricular areas, chin, mandible, lower lip, anterior neck	Risk of upper airway (especially subglottic) IH May present with biphasic stridor, barky cough	Otolaryngology referral if concern; endoscopy usually performed; imaging (US, CT, MRI) may be helpful	Oral propranolol treatment of choice; laser ablation, excision rarely used in current era
Lumbosacral IH (Fig. 16)	Large (>2.5 cm) midline IH of the lumbosacral region	Risk of spinal dysraphism, spinal cord defects Presence of additional cutaneous findings (lipoma, hair tuft, gluteal cleft deviation, prominent dimple) increases risk	Spinal US can be considered if <3 mo of age (but may be false-negatives); spinal MRI diagnostic modality of choice	Treatment of IH as clinically indicated; referral to neurosurgery if spine/cord abnormalities noted

Abbreviations: CHF, congestive heart failure; CT, computed tomography; CVA, cerebrovascular accident; free T4, free thyroxine; LUMBAR, lower body hemangioma and other cutaneous defects, urogenital anomalies, ulceration, myelopathy, bony deformities, anorectal malformations, arterial anomalies, and renal anomalies; MRA, magnetic resonance angiography; MRI, magnetic resonance imaging; PELVIS, perineal hemangioma, external genital malformations, lipomyelomeningocele, vesicorenal abnormalities, imperforate anus, skin tag; PHACES, posterior fossa defects, hemangiomas, arterial anomalies, cardiac anomalies/coarctation of the aorta, eye anomalies, sternal defect/supraumbilical raphe; reverse T3, reverse triiodothyronine; TSH, thyroid stimulating hormone; US, ultrasonography; US, ultrasound.
Data from Refs. [5,14,57,58,66–74]

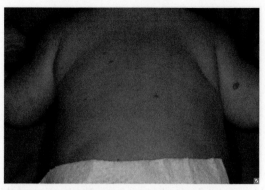

Fig. 13. Diffuse cutaneous hemangiomatosis. This male infant warranted hepatic ultrasound given the presence of more than 5 cutaneous hemangiomas. Imaging revealed multiple hepatic lesions, and he was also found to have acquired hypothyroidism.

Two formulations of propranolol are available, the FDA-approved Hemangeol (propranolol hydrochloride 4.28 mg/mL solution, Pierre Fabre, Parsippany, NJ) and generic propranolol (propranolol hydrochloride 20 mg/5 mL or 40 mg/5 mL, West-War Pharmaceuticals Corp, Eatontown, NJ). Potential benefits of use of the branded formulation include the flavor profile and lack of added alcohol, sugar, or paraben. Although the FDA approval of Hemangeol suggests a target dose of 3.4 mg/kg/d, there is variability in dosing by hemangioma experts, typically ranging between 1.5 and 3 mg/kg/d. Propranolol initiation guidelines were published in 2013 (and are summarized in **Table 7**), but were published before the FDA approval and will be revised in the near future (A.J. Mancini, personal communication, 2018).

Given propranolol's potential effects of lowering heart rate and blood pressure, initial recommendations included a screening electrocardiogram (ECG) before initiation of therapy. Several published studies have reported that this practice, when applied to the general population, is not useful in detecting abnormalities that would alter the decision to start propranolol, nor does it identify patients at greater risk of having adverse events during treatment. Routine ECG screening is thus not recommended; however, it is used in certain high-risk situations (see **Table 7**).[28–31]

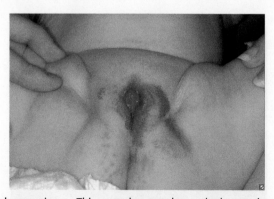

Fig. 14. Perineal hemangioma. Thin vascular papules and plaques involving the vulva, gluteal region, and perineum; segmental hemangiomas with this distribution warrant evaluation for PELVIS/LUMBAR syndrome (see text).

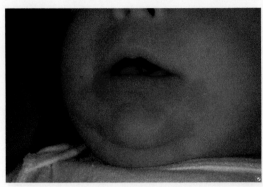

Fig. 15. Segmental beard-distribution hemangioma. The location of this large segmental lesion warranted airway evaluation, which revealed a subglottic hemangioma.

Possible adverse events associated with propranolol therapy are listed in **Table 8**.

Other beta-blocking agents have been reported for treatment of IH, although they are used far less commonly in clinical practice. Atenolol is a selective β1-antagonist, which is proposed to have a lower risk of bronchial hyper-reactivity owing to its selective nature of beta-blockade.[32–34] Atenolol is dosed once daily and does not cross the blood-brain barrier, in contrast to propranolol. Nadolol is a non-selective beta-blocker, dosed twice daily, which also does not cross the blood-brain barrier. This property is theorized to underlie the reduction in sleep disturbances when compared with propranolol.[35–37] Nadolol was demonstrated to be safe and effective in the treatment of IH in a small comparative trial with propranolol.[6,35,37]

There are multiple reports on the use of ophthalmic topical timolol (usually the gel-forming solution) for the treatment of IH since it was initially described in 2010.[35,38] Timolol is FDA approved for treatment of glaucoma in infants, but has been shown to be helpful in treating thin, superficial, localized IH when used in an off-label fashion.[34,39] There are few data on pharmacokinetics of topical timolol in this setting, with some studies showing undetectable or clinically insignificant serum levels; further studies are currently underway. Systemic absorption after cutaneous application remains a potential concern (especially in preterm infants, see below under "Special Considerations in the Premature Infant"), as timolol has significantly greater potency

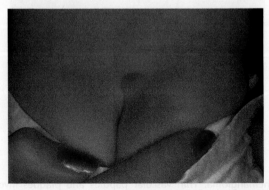

Fig. 16. Lumbosacral hemangioma. Given the presence of both a hemangioma and a deviated gluteal cleft, imaging was performed and was unrevealing in this patient.

Table 5
High-risk IH/indications for possible therapy

Feature	Comment
Risk of functional impairment	Periocular IH • Obstruction of visual axis • Astigmatism, light-deprivation amblyopia Nasal tip and periauricular IH • Cartilaginous destruction Perioral or lip IH • Ulceration, feeding difficulties
Ulceration	Greater risk with: • Segmental distribution • Large size • Perioral, perineal/anogenital, neck locations
Risk of permanent disfigurement	Large facial IH Nasal tip IH Breast IH
Life-threatening IH	Hemodynamically significant liver IH • High-output cardiac failure Beard-distribution IH with airway obstruction

Data from Refs.[5,11,14,16,59–63,75]

in beta receptor blockade than propranolol, and has been found in the urine and serum of treated infants, albeit at low levels.[14,40] The current consensus is that timolol has a favorable safety profile overall, without severe systemic adverse events.[39–41] It is typically applied as 1 drop 2–3 times daily.

Corticosteroids
Before the discovery of the efficacy of propranolol in the treatment of IH, systemic prednisone or prednisolone at a dose of 2 to 3 mg/kg/d was considered first-line treatment for complicated IH. However, their use has now been largely replaced by oral propranolol. Potential side effects of long-term corticosteroid therapy include growth impairment, behavioral changes, sleep disturbance, Cushingoid changes,

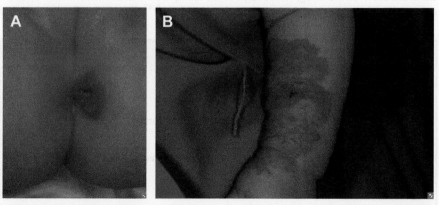

Fig. 17. Ulcerated IH. (*A*) Superficial ulceration in a focal perianal hemangioma. (*B*) This IH-MAG (infantile hemangioma with minimal to arrested growth) on the forearm developed ulceration centrally.

Table 6
Options for treatment of ulcerated IH

Treatment	Comment/Examples
Barrier products	Petrolatum, zinc oxide, dimethicone
Antimicrobial therapy	Metronidazole 0.75% gel Mupirocin 2% ointment
Non-adhesive wound dressings	Petrolatum-impregnated gauze Tegaderm (TM 3-M, London, ON) Mepilex Border (Mölinlycke Health Care, Gothenberg, Sweden) Telfa (Covidien, Minneapolis, MN) DuoDerm (Convatec, Skilman, NJ)
Topical IH therapy	Timolol 0.25% or 0.5% gel-forming solution (see discussion in text)
Recombinant growth factor	Becaplermin 0.01% gel (recombinant platelet-derived growth factor)
Pain control	Acetaminophen, NSAIDs, opioid analgesics (rarely indicated) Topical lidocaine 5% cream (rarely used)
Other medical therapies	Oral propranolol Oral corticosteroids
Laser/surgical therapies	PDL Excision (when feasible, in the right setting)

Abbreviations: NSAIDs, non-steroidal anti-inflammatory drugs; PDL, pulsed-dye laser.
Data from Refs.[14,24,44]

gastrointestinal upset, osteoporosis, and opportunistic infection. Systemic steroids are now primarily used as an alternative treatment in patients with contraindications (or lack of response) to propranolol therapy, as well as occasionally as an adjunct in the treatment of some ulcerated IH, or in conjunction with propranolol for rapidly progressive IH in which monotherapy has not led to adequate response.[5,14,42]

Intralesional corticosteroids are still used in the treatment of primarily small, bulky, localized IH that are not good candidates for oral propranolol or topical timolol therapy.[43] Intralesional therapy is most often used for mixed or deep IH of the nasal tip or lip.[34,44] Local complications of intralesional steroids include atrophy, dyspigmentation, and/or ulceration. Systemic adverse effects are rare given the local administration of the drug; however, retinal artery embolization has been reported as a side effect after treatment of upper eyelid IH.[5,43] This latter finding has led

Box 2
Contraindications to oral propranolol therapy

Premature infants with corrected age less than 5 weeks

Infants weighing less than 2 kg

Known hypersensitivity to propranolol or any of the excipients

Asthma or history of bronchospasm

Heart rate less than 80 beats per minute, greater than first-degree heart block, or decompensated heart failure

Blood pressure less than 50/30 mm Hg

Pheochromocytoma

Data from Hemangeol [package insert]. Parsippany, NJ: Pierre Fabre; 2014.

Table 7 Propranolol initiation guidelines[a]	
Outpatient Initiation	**Inpatient Initiation**
Corrected gestational age >8 wk	Corrected gestational age <8 wk
Adequate social support	Poor social support network
	Cardiac or pulmonary comorbidities
Normal cardiopulmonary examination	Normal cardiopulmonary examination
Normal baseline VS	Normal baseline VS
Normal ECG, if indicated[b]	Normal ECG, if indicated[b]
Single dose of propranolol given at 1 mg/kg/d divided 3 times daily	Single dose of propranolol given at 1 mg/kg/d divided 3 times daily
HR/BP checked 1 and 2 h after first dose, and with each dose escalation	HR/BP checked 1 and 2 h after first 1–3 doses
If tolerated, discharge home on 1 mg/kg/d divided 3 times daily[c]	If tolerated, increase to target dose of 2 mg/kg/d divided 3 times daily[c]
After 3–7 d, increase to 1.5 mg/kg/d divided 3 times daily according to above algorithm	If tolerated, discharge home on 2 mg/kg/d divided 3 times daily
After 3–7 d, increase to 2 mg/kg/d divided 3 times daily according to above algorithm	

Abbreviations: BP, blood pressure; ECG, electrocardiogram; HR, heart rate; VS, vital signs.

[a] Notes from authors: (1) significant variability exists among clinicians who treat infantile hemangioma in terms of initiation dose, dose escalation, goal dose (typically ranges between 1.5 and 3 mg/kg/d), and dosing frequency (BID vs TID). (2) The FDA-approved labeling of Hemangeol includes outpatient therapy initiation for infants 5 wk of age and older, with dosing on a BID basis.

[b] Screening electrocardiography recommended for: personal history of cardiac arrhythmia or arrhythmia auscultated on examination. Family history of congenital heart disease, sudden cardiac death, arrhythmia, or unknown family history. Maternal history of connective tissue disease. HR below normal for age.

[c] If dose not tolerated, reduce dose or reduce to previously tolerated dose, and then slowly escalate.

Data from Drolet BA, Frommelt PC, Chamlin SL, et al. Initiation and use of propranolol for infantile hemangioma: report of a consensus conference. Pediatrics 2013;131(1):128–40.

many clinicians to abandon intralesional steroid injections for IH in this location, and most now typically use oral propranolol.

Other treatments

Historically, patients with severe, ulcerating, or life-threatening IH that did not respond to oral corticosteroids were treated with alternative agents, mostly interferon α2a or vincristine therapy. Vincristine is a chemotherapeutic agent with antimitotic and anti-angiogenic activity. It is administered intravenously over multiple weekly treatments, with potential side effects including myelosuppression and neurotoxicity with sensory-motor neuropathy.[21] Interferon α2a was proposed to treat IH via antiangiogenic effects, and is given via daily subcutaneous injection. Serious adverse effects include fever, leukopenia, and risk of irreversible spastic diplegia. Given their associated significant toxicities, and the availability of oral propranolol, these 2 agents are now rarely used for treatment of IH.[14,45–47]

Laser Therapy

Pulse-dye laser (PDL) may be employed in the treatment of IH in certain instances. Although it has traditionally been used for superficial or very early lesions, its use in the propranolol era is typically limited to ulcerated IH, in which case PDL therapy seems to accelerate re-epithelialization and diminish pain. It is also used later in life

Table 8
Potential adverse events associated with oral propranolol therapy

Potential Adverse Event	Comment
Sleep disturbances • Nightmares, night terrors, insomnia, hypersomnolence	Common • Avoid giving late evening dose • May occasionally require dose reduction
Cool extremities/acrocyanosis	Mild/usually asymptomatic
Agitation	Uncommon
Atrioventricular block	Rare
Decreased heart rate Decreased blood pressure	Mild/typically asymptomatic Rarely clinically significant
GI disturbance • Diarrhea, constipation	Typically mild when present
Bronchospasm/bronchial hyper-reactivity	Most significant during intercurrent viral illness May necessitate holding therapy until illness resolved
Hypoglycemia/hypoglycemia-induced seizure	Rare Greater risk in infants <3 mo old Best minimized by dosing medication with food and avoidance of prolonged fasting
Cognitive impairment	Controversial Most studies to date reassuring

Abbreviation: GI, gastrointestinal.
Data from Refs.[14,27,36,49,51,76–80]

following involution of IH, for residual telangiectasias. When used to treat ulcerated IH, PDL has been shown to be most effective in conjunction with other therapies, such as topical timolol or a systemic agent (propranolol or corticosteroids).[5,24,48]

Surgical Therapy

Surgical excision of IH is typically limited to fibrofatty residua, scars that persist in the post-involution phase, or for reconstruction of deformed areas. Surgery may occasionally be considered during the proliferative phase for IH that are surgical candidates (and in anatomically feasible locations) but are not responding to medical therapy; if there is a treatment contraindication; or when there is concern about compromise in function of a vital organ.[5,14]

SPECIAL CONSIDERATIONS IN THE PREMATURE INFANT

The literature is sparse with regard to treatment of IH specifically in premature and low-birth-weight infants, and most recommendations for this patient population are extrapolated from published studies and clinical experiences in older and larger infants.[49–51] There are, however, several publications attesting to propranolol's effectiveness and safety in this population.

In one report of 4 extremely low-birth-weight (582–814 g) neonates with IH treated with propranolol, the authors reported good efficacy and lack of adverse events in all 4.[49] Erbay and colleagues[52] reported on oral propranolol therapy in 9 preterm and very low-birth-weight infants, with regression noted in all infants within 2 months of therapy without serious adverse effects. In addition, somatic growth was normal in these infants during propranolol treatment. A retrospective observational study in 24 infants with IH treated with propranolol included 16 premature infants, and found improvement with treatment and lack of significant side effects during therapy.[51]

Several studies have addressed the issue of topical timolol for IH in premature infants. Moehrle and colleagues[53] evaluated application of topical timolol 0.5% gel under an occlusive dressing in 9 children, including 6 preterm infants. There was positive effect in all patients, with near complete resolution in greater than 80%, and no adverse effects. Frommelt and colleagues[54] performed Holter monitoring during topical timolol therapy for infants deemed at high risk of systemic absorption or adverse events. Two patients with symptomatic bradycardia were the lowest weight infants (both <2500 g) in the study, both were premature (26 and 33 weeks' gestation), had a history of bradycardia, and had received timolol doses above the average exposure for the cohort. In addition, the lesions treated would not be considered appropriate candidates for timolol therapy by the authors of this report, given their size, depth, and location. The authors of that study propose that very young and low-birth-weight infants, especially those with history of prematurity, apnea, or bradycardia, may be at greater risk of adverse events. In this cohort, they recommend monitoring of vital signs (and Holter monitoring) during timolol therapy, and limiting the total dose of timolol to 0.25 mg/kg/d.[54]

SUMMARY

IH are the most common benign tumors of infancy, with most being uncomplicated and not requiring intervention. The pediatric provider must be familiar with the morphology, distribution, and natural history of IH to provide appropriate counseling and expectant management. Location, size, and presence of complicating factors all influence the decision to treat IH, including when to initiate therapy and what modality to use. Early recognition of IH-associated syndromes is key to prompt initiation of diagnostic imaging and laboratory studies, when indicated. Propranolol therapy has revolutionized the treatment of IH and become the standard of care in treating ulcerated, life- or function-threatening, or potentially disfiguring IH. Propranolol has demonstrated an excellent safety profile in neonates and infants thus far, but must be administered after appropriate and thorough evaluation, with diligent parent/caretaker education. In certain cases, alternative or adjunctive therapies are employed, including specialized wound care for ulcerated IH; topical beta-blockers for small, superficial IH; and PDL treatment and/or surgical intervention for IH residua. Early and appropriate treatment of IH may also be indicated for its role in minimizing potential psychosocial morbidity down the road.

REFERENCES

1. Smith CJF, Friedlander SF, Guma M, et al. Infantile hemangiomas: an updated review on risk factors, pathogenesis, and treatment. Birth Defects Res 2017; 109(11):809–15.

2. Janmohamed SR, Madern GC, de Laat PC, et al. Educational paper: pathogenesis of infantile haemangioma, an update 2014 (part I). Eur J Pediatr 2015;174(1): 97–103.

3. Wassef M, Blei F, Adams D, et al. Vascular anomalies classification: recommendations from the International Society for the Study of Vascular Anomalies. Pediatrics 2015;136(1):e203–14.

4. Stringari G, Barbato G, Zanzucchi M, et al. Propranolol treatment for infantile hemangioma: a case series of sixty-two patients. Pediatr Med Chir 2016; 38(2):113.
5. Darrow DH, Greene AK, Mancini AJ, et al, Section on Dermatology, Section on Otolaryngology–Head and Neck Surgery, and Section on Plastic Surgery. Diagnosis and management of infantile hemangioma. Pediatrics 2015;136(4): e1060–104.
6. Léauté-Labrèze C, Harper JI, Hoeger PH. Infantile haemangioma. Lancet 2017; 390(10089):85–94.
7. Mancini AJ, Smoller BR. Proliferation and apoptosis within juvenile capillary hemangiomas. Am J Dermatopathol 1996;18(5):505–14.
8. Ma EH, Robertson SJ, Chow CW, et al. Infantile hemangioma with minimal or arrested growth: further observations on clinical and histopathologic findings of this unique but underrecognized entity. Pediatr Dermatol 2017;34(1):64–71.
9. Suh KY, Frieden IJ. Infantile hemangiomas with minimal or arrested growth: a retrospective case series. Arch Dermatol 2010;146(9):971–6.
10. Chiller KG, Passaro D, Frieden IJ. Hemangiomas of infancy: clinical characteristics, morphologic subtypes, and their relationship to race, ethnicity, and sex. Arch Dermatol 2002;138(12):1567–76.
11. Liang MG, Frieden IJ. Infantile and congenital hemangiomas. Semin Pediatr Surg 2014;23(4):162–7.
12. Chang LC, Haggstrom AN, Drolet BA, et al. Growth characteristics of infantile hemangiomas: implications for management. Pediatrics 2008;122(2):360–7.
13. Brandling-Bennett HA, Metry DW, Baselga E, et al. Infantile hemangiomas with unusually prolonged growth phase: a case series. Arch Dermatol 2008;144(12): 1632–7.
14. Cheng CE, Friedlander SF. Infantile hemangiomas, complications and treatments. Semin Cutan Med Surg 2016;35(3):108–16.
15. Castrén E, Salminen P, Gissler M, et al. Risk factors and morbidity of infantile haemangioma: preterm birth promotes ulceration. Acta Paediatr 2016;105(8):940–5.
16. Haggstrom AN, Drolet BA, Baselga E, et al. Prospective study of infantile hemangiomas: clinical characteristics predicting complications and treatment. Pediatrics 2006;118(3):882–7.
17. Baselga E, Roe E, Coulie J, et al. Risk factors for degree and type of sequelae after involution of untreated hemangiomas of infancy. JAMA Dermatol 2016; 152(11):1239–43.
18. Chamlin SL, Mancini AJ, Lai JS, et al. Development and validation of a quality-of-life instrument for infantile hemangiomas. J Invest Dermatol 2015;135(6):1533–9.
19. Tanner JL, Dechert MP, Frieden IJ. Growing up with a facial hemangioma: parent and child coping and adaptation. Pediatrics 1998;101(3 Pt 1):446–52.
20. Krowchuk DP, Frieden IJ, Mancini AJ, et al. Clinical practice guideline for the management of infantile hemangiomas. Pediatrics 2019;143(1):e20183475.
21. Janmohamed SR, Madern GC, de Laat PC, et al. Educational paper: therapy of infantile haemangioma – history and current state (part II). Eur J Pediatr 2015; 174(2):259–66.
22. Grzesik P, Wu JK. Current perspectives on the optimal management of infantile hemangioma. Pediatric Health Med Ther 2017;8:107–16.
23. Garzon MC, Frieden IJ. Hemangiomas: when to worry. Pediatr Ann 2000;29(1): 58–67.
24. McCuaig CC, Cohen L, Powell J, et al. Therapy of ulcerated hemangiomas. J Cutan Med Surg 2013;17(4):233–42.

25. Léauté-Labrèze C, Dumas de la Roque E, Hubiche T, et al. Propranolol for severe hemangiomas of infancy. N Engl J Med 2008;358(24):2649–51.
26. Ji Y, Chen S, Xu C, et al. The use of propranolol in the treatment of infantile hae-mangiomas: an update on potential mechanisms of action. Br J Dermatol 2015; 172(1):24–32.
27. Admani S, Feldstein S, Gonzalez EM, et al. Beta blockers: an innovation in the treatment of infantile hemangiomas. J Clin Aesthet Dermatol 2014;7(7):37–45.
28. Yarbrough KB, Tollefson MM, Krol AL, et al. Is Routine electrocardiography necessary before initiation of propranolol for treatment of infantile hemangiomas? Pediatr Dermatol 2016;33(6):615–20.
29. Streicher JL, Riley EB, Castelo-Soccio LA. Reevaluating the need for electrocar-diograms prior to initiation of treatment with propranolol for infantile hemangi-omas. JAMA Pediatr 2016;170(9):906–7.
30. Raphael MF, Breugem CC, Vlasveld FA, et al. Is cardiovascular evaluation neces-sary prior to and during beta-blocker therapy for infantile hemangiomas?: a cohort study. J Am Acad Dermatol 2015;72(3):465–72.
31. Lund EB, Chamlin SL, Mancini AJ. Utility of routine electrocardiographic screening before initiation of propranolol for infantile hemangiomas. Pediatr Der-matol 2018;35(4):e233–4.
32. Bayart CB, Tamburro JE, Vidimos AT, et al. Atenolol versus propranolol for treat-ment of infantile hemangiomas during the proliferative phase: a retrospective noninferiority study. Pediatr Dermatol 2017;34(4):413–21.
33. Ji Y, Wang Q, Chen S, et al. Oral atenolol therapy for proliferating infantile hem-angioma: a prospective study. Medicine (Baltimore) 2016;95(24):e3908.
34. Frieden IJ, Spring S. Infantile hemangiomas. J Drugs Dermatol 2015;14(5):443–5.
35. Pope E, Chakkittakandiyil A, Lara-Corrales I, et al. Expanding the therapeutic repertoire of infantile haemangiomas: cohort-blinded study of oral nadolol compared with propranolol. Br J Dermatol 2013;168(1):222–4.
36. Ji Y, Chen S, Wang Q, et al. Intolerable side effects during propranolol therapy for infantile hemangioma: frequency, risk factors and management. Sci Rep 2018; 8(1):4264.
37. Bernabeu-Wittel J, Narváez-Moreno B, de la Torre-García JM, et al. Oral nadolol for children with infantile hemangiomas and sleep disturbances with oral propran-olol. Pediatr Dermatol 2015;32(6):853–7.
38. Guo S, Ni N. Topical treatment for capillary hemangioma of the eyelid using beta-blocker solution. Arch Ophthalmol 2010;128(2):255–6.
39. Püttgen K, Lucky A, Adams D, et al. Topical timolol maleate treatment of infantile hemangiomas. Pediatrics 2016;138(3) [pii:e20160355].
40. Painter SL, Hildebrand GD. Review of topical beta blockers as treatment for infan-tile hemangiomas. Surv Ophthalmol 2016;61(1):51–8.
41. Ovadia SA, Landy DC, Cohen ER, et al. Local administration of β-blockers for in-fantile hemangiomas: a systematic review and meta-analysis. Ann Plast Surg 2015;74(2):256–62.
42. Lie E, Püttgen KB. Corticosteroids as an adjunct to propranolol for infantile hae-mangiomas complicated by recalcitrant ulceration. Br J Dermatol 2017;176(4): 1064–7.
43. Couto JA, Greene AK. Management of problematic infantile hemangioma using intralesional triamcinolone: efficacy and safety in 100 infants. J Plast Reconstr Aesthet Surg 2014;67(11):1469–74.
44. Luu M, Frieden IJ. Haemangioma: clinical course, complications and manage-ment. Br J Dermatol 2013;169(1):20–30.

45. Yeh I, Bruckner AL, Sanchez R, et al. Diffuse infantile hepatic hemangiomas: a report of four cases successfully managed with medical therapy. Pediatr Dermatol 2011;28(3):267–75.
46. Michaud AP, Bauman NM, Burke DK, et al. Spastic diplegia and other motor disturbances in infants receiving interferon-alpha. Laryngoscope 2004;114(7): 1231–6.
47. Fawcett SL, Grant I, Hall PN, et al. Vincristine as a treatment for a large haemangioma threatening vital functions. Br J Plast Surg 2004;57(2):168–71.
48. Chinnadurai S, Sathe NA, Surawicz T. Laser treatment of infantile hemangioma: a systematic review. Lasers Surg Med 2016;48(3):221–33.
49. Kado M, Shimizu A, Matsumura T, et al. Successful treatment of infantile hemangiomas with propranolol in low-birth-weight infants. J Craniofac Surg 2017;28(3): 789–93.
50. Goelz R, Poets CF. Incidence and treatment of infantile haemangioma in preterm infants. Arch Dis Child Fetal Neonatal Ed 2015;100(1):F85–91.
51. Brazzelli V, Giorgini C, Barruscotti S, et al. Efficacy of propranolol for cutaneous hemangiomas in premature children. G Ital Dermatol Venereol 2016;151(5): 485–91.
52. Erbay A, Sarialioglu F, Malbora B, et al. Propranolol for infantile hemangiomas: a preliminary report on efficacy and safety in very low birth weight infants. Turk J Pediatr 2010;52(5):450–6.
53. Moehrle M, Léauté-Labrèze C, Schmidt V, et al. Topical timolol for small hemangiomas of infancy. Pediatr Dermatol 2013;30(2):245–9.
54. Frommelt P, Juern A, Siegel D, et al. Adverse events in young and preterm infants receiving topical timolol for infantile hemangioma. Pediatr Dermatol 2016;33(4): 405–14.
55. Chen XD, Ma G, Chen H, et al. Maternal and perinatal risk factors for infantile hemangioma: a case-control study. Pediatr Dermatol 2013;30(4):457–61.
56. Hunjan MK, Schoch JJ, Anderson KR, et al. Prenatal risk factors for infantile hemangioma development. J Invest Dermatol 2017;137(4):954–7.
57. Huang SA, Tu HM, Harney JW, et al. Severe hypothyroidism caused by type 3 iodothyronine deiodinase in infantile hemangiomas. N Engl J Med 2000;343(3): 185–9.
58. Konrad D, Ellis G, Perlman K. Spontaneous regression of severe acquired infantile hypothyroidism associated with multiple liver hemangiomas. Pediatrics 2003; 112(6 Pt 1):1424–6.
59. Broeks IJ, Hermans DJ, Dassel AC, et al. Propranolol treatment in life-threatening airway hemangiomas: a case series and review of literature. Int J Pediatr Otorhinolaryngol 2013;77(11):1791–800.
60. Perkins JA, Chen BS, Saltzman B, et al. Propranolol therapy for reducing the number of nasal infantile hemangioma invasive procedures. JAMA Otolaryngol Head Neck Surg 2014;140(3):220–7.
61. Koka K, Mukherjee B, Agarkar S. Effect of oral propranolol on periocular capillary hemangiomas of infancy. Pediatr Neonatol 2018;59(4):390–6.
62. Ben-Amitai D, Halachmi S, Zvulunov A, et al. Hemangiomas of the nasal tip treated with propranolol. Dermatology 2012;225(4):371–5.
63. Ceisler EJ, Santos L, Blei F. Periocular hemangiomas: what every physician should know. Pediatr Dermatol 2004;21(1):1–9.
64. Vigone MC, Cortinovis F, Rabbiosi S, et al. Difficult treatment of consumptive hypothyroidism in a child with massive parotid hemangioma. J Pediatr Endocrinol Metab 2012;25(1–2):153–5.

65. De Corti F, Crivellaro C, Zanon GF, et al. Consumptive hypothyroidism associated with parotid infantile hemangioma. J Pediatr Endocrinol Metab 2015;28(3–4): 467–9.
66. Dotan M, Lorber A. Congestive heart failure with diffuse neonatal hemangiomatosis – case report and literature review. Acta Paediatr 2013;102(5):e232–8.
67. Drolet BA, Chamlin SL, Garzon MC, et al. Prospective study of spinal anomalies in children with infantile hemangiomas of the lumbosacral skin. J Pediatr 2010; 157(5):789–94.
68. Iacobas I, Burrows PE, Frieden IJ, et al. LUMBAR: association between cutaneous infantile hemangiomas of the lower body and regional congenital anomalies. J Pediatr 2010;157(5):795–801.e1-7.
69. Girard C, Bigorre M, Guillot B, et al. PELVIS syndrome. Arch Dermatol 2006; 142(7):884–8.
70. Garzon MC, Epstein LG, Heyer GL, et al. PHACE syndrome: consensus-derived diagnosis and care recommendations. J Pediatr 2016;178:24–33.e2.
71. de Graaf M, Pasmans SG, van Drooge AM, et al. Associated anomalies and diagnostic approach in lumbosacral and perineal haemangiomas: case report and review of the literature. J Plast Reconstr Aesthet Surg 2013;66(1):e26–8.
72. Orlow SJ, Isakoff MS, Blei F. Increased risk of symptomatic hemangiomas of the airway in association with cutaneous hemangiomas in a "beard" distribution. J Pediatr 1997;131(4):643–6.
73. Piram M, Hadj-Rabia S, Boccara O, et al. Beard infantile hemangioma and subglottic involvement: are median pattern and telangiectatic aspect the clue? J Eur Acad Dermatol Venereol 2016;30(12):2056–9.
74. Schumacher WE, Drolet BA, Maheshwari M, et al. Spinal dysraphism associated with the cutaneous lumbosacral infantile hemangioma: a neuroradiological review. Pediatr Radiol 2012;42(3):315–20.
75. Paller A, Mancini AJ, Hurwitz S. Hurwitz clinical pediatric dermatology. New York: Elsevier Saunders; 2016.
76. Drolet BA, Frommelt PC, Chamlin SL, et al. Initiation and use of propranolol for infantile hemangioma: report of a consensus conference. Pediatrics 2013; 131(1):128–40.
77. Léaute-Labrèze C, Boccara O, Degrugillier-Chopinet C, et al. Safety of oral propranolol for the treatment of infantile hemangioma: a systematic review. Pediatrics 2016;138(4) [pii:e20160353].
78. Moyakine AV, Kerstjens JM, Spillekom-van Koulil S, et al. Propranolol treatment of infantile hemangioma (IH) is not associated with developmental risk or growth impairment at age 4 years. J Am Acad Dermatol 2016;75(1):59–63.e1.
79. Moyakine AV, Spillekom-van Koulil S, van der Vleuten CJM. Propranolol treatment of infantile hemangioma is not associated with psychological problems at 7 years of age. J Am Acad Dermatol 2017;77(1):105–8.
80. Martin K, Blei F, Chamlin SL, et al. Propranolol treatment of infantile hemangiomas: anticipatory guidance for parents and caretakers. Pediatr Dermatol 2013;30(1):155–9.

Gastroesophageal Reflux Disease in the Neonatal Intensive Care Unit Infant

Who Needs to Be Treated and What Approach Is Beneficial?

Ish K. Gulati, MD[a,b],
Sudarshan R. Jadcherla, MD, FRCP (Irel), DCH[a,b,c,d],*

KEYWORDS

• GER • GERD • Preterm • Neonate • NICU

KEY POINTS

• Gastroesophageal reflux (GER) is defined as the retrograde passage of gastric contents into the esophagus and possibly the oral cavity, and when "troublesome symptoms" persist because of these events, it is called gastroesophageal reflux disease (GERD).

• Transient lower esophageal sphincter relaxation remains the most common mechanism of GER in neonates and infants.

• Neonatal presentations are distinct from clinical findings in older infants and children with GERD.

• Symptom-based diagnosis and empirical pharmacologic therapies are not appropriate in the management of neonates with GERD.

Disclosures: S.R. Jadcherla's efforts are supported in part by NIH R01 DK 068158.
[a] Innovative Research Program in Neonatal Feeding Disorders; [b] The Neonatal and Infant Feeding Disorders Program, Nationwide Children's Hospital, Columbus, OH, USA; [c] Division of Neonatology, Department of Pediatrics, Center for Perinatal Research, WB 5211, The Research Institute at Nationwide Children's Hospital, The Ohio State University College of Medicine, 575 Children's Cross Roads, Columbus, OH 43215, USA; [d] Division of Pediatric Gastroenterology and Nutrition, Department of Pediatrics, Center for Perinatal Research, WB 5211, The Research Institute at Nationwide Children's Hospital, The Ohio State University College of Medicine, 575 Children's Cross Roads, Columbus, OH 43215, USA
* Corresponding author. Division of Neonatology, Center for Perinatal Research, WB 5211, The Research Institute at Nationwide Children's Hospital, 575 Children's Cross Roads, Columbus, OH 43215.
E-mail address: Sudarshan.Jadcherla@nationwidechildrens.org

Pediatr Clin N Am 66 (2019) 461–473
https://doi.org/10.1016/j.pcl.2018.12.012
0031-3955/19/© 2018 Elsevier Inc. All rights reserved.

INTRODUCTION
Definition

Gastroesophageal reflux (GER) is defined as the retrograde passage of gastric contents into the esophagus and possibly the oral cavity, and when "troublesome symptoms" persist because of these events, it is called gastroesophageal reflux disease (GERD).[1–3] Infants in the neonatal intensive care unit (NICU) present with a multitude of aerodigestive, cardiorespiratory, and somatic symptoms; it is often unclear whether these symptoms can be attributed to GER. In infants in the NICU or in nonverbal developmentally challenged patients, it is common to associate the troublesome symptoms or cues that are witnessed by an observer with GERD; however, the definition of "troublesome" can be challenging. Based on subjective definitions, the use of pharmacologic and nonpharmacologic therapies to mitigate these symptoms has become a common practice, although there is significant practice variation among providers. Many infants in the NICU are prescribed acid-suppressive therapies to treat a presumed diagnosis of GERD.[4,5] These and other pharmacologic approaches, including prokinetics and antacids, have all been associated with serious short-term and long-term consequences.[5–9] Furthermore, empirical and over-the-counter approved and unapproved therapies are commonly used, adding to the expense and contributing to unintended long-term consequences.[10]

Epidemiology and Burden

The exact burden of GERD in the NICU infant is not known, partly as a result of diverse definitions. To complicate matters, GER is a normal occurrence in the neonate with 2 to 3 episodes of reflux per hour,[11] and is related to the infants' frequent feeding cycles. The composition of gastric contents varies with feeding methods, and therefore the physical and chemical properties of the gastric contents, vary within an infant's feeding cycle.[12] Symptoms are based on the state of activity of the infant (ie, sleep-awake-activity states), with infants spending a considerable amount of time sleeping. Interventions that alter the sleep-awake-activity states may include, but are not limited to, routine examination and providing care, nasogastric tube placement and feeding methods, checking residuals, and suctioning aerodigestive tract secretions in sicker infants. Therefore, changes in sleep patterns and interventions in NICU infants may modify the symptoms and responses to reflux events.[13,14]

In an attempt to determine the burden of GERD, the authors studied 33 academic freestanding children's hospital NICUs in the United States. Using the definition of GERD based on symptoms, they noted a 13-fold variation (2%–26%) in the diagnosis of GERD and found that infants with a diagnosis of GERD stayed 1 month longer in the NICU.[12] Preterm infants who are diagnosed with GERD have longer hospital stays and higher hospital costs than infants without this diagnostic label.[12] It is estimated that the diagnosis of GERD in an NICU infant increases the NICU costs by ~US$70,000.[12] Furthermore, many infants continue to be treated after they are discharged from the NICU.[5,15]

CONTROVERSIES SURROUNDING GASTROESOPHAGEAL REFLUX DISEASE IN THE NEONATAL INTENSIVE CARE UNIT INFANT

Ambiguity in the diagnosis of GER or GERD in the NICU may be related to lack of proper understanding and inability to differentiate normal (physiologic) from disease (pathologic) processes. In the absence of physiologic evidence, the diagnosis and management approaches are often influenced by 4 factors.

1. *Symptoms and cues of the patient.* In general, NICU infants have many types of presenting symptoms and cues; these can be classified into 4 groups: (a) *gastrointestinal* (regurgitation, emesis, abdominal distention), (b) *cardiorespiratory* (spells characterized with bradycardia, tachycardia, apnea, periodic breathing, tachypnea, increased respiratory effort, desaturations), (c) *somatosensory* (irritability, back arching, crying, and grimace), and (d) *aerodigestive* (swallowing and feeding difficulties, sneezing, coughing and choking, breathing disturbances) systems. Attributing such troublesome symptoms to reflux events in the absence of evidence remains controversial. Often there is more than one category of presenting symptoms and cues, which can occur with any provocation from within the airway, pulmonary, digestive, cardiac, or neurologic systems. However, the vagal response is a common attribute that can possibly link all of these 4 categories with nerve-mediated aggravating and ameliorating sensorimotor mechanisms that involve sympathetic and parasympathetic responses.

2. *Perceptions of parents and providers.* Parents and bedside care providers are often the first responders to symptoms and clinical signs, and an initial workup for GERD is often based on their reports. Parental perception of GERD may be influenced by individual experiences or readings from older literature. The presence or magnitude of symptoms as a significant predictor of GERD has been evaluated in a survey, the Infant Gastroesophageal Reflux Questionnaire Revised (I-GERQ-R).[16] The I-GERQ-R is a brief 12-item validated questionnaire completed by parents and physician providers to measure GERD symptoms in infants. This questionnaire validates the diagnosis of GERD in children aged 1 to 14 months by using abnormal pH-probe studies and abnormal esophageal biopsies as gold standards. An I-GERQ-R score greater than 16 is suggestive of acid GERD. However, Salvatore and colleagues[17] found that the I-GERQ-R questionnaire is not reliable for predicting the severity of GERD. The questionnaire had no correlation with esophageal acid exposure as measured by pH-metry and with esophagitis as evaluated by histology of esophageal biopsies. The questionnaire also does not assess the anticipated response to therapeutic interventions.[17]

3. *NICU operational systems and processes.* The NICU operating systems also play an important role in the supply chain of diet and feeding methods provided to hospitalized infants. For example, the processes involving infant diet, volume intake, milk type, position during feeding, caloric density, osmolality of feedings, use of feeding pumps and gavage tube, or transitional or oral feeding methods can influence GER.[12,18]

4. *Physician's role in the definition of the GERD.* Responsibility ultimately rests with the physician as to whether to treat GERD empirically or wait, or to consider tests for persistent feeding difficulties or troublesome symptoms, and seek alternative diagnoses. Such a determination can be challenging when several factors, as described earlier, are at play. The absence of a highly sensitive and specific, easily available crib-side test makes it more difficult to make a diagnosis based on objective criteria.

DEVELOPMENTAL ANATOMY AND PHYSIOLOGY OF THE GASTROESOPHAGEAL JUNCTION

The neonatal period is the only time when anatomic development and functional physiologic maturation of individual systems are rapidly evolving ex utero. This process further depends on the birth gestation, efficient nutrition and feeding methods, and interventions associated with coexisting morbidities. For the purpose of delineating the pathophysiological basis of GERD as related to NICU infants, it is important to understand the development and maturation of the gastroesophageal junction (GEJ) in early infancy, because structural and functional abnormalities can influence the GERD diagnosis particularly in the NICU setting.

Embryology and Clinical Implications

The neuroanatomic relationship between the airway and foregut can be explained by their embryologic origins from adjacent segments of the primitive foregut.[19–22] The tracheobronchial diverticulum, the pharynx, the esophagus, the stomach, and the diaphragm are all derived from the primitive foregut or its mesenchyme and share similar control systems. By 4 weeks' gestation, the tracheobronchial diverticulum appears at the ventral wall of the foregut, with the left vagus located anterior and the right vagus located posterior. The stomach is a fusiform tube with a growth rate of the dorsal side that is greater than the ventral side, thus creating greater and lesser curvatures. At 7 weeks' gestation, the stomach also rotates 90° clockwise, with the greater curvature displaced to the left. By the sixth or seventh week of gestation, a structure superior to the true vocal cords evolves to protect the vocal cords and lower airway. This superior structure consists of the epiglottis, aryepiglottic folds, false vocal cords, and the laryngeal ventricles. The epiglottis starts as a hypobranchial eminence behind the future tongue. By week 7, the epiglottis is separated from the tongue and 2 lateral folds are connected to the base of the epiglottis, and the distal end of the lateral folds develops into the arytenoids cartilages. The larynx begins as a groove in the primitive foregut, which folds on itself to become the laryngotracheal bud, the subsequent divisions of which form the bronchopulmonary segments. From this phase, 20 generations of conducting airways form. The first 8 generations constitute bronchi and acquire cartilaginous walls; the next 9 to 20 generations constitute the nonrespiratory bronchioles, which are not cartilaginous and contain smooth muscle. Subsequent divisions form the bronchopulmonary segments. At 10 weeks' gestation, the esophagus and the stomach are properly positioned; the circular and longitudinal muscle layers and the ganglion cells are in place. The true vocal cords begin as glottal folds.

Thus, from 4 weeks to 24 weeks of intrauterine growth, rapid changes in development, maturation, and functioning of the organs related to the pharyngoesophageal and cardiorespiratory apparatus occur. In the premature infant developing ex utero, further development and maturation of these inadequately developed organ systems can influence the overlapping reflexes involving the 4 categories of symptoms described earlier. Therefore, the structural maldevelopment of the aerodigestive tract and GEJ can result in situations predisposing to GER. Such predisposing conditions for a causal increase in GER events or maladaptive presenting symptoms may include, but are not limited to, craniofacial anomalies, airway anomalies, esophageal atresia and tracheoesophageal fistula, congenital diaphragmatic hernia, hiatal hernia, abdominal wall defects, malrotation, pyloric stenosis, atresia and stricture, and duplication of the small intestine.

Neuromuscular Physiology of Gastroesophageal Junction and Clinical Implications

The pharynx, upper esophageal sphincter (UES), and proximal esophagus are composed of striated muscle. The UES is a high-pressure zone generated by the cricopharyngeus, proximal cervical esophagus, and inferior pharyngeal constrictor, and is located between the pharynx and the esophagus.[23] The UES is innervated by the vagus nerve via the branches of the pharyngoesophageal, superior laryngeal, and recurrent laryngeal nerve, the glossopharyngeal nerve, and the sympathetic nerve fibers via the cranial nerve ganglia. The distal esophagus and the lower esophageal sphincter (LES) are composed of smooth muscle with an inner layer consisting of circular muscle cells and an outer layer consisting of longitudinal muscle cells with a myenteric plexus in between. The LES is an autonomous contractile apparatus that is tonically active and relaxes periodically to facilitate bolus transit. The integrity of the GEJ is augmented by the LES, diaphragmatic crural fibers, intra-abdominal esophagus, and sling fibers of the stomach.[2]

The high-pressure zone at the GEJ relaxes via inhibitory neural pathways to allow the passage of contents into the stomach during swallowing or into the proximal esophagus and higher structures, as in GER. As shown in the high-resolution impedance manometry recording (**Fig. 1**), the high-pressure zone at the LES abruptly drops, and this reflex is known as transient LES relaxation (TLESR), the most common mechanism of GER.[24–26] The LES relaxes during basal swallowing, pharyngeal stimulation, esophageal distention, abdominal strain, and GER.[27] In general, the clearance of the refluxate occurs via peristaltic reflexes, and retrograde movement is abruptly halted through the contraction of the UES (see **Fig. 1**); this barrier function matures with postnatal development. The retrograde movement and clearance of refluxate is captured on the pH-impedance recording (**Fig. 2**).

In summary, the high-pressure zone at the GEJ depends on the tone generated by the intrinsic LES and also on the magnitude of crural diaphragmatic contraction.

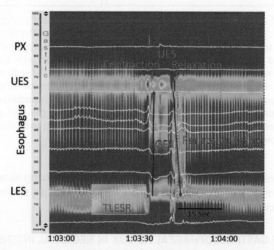

Fig. 1. GER event in a neonate recorded by high-resolution manometry capturing the actual occurrence of a GER event in a neonate. The blue zone reflects 0 mm Hg, whereas the purple zone reflects 100 mm Hg (*designated on the left*). The white horizontal lines represent impedance lines that detect bolus presence, directionality, and characteristic of the bolus (air, liquid, and mixed). As the liquid refluxate moves retrograde (decrease in impedance), it drags air with it (shown as increase in impedance). Note that the most proximal extent of reflux stops at the upper esophageal sphincter (UES). At that point there is an increase in UES contractility (protective UES contractile reflex), immediately followed by relaxation of UES associated with swallowing and the peristaltic reflex. Note also that the UES barrier maintains integrity after swallowing (UES relaxation). PX stands for pharynx. The peristaltic reflex is the mechanism for clearance of the bolus. TLESR is the transient relaxation of lower esophageal sphincter wherein the LES resting pressure drops abruptly (relaxes), during which time the ascent of the reflux material occurs. TLESR is the most common mechanism for a GER event. The burdensome symptoms that result as a consequence of GER events contribute toward the diagnosis of GERD.

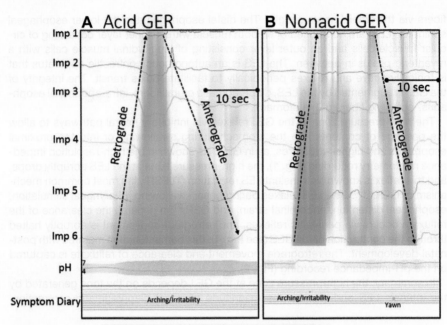

Fig. 2. Example of pH-impedance recordings. There are 6 impedance (Imp) channels, and 1 and 6 refer to the proximal channel and the distal channel, respectively. During this measurement, the pH sensor records the degree of acid exposure over a period of time. (*A*) During an acid-related GER event, the acid exposure at the distal channel is shown by a drop in pH at the acid sensor, and a decrease in impedance is also associated with retrograde migration of acid reflux material. This is followed by clearance of the refluxate, which is mediated via anterograde peristalsis, as evidenced by the return of the impedance to baseline. Of note, this infant presented with arching and irritability during the GER event. (*B*) During a nonacid GER event, the pH is not in the acidic range and liquid material is moving retrograde, and is followed by anterograde clearance and peristalsis.

Transit of material through the GEJ is most likely to occur during simultaneous relaxation of the LES and inhibition of the crural diaphragm, and also depends on the pressure gradients across the stomach and esophageal lumen.

PHYSIOLOGY OF GASTROESOPHAGEAL REFLUX IN NEONATAL INTENSIVE CARE UNIT INFANTS

TLESR (see **Fig. 1**) remains the most common mechanism of GER in neonates and infants.[25,28,29] Regurgitation is very common in this age group; 40% to 60% of normal 0- to 4-month-old infants regurgitate some amount of their feedings. Basic mechanical considerations provide some explanation for the high frequency of regurgitation in infants.[1,30–34] Newborns sleep or spend most of their time in the supine position, a position that is protective against sudden infant death syndrome (SIDS). Supine and right lateral positions increase the risk for GER, whereas prone and left lateral positions are associated with less GER but an increased rate of SIDS.[1,35–37] Preterm infants are noted to have GER immediately following their feeding, which is most likely due to gastric distension rather than delayed gastric emptying. Studies have shown a normal gastric emptying pattern in both infants with symptomatic GER and those without symptoms.[25,38] Preterm infants who receive tube feedings may have increased episodes of GER because of incomplete closure of the LES secondary to the presence of a feeding tube.[39] However, on the contrary, in symptomatic dysphagic neonates evaluated for suspected GERD using pH-impedance methods, the authors showed that tube-fed infants had fewer GER events than the exclusively oral-fed group.[12] The length of the infant's esophagus and LES are short and increase with maturation.[40] A term infant's esophagus may be only 8 to 10 cm; the intra-abdominal esophagus develops during the first 6 months of life after full-term birth. Thus, refluxed material has a greater chance of extending to a more proximal extent in preterm infants who are at 6 months corrected age.

Manometric studies in both premature and term neonates have confirmed normal primary esophageal peristalsis. However, premature infants at 30 to 34 weeks' gestational age have lower esophageal peristaltic velocity and amplitude than term infants,[41,42] and preterm infants as young as 33 weeks' postmenstrual age have a reduced esophageal high-pressure zone, which increases with age.[43–45] In response to midesophageal liquid stimulus provocations, premature infants have a longer delay to LES relaxation, but once relaxation occurs it is of longer duration than that found in term infants.[27] Premature infants have an elevated frequency of nonperistaltic esophageal contractions in the absence of a swallow, and this lack of coordination may lead to inadequate clearance of refluxed material.[43,45] As in adults, it seems that transient relaxations of the high-pressure zone are the primary mechanism of GER in neonates.[43,45,46]

In summary, the most frequent mechanism for GER is TLESR, a common mechanism in neonates and adults. Factors unique to neonates include anatomic factors, position, feeding methods, immaturity, esophageal clearance mechanisms, and presence of inflammation or anomalies.

PATHOPHYSIOLOGY OF GASTROESOPHAGEAL REFLUX DISEASE

The esophageal and laryngeal reflexes that protect the esophagus and airway from damage caused by GER appear to be present in healthy preterm infants. Esophageal distension from the reflux of gastric contents activates anterograde peristalsis reflex of the esophagus along with closure of the UES. This prevents the refluxate from reaching the pharynx. However, if the UES relaxes to allow the refluxate to reach the pharynx, the laryngeal chemosensitive receptors trigger the initiation of the laryngeal chemoreflex to prevent aspiration of gastric contents by glottis closure, which is always accompanied by a period of apnea (glottal closure reflex), although the duration of pause in breathing varies. In addition, primary peristalsis is triggered when the refluxate is present in the pharynx. Theoretically, GERD and retrograde aspiration could result from the failure of these mechanisms. Abnormalities of all of these reflexes are unlikely in physiologically healthy infants, which is why most healthy infants are asymptomatic despite having frequent episodes of GER.[47–49]

RISK FACTORS FOR GASTROESOPHAGEAL REFLUX DISEASE

Several risk factors for GERD have been identified in infants, and the most common causes are listed in **Fig. 3**. Apart from the congenital causes and physiologic consequences of prematurity, it is important to analyze the causes of GER events that arise from complications of prematurity. Bronchopulmonary dysplasia is a major complication of prematurity that affects 30% of extremely low birth weight infants.[50] These infants have an increased risk of GER events secondary to increased respiratory effort and transient increase in intra-abdominal pressure resulting from coughing, airflow obstruction, and crying. This causes the LES tone to decrease and in turn contributes

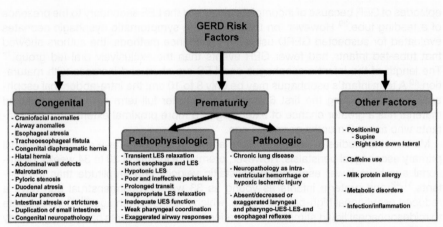

Fig. 3. Risk factors for GERD in the NICU infant. Owing to embryologic and neuroanatomic considerations on the aerodigestive functions, the neonate in the NICU is in a much more vulnerable state than at any other periods of life. The risk factors are classified into 4 domains as stated in the text.

to TLESR.[1,46,51] In addition, these infants are usually treated with respiratory stimulants such as caffeine, which may exacerbate GER events because of an increase in secretion of gastric acid and lowering of LES pressure.[52,53] Neuropathology such as intraventricular hemorrhage, noted in 30% to 40% of preterm infants,[54,55] and hypoxic-ischemic encephalopathy[56] are some of the common risk factors likely to alter the causal or ameliorating mechanisms for reflux events and resulting troublesome symptoms. The incidence of GERD is about 15% to 75% in children with

---

Box 1
Screening history for GERD in NICU infants

- Age at symptom onset
- Length of feeding periods
- Volume of each feeding
- Type of milk
- Methods of mixing the formula
- Additives to the feedings
- Attention to food allergens
- Time interval between feeding
- Pattern of regurgitation/spitting/vomiting
- Family medical history
- Environmental triggers—position
- Infant's growth trajectory
- Prior pharmacologic and dietary interventions
- Presence of warning signs such as failure to thrive, back arching and irritability, airway signs, poor oral intake, coughing, and choking spells

neurologic impairment, and the prevalence of GERD in the presence of neuropathology is estimated to be 50%.[57] Neuropathology contributes to GERD through dysregulation of aerodigestive reflexes. Several other causes may contribute to GERD, including metabolic disorders, body positioning, milk protein allergy, and infections, to name a few. These conditions must be investigated in preterm infants who present with signs concerning GERD.

APPROACH TO THE PROBLEM THOUGHT TO BE DUE TO GASTROESOPHAGEAL REFLUX DISEASE IN INFANTS IN THE NEONATAL INTENSIVE CARE UNIT

In 2018, the North American Society for Pediatric Gastroenterology, Hepatology and Nutrition and the European Society for Pediatric Gastroenterology Hepatology and Nutrition[1] published guidelines on the approach to children presenting with GER or GERD. However, further research is needed because these guidelines are not entirely clear about applicability to infants in the NICU. Infants in the NICU presenting with

---

Box 2
Signs and symptoms that may be associated with GERD in NICU infants

Symptoms

Gastrointestinal
- Regurgitation
- Spitting
- Emesis
- Abdominal distension

Aerodigestive
- Swallowing problems
- Feeding problems
- Sneezing
- Coughing
- Choking
- Wheezing
- Stridor

Cardiorespiratory Spells
- Bradycardia
- Tachycardia
- Apneas
- Periodic breathing
- Tachypnea
- Increased respiratory effort
- Desaturations

Somatosensory
- Irritability
- Back arching
- Crying
- Grimace

Signs

Aerodigestive
- Esophagitis
- Recurrent pneumonia with aspiration
- Recurrent otitis media

General
- Anemia
- Failure to thrive

troublesome signs and symptoms suspected to be due to GERD should be evaluated thoroughly for any findings suggestive of disorders other than GERD. A wide range of clinical symptoms are attributed to GERD in NICU infants; however, the reliability of these symptoms as a manifestation of GERD is not clear. The evaluation of a neonate with a suspicion for GERD begins with a thorough focused history (**Box 1**) and physical examination while paying attention to the pharyngoesophageal, cardiorespiratory, and neurologic systems, nutrition, feeding methods, and growth characteristics. In particular, the evaluation should pay attention to signs and symptoms of aerodigestive problems, nonspecific behavioral signs including arching and irritability, and feeding problems that may be associated with GERD (**Box 2**). Additionally it is imperative to exclude any symptoms and signs that masquerade as GERD. Relevant risk factors (see **Fig. 3**) must be addressed. Initial management should include paying attention to optimal nutrition and feeding methods, and continued breastfeeding. However, if there are no improvements a trial of protein hydrolysate or amino acid–based formula or, in breastfed infants, elimination of cow's milk in the maternal diet should be considered for 2 to 4 weeks. If there are no improvements despite these interventions, gastrointestinal specialty testing using pH impedance with symptom correlation methods, and/or manometry for pharyngoesophageal functional abnormalities, may be considered when available to ascertain the causal and ameliorating mechanisms. In such situations, or if a referral for specialty testing is not possible, 4 to 8 weeks' trial of acid suppression using proton-pump inhibitors may be considered with extreme caution, while weighing the benefits versus risks, and this can only be considered when infants are at and beyond full term age.[10] There are no safe prokinetic agents for use in premature infants. The role of antacids remains uncertain in the premature infant population.

SUMMARY

Diagnosis and management considerations for GER and GERD in the NICU infant can be challenging. Neonatal presentations are not as typical as those seen in older infants and children with GERD. Symptom-based diagnosis and empirical pharmacologic therapies are not appropriate. Developmental pathologies and maturational deficits in the causal and ameliorating mechanisms of GER may be associated with GERD risks. When relevant, structural anomalies and risk factors of GERD must be addressed. Emphasis must first be placed on optimal nutrition, feeding methods, growth, conservative management, and reassurance. Because symptoms are nonspecific, other causes and diagnoses that masquerade as GERD must be considered. Minimizing the use and duration of acid-suppressive therapies is appropriate while weighing benefits and risks. Further research is critically needed in this high-risk population of NICU infants, with relevance to screening, diagnostic algorithms, objective criteria, and nonpharmacologic and pharmacologic approaches, to manage objectively determined acid and nonacid GERD and their consequences.

ACKNOWLEDGMENTS

The authors are thankful to Nour Hanandeh, BS, BME for help with figures, and Kathryn A. Hasenstab, BS, BME for help with tables and references.

REFERENCES

1. Rosen R, Vandenplas Y, Singendonk M, et al. Pediatric gastroesophageal reflux clinical practice guidelines: joint recommendations of the North American Society

for Pediatric Gastroenterology, Hepatology, and Nutrition and the European Society for Pediatric Gastroenterology, Hepatology, and Nutrition. J Pediatr Gastroenterol Nutr 2018;66(3):516–54.

2. Jadcherla SR. Pathophysiology of gastroesophageal reflux. In: Polin RA, Abman SH, Rowitch D, et al, editors. Fetal and neonatal physiology. 5th edition. Philadelphia: Elsevier; 2017. p. 1643–52.

3. Eichenwald EC. Committee on fetus and newborn. Diagnosis and management of gastroesophageal reflux in preterm infants. Pediatrics 2018;142(1):e20181061.

4. Slaughter JL, Stenger MR, Reagan PB, et al. Neonatal histamine-2 receptor antagonist and proton pump inhibitor treatment at United States Children's Hospitals. J Pediatr 2016;174:63–70.

5. Malcolm WF, Cotton CM. Metoclopramide, H2 blockers, and proton pump inhibitors: pharmacotherapy for gastroesophageal reflux in neonates. Clin Perinatol 2012;39(1):99–109.

6. Hibbs AM, Lorch SA. Metoclopramide for the treatment of gastroesophageal reflux disease in infants: a systematic review. Pediatrics 2006;118(2):746–52.

7. Guillet R, Stoll BJ, Cotton CM, et al. Association of H2-blocker therapy and higher incidence of necrotizing enterocolitis in very low birth weight infants. Pediatrics 2006;117(2):e137–42.

8. Terrin G, Passariello A, DeCurtis M, et al. Ranitidine is associated with infections, necrotizing enterocolitis, and fatal outcome in newborns. Pediatrics 2012;129(1): e40–5.

9. Orenstein SR, Hassall E, Furmaga-Jablonska W, et al. Multicenter, double-blind, randomized, placebo-controlled trial assessing the efficacy and safety of proton pump inhibitor lansoprazole in infants with symptoms of gastroesophageal reflux disease. J Pediatr 2009;154(4):514–20.

10. El-Mahdy MA, Mansoor FA, Jadcherla SR. Pharmacological management of gastroesophageal reflux disease in infants: current opinions. Curr Opin Pharmacol 2017;37:112–7.

11. Lopez-Alonso M, Moya MJ, Cabo JA, et al. Twenty-four-hour esophageal impedance-pH monitoring in healthy preterm neonates: rate and characteristics of acid, weakly acidic, and weakly alkaline gastroesophageal reflux. Pediatrics 2006;118(2):e299–308.

12. Jadcherla SR, Slaughter JL, Stenger MR, et al. Practice variance, prevalence, and economic burden of premature infants diagnosed with GERD. Hosp Pediatr 2013;3(4):335–41.

13. Qureshi A, Malkar M, Splaingard M, et al. The role of sleep in the modulation of gastroesophageal reflux and symptoms in NICU neonates. Pediatr Neurol 2015;53(3):226–32.

14. Sankaran J, Qureshi AH, Woodley F, et al. Effect of severity of esophageal acidification on sleep vs wake periods in infants presenting with brief resolved unexplained events. J Pediatr 2016;179:42–8.

15. Golski CA, Rome EW, Martin RJ, et al. Pediatric specialists' beliefs about gastroesophageal reflux disease in premature infants. Pediatrics 2010;125(1):96–104.

16. Kleinman L, Rothman M, Strauss R, et al. The infant gastroesophageal reflux questionnaire revised: development and validation as an evaluative instrument. Clin Gastroenterol Hepatol 2006;4(5):588–96.

17. Salvatore S, Hauser B, Vandemaele K, et al. Gastroesophageal reflux disease in infants: how much is predictable with questionnaires, pH-metry, endoscopy and histology? J Pediatr Gastroenterol Nutr 2005;40(2):210–5.

18. Levy DS, Osborn E, Hasenstab KA, et al. The effect of additives for reflux or dysphagia management on osmolality in ready-to-feed preterm formula: practice implications. JPEN J Parenter Enteral Nutr 2018. https://doi.org/10.1002/jpen.1418.

19. Mansfield LE. Embryonic origins of the relation of gastroesophageal reflux disease and airway disease. Am J Med 2001;111(Suppl 8A):3S–7S.

20. Miller JL, Sonies BC, Macedonia C. Emergence of oropharyngeal, laryngeal and swallowing activity in the developing fetal upper aerodigestive tract: an ultrasound evaluation. Early Hum Dev 2003;71(1):61–87.

21. Sadler TW. Respiratory system. In: Sadler TW, editor. Langman's medical embryology. Baltimore (MD): Williams & Wilkins; 1995. p. 232–41.

22. Sadler TW. Digestive system. In: Sadler TW, editor. Langman's medical embryology. Baltimore (MD): Williams & Wilkins; 1995. p. 208–29.

23. Lang IM, Shaker R. Anatomy and physiology of the upper esophageal sphincter. Am J Med 1997;103(5A):50S–5S.

24. Werlin SL, Dodds WJ, Hogan WJ, et al. Mechanisms of gastroesophageal reflux in children. J Pediatr 1980;97(2):244–9.

25. Omari TI, Barnett CP, Benninga MA, et al. Mechanisms of gastro-oesophageal reflux in preterm and term infants with reflux disease. Gut 2002;51(4):475–9.

26. Dent J, Dodds WJ, Friedman RH, et al. Mechanism of gastroesophageal reflux in recumbent asymptomatic human-subjects. J Clin Invest 1980;65(2):256–67.

27. Pena EM, Parks VN, Peng J, et al. Lower esophageal sphincter relaxation reflex kinetics: effects of peristaltic reflexes and maturation in human premature neonates. Am J Physiol Gastrointest Liver Physiol 2010;299(6):G1386–95.

28. Omari TI, Barnett C, Snel A, et al. Mechanisms of gastroesophageal reflux in healthy premature infants. J Pediatr 1998;133(5):650–4.

29. Omari TI, Benninga MA, Barnett CP, et al. Characterization of esophageal body and lower esophageal sphincter motor function in the very premature neonate. J Pediatr 1999;135(4):517–21.

30. Hyman PE, Milla PJ, Benninga MA, et al. Childhood functional gastrointestinal disorders: neonate/toddler. Gastroenterology 2006;130(5):1519–26.

31. Orenstein SR. Prone positioning in infant gastroesophageal reflux: is elevation of the head worth the trouble? J Pediatr 1990;117(2 Pt 1):184–7.

32. Sondheimer JM. Gastroesophageal reflux: update on pathogenesis and diagnosis. Pediatr Clin North Am 1988;35(1):103–16.

33. Corvaglia L, Rotatori R, Ferlini M, et al. The effect of body positioning on gastroesophageal reflux in premature infants: evaluation by combined impedance and pH monitoring. J Pediatr 2007;151(6):591–6.

34. Omari TI, Rommel N, Staunton E, et al. Paradoxical impact of body positioning on gastroesophageal reflux and gastric emptying in the premature neonate. J Pediatr 2004;145(2):194–200.

35. Jadcherla SR, Rudolph CD. Gastroesophageal reflux in the preterm neonate. Neoreviews 2005;6(2):e87–98.

36. Jadcherla SR. Gastroesophageal reflux in the neonate. Clin Perinatol 2002;29(1):135–58.

37. Jadcherla SR. Pathophysiology of aerodigestive pulmonary disorders in the neonate. Clin Perinatol 2012;39(3):639–54.

38. Ewer AK, Durbin GM, Morgan ME, et al. Gastric emptying and gastro-oesophageal reflux in preterm infants. Arch Dis Child Fetal Neonatal Ed 1996;75(2):F117–21.

39. Peter CS, Sprodowski N, Bohnhorst B, et al. Gastroesophageal reflux and apnea of prematurity: no temporal relationship. Pediatrics 2002;109(1):8–11.
40. Gupta A, Jadcherla SR. The relationship between somatic growth and in vivo esophageal segmental and sphincteric growth in human neonates. J Pediatr Gastroenterol Nutr 2006;43(1):35–41.
41. Gupta A, Gulati P, Kim W, et al. Effect of postnatal maturation on the mechanisms of esophageal propulsion in preterm human neonates: primary and secondary peristalsis. Am J Gastroenterol 2009;104(2):411–9.
42. Jadcherla SR, Duong HQ, Hofmann C, et al. Characteristics of upper oesophageal sphincter and oesophageal body during maturation in healthy human neonates compared with adults. Neurogastroenterol Motil 2005;17(5):663–70.
43. Omari TI, Miki K, Davidson G, et al. Characterisation of relaxation of the lower oesophageal sphincter in healthy premature infants. Gut 1997;40(3):370–5.
44. Kawahara H, Dent J, Davidson G. Mechanisms responsible for gastroesophageal reflux in children. Gastroenterology 1997;113(2):399–408.
45. Omari TI, Miki K, Fraser R, et al. Esophageal body and lower esophageal sphincter function in healthy premature infants. Gastroenterology 1995;109(6): 1757–64.
46. Omari T, Barnett C, Snel A, et al. Mechanism of gastroesophageal reflux in premature infants with chronic lung disease. J Pediatr Surg 1999;34(12):1795–8.
47. Thach BT. Reflux associated apnea in infants: evidence for a laryngeal chemoreflex. Am J Med 1997;103:120s–4s.
48. Jadcherla SR, Hoffmann RG, Shaker R. Effect of maturation of the magnitude of mechanosensitive and chemosensitive reflexes in the premature human esophagus. J Pediatr 2006;149(1):77–82.
49. Jadcherla SR, Gupta A, Coley BD, et al. Esophago-glottal closure reflex in human infants: a novel reflex elicited with concurrent manometry and ultrasonography. Am J Gastroenterol 2007;102(10):2286–93.
50. Nobile S, Noviello C, Cobellis G, et al. Are infants with bronchopulmonary dysplasia prone to gastroesophageal reflux? a prospective observational study with esophageal ph-impedance monitoring. J Pediatr 2015;167(2):279–85.
51. Orenstein SR, Orenstein DM. Gastroesophageal reflux and respiratory-disease in children. J Pediatr 1988;112(6):847–58.
52. Foster LJ, Trudeau WL, Goldman AL. Bronchodilator effects on gastric acid secretion. JAMA 1979;241(24):2613–5.
53. Stein MR, Towner TG, Weber RW, et al. The effect of theophylline on the lower esophageal sphincter pressure. Ann Allergy 1980;45(4):238–41.
54. Ballabh P. Intraventricular hemorrhage in premature infants: mechanism of disease. Pediatr Res 2010;67(1):1–8.
55. Payne AH, Hintz SR, Hibbs AM, et al. Neurodevelopmental outcomes of extremely low-gestational-age neonates with low-grade periventricular-intraventricular hemorrhage. JAMA Pediatr 2013;167(5):451–9.
56. Hill CD, Jadcherla SR. Esophageal mechanosensitive mechanisms are impaired in neonates with hypoxic-ischemic encephalopathy. J Pediatr 2013;162(5): 976–82.
57. Del Buono R, Wenzl TG, Rawat D, et al. Acid and nonacid gastro-oesophageal reflux in neurologically impaired children: investigation with the multiple intraluminal impedance procedure. J Pediatr Gastroenterol Nutr 2006;43(3):331–5.

Stridor in the Newborn

Andrew E. Bluher, MD, David H. Darrow, MD, DDS*

KEYWORDS

- Stridor • Newborn • Neonate • Neonatal • Laryngomalacia • Larynx • Trachea

KEY POINTS

- *Stridor* originates from laryngeal subsites (supraglottis, glottis, subglottis) or the trachea; a snoring sound originating from the pharynx is more appropriately considered *stertor*.
- Stridor is characterized by its volume, pitch, presence on inspiration or expiration, and severity with change in state (awake vs asleep) and position (prone vs supine).
- Laryngomalacia is the most common cause of neonatal stridor, and most cases can be managed conservatively provided the diagnosis is made with certainty.
- Premature babies, especially those with a history of intubation, are at risk for subglottic pathologic condition,
- Changes in voice associated with stridor suggest glottic pathologic condition and a need for otolaryngology referral.

INTRODUCTION

Families and practitioners alike may understandably be alarmed by stridor occurring in a newborn. An understanding of the presentation and differential diagnosis of neonatal stridor is vital in determining whether to manage the child with further observation in the primary care setting, specialist referral, or urgent inpatient care. In most cases, the management of neonatal stridor is outside the purview of the pediatric primary care provider. The goal of this review is not, therefore, to present an exhaustive review of causes of neonatal stridor, but rather to provide an approach to the stridulous newborn that can be used effectively in the assessment and triage of such patients.

Definitions

The *neonatal period* is defined by the World Health Organization as the first 28 days of age. For the purposes of this discussion, the newborn period includes the first 3 months of age.

Stridor consists of a harsh whistle that is classically produced when air emanates from a narrowed portion of the airway. It can be low or high pitched, depending on the caliber and shape of the airway and the amount of respiratory effort. In most

Disclosure Statement: The authors declare that they have no relevant or material financial interests that relate to the research described in this paper.
Department of Otolaryngology–Head and Neck Surgery, Children's Hospital of The King's Daughters, Eastern Virginia Medical School, 600 Gresham Drive, Norfolk, VA 23507, USA
* Corresponding author.
E-mail address: David.Darrow@chkd.org

cases, it is readily distinguished from *stertor*, which is a flapping or snoring sound generated by redundant soft tissue or secretions in the nasal passages, nasopharynx, oral cavity, or oropharynx. The only location in which stridor and/or stertor often present together is the supraglottis. Although stridor may be inspiratory or expiratory, most clinicians refer to expiratory stridor as *wheezing*, which is generally softer, higher pitched, multitoned, and most audible over the lower lung fields.

Operative endoscopy refers to endoscopic evaluation of the airway under anesthesia in the operating room. *Flexible fiber-optic laryngoscopy* (FFL) is usually performed in the office or at the bedside and does not require anesthesia; however, the examination is usually limited to the supraglottis and glottis.

Anatomy

The airway can be broadly divided into clinically relevant segments. Obstruction of the nasal passages, nasopharynx, oral cavity, and oropharynx can produce obstructive breathing sounds that are usually stertorous in nature and are beyond the scope of this review. This discussion focuses on the anatomic regions that produce classic stridor; namely, the larynx and trachea (**Fig. 1**). The larynx is divided into the supraglottis (including the cartilages and folds above the true vocal folds), the glottis (true vocal folds), and the subglottis (1 cm of airway below the vocal folds). The trachea begins below the subglottis at the inferior border of the cricoid cartilage and ends by branching into the right and left main bronchi.

CLINICAL EVALUATION
History

The history of a neonate's stridor is critical in considering its likely cause and the need for potential operative endoscopy. The following are features of the stridor about which caregivers should be questioned:

Time of initial onset
In most cases, stridor in a newborn will be due to a congenital anomaly and therefore presents at birth. Even laryngomalacia, which may be reported as manifesting in

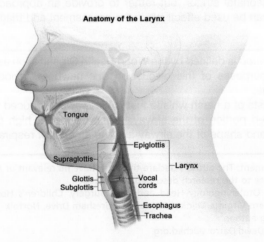

Anatomy of the Larynx

Fig. 1. Anatomy of the larynx and trachea. Note division of larynx into supraglottis, glottis, and subglottis. (For the National Cancer Institute © 2012 Terese Winslow LLC, U.S. Govt. has certain rights.)

the first week or 2 after birth, is usually present to some degree soon after delivery. In rare cases, masses or vascular compression of the airway, brainstem abnormalities, or perinatal iatrogenic injury to the recurrent laryngeal nerve may result in stridor in the newborn that presents postnatally. Examples include masses within the airway, mediastinal masses, vascular compression of the trachea, Chiari malformation, and recurrent nerve injury during congenital heart surgery or ligation of a patent ductus.

Quality of the stridor

In general, extrathoracic pathologic condition presents with inspiratory stridor, whereas intrathoracic pathologic condition presents with expiratory stridor (also known as wheezing). This rule holds up well in differentiating laryngeal abnormalities from those in the trachea. However, lesions of the glottis and subglottis both may present with biphasic (inspiratory and expiratory) stridor, making it difficult to distinguish lesions within the larynx based on phase of breathing alone. Diagnosing laryngeal pathologic condition is further complicated by the fact that some supraglottic pathologic conditions (primarily laryngomalacia and vallecular cysts) can present with stertor rather than, or in addition to, stridor. Most lesions below the supraglottis present with coarse stridor, whereas laryngomalacia and vallecular cysts may present with a more musical ("ascending glissando") quality.

Progression of the stridor

Stridor that increases in severity or frequency over time implies an evolving pathologic condition, such as compression from growing mass (most commonly subglottic infantile hemangiomas or cysts), progressive stenosis following endolaryngeal or endotracheal injury, or increasing vascular compression of the airway. Stridor that is improving is more likely due to inflammation, or to laryngomalacia that is spontaneously resolving.

Changes with position (prone vs supine) or state (sleep vs awake)

Changes due to position and/or state are usually associated with lesions in dynamic, as opposed to static, portions of the airway, namely the supraglottis and trachea. When changes occur with positioning, the stridor is usually worse supine; this occurs primarily with laryngomalacia and supraglottic pathologic conditions, in which the symptoms are exacerbated by retropositioning of the tongue due to gravity. Stridor that changes with state is usually worse awake than asleep, and due to dynamic disorders such as laryngomalacia and tracheomalacia. Obstruction at the tongue base is generally worse asleep.

Changes in voice

Dysphonia, manifested as a hoarse cry, is associated almost exclusively with glottic pathologic conditions, such as vocal fold paralysis or laryngeal web.

Associated symptoms

Cough may be present in a variety of pathologic conditions, but is seen most commonly in lesions that narrow the subglottis or trachea. Cough with feeding is often suggestive of abnormalities of vocal fold mobility or dyscoordination between swallowing and breathing as is seen in laryngomalacia, but may also suggest a cleft of the larynx or tracheoesophageal fistula. Gastroesophageal reflux has been implicated as both a cause and a sequela of airway pathologic condition and is commonly associated with laryngomalacia.[1]

Additional history is useful in decision-making regarding the need for operative endoscopy or surgical intervention. Many practitioners may be familiar with the

"SPECS" algorithm, as delineated in **Table 1**.[2] The presence of sternal retractions, progression, feeding difficulty or failure to thrive, and/or acute life-threatening episodes often suggests a need for further intervention. Birth history, intubation history, medical and surgical history, and family history are also helpful in determining possible causes.

Physical Examination

Assessment should first rule out severe respiratory distress, focusing on vital signs, and noninvasive assessment of level of consciousness, skin color, and accessory muscle use. If the patient is unstable, further management will focus on assessing and supporting the patient's airway, breathing, and circulation, with urgent transfer to a higher level of care once secure.

Most patients will present in a far less urgent manner. Examination of the stable newborn with stridor should focus on nasal and oral patency as well as many of the features previously discussed: the quality of breathing sounds on inspiration and expiration, the presence of retractions, changes in the pattern of breathing with positioning, and assessment of voice. A complete neonatal examination, including recognition of syndromic features, overall neuromuscular tone, and auscultation of the heart and lungs, may provide important additional information regarding possible cause of the stridor. Assessment of the child's growth will provide further information about the child's overall functioning and ability to balance feeding with respiratory effort and caloric consumption.

Imaging

Imaging is rarely necessary in the assessment of newborn stridor, with the exception of those cases in which intrathoracic pathologic condition is suspected. In such cases, the imaging can usually be deferred to specialist assessment, but should be a part of the evaluation. A chest radiograph will occasionally demonstrate vascular compression of the trachea or mediastinal masses. A plain radiograph of the larynx is more useful beyond the newborn period, particularly in the diagnosis of croup, subglottic masses, supraglottitis, and foreign bodies; however, the utility of laryngeal plain films is very dependent on technique. Computed tomography (CT) scans with contrast can be used in the assessment of suspected masses of the airway, neck, or mediastinum, and CT angiography is diagnostic in cases of vascular compression of the airway. MRI is particularly helpful in the assessment of vascular anomalies, or if there is concern for Chiari malformation in the case of bilateral vocal fold paralysis. Some practitioners also recommend MRI to image the course of the recurrent laryngeal nerve in cases of unilateral vocal fold paralysis. The primary care provider should consider that an inappropriately ordered scan will subject the patient to unnecessary expense and/or radiation, without providing clinically relevant information.

Table 1		
SPECS algorithm for evaluation of stridor		
S	Severity	Retractions, respiratory effort
P	Progression	Changes in quality and severity over time
E	Eating difficulties	Prolonged feeding time, aspiration, failure to thrive, gastroesophageal reflux
C	Cyanosis or apneic events	Acute life-threatening episodes
S	Sleep disturbance	Changes in stridor during sleep; note position during sleep

Endoscopic Assessment

In most cases, initial endoscopic assessment of the neonatal airway may be performed with a flexible endoscope in the otolaryngology office or at the hospital bedside. The procedure does not require anesthesia and, in most cases, can be performed in less than 2 minutes. Flexible fiber-optic endoscopy allows the examiner to visualize the pharynx as well as the supraglottic and glottic larynx. Examination of the subglottic larynx and trachea is more safely and accurately performed as an operative endoscopy procedure under anesthesia in the operating room. Operative endoscopy uses rigid endoscopes that provide excellent visualization and high-resolution images of the larynx and trachea (**Fig. 2**). The procedure is usually performed with the child ventilating spontaneously to allow the child to protect the airway during the procedure and to better simulate the conditions under which the stridor is observed.

CAUSES OF NEWBORN STRIDOR

Stridor classically originates from the larynx and/or the trachea. **Table 2** lists the most common causes of neonatal stridor by anatomic subsite.

Supraglottic Obstruction

Supraglottic obstruction is characterized by inspiratory stridor, because the negative pressure generated during inspiration tends to collapse relatively soft supraglottic structures. Laryngomalacia is the most common cause of supraglottic obstruction and the most common cause of neonatal stridor in general. The cause of laryngomalacia remains unestablished, although most investigators implicate neuromuscular immaturity as the likely cause.[3,4] Mild laryngomalacia is the only cause of newborn stridor that can be appropriately managed without specialist referral, but must be diagnosed with a high degree of certainty. Symptoms classically include a high-pitched, sometimes staccato stridor that worsens when the child is agitated and/or supine. Endoscopic evaluation typically reveals prolapse of the epiglottis and/or the

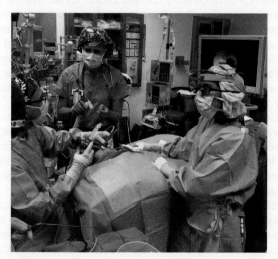

Fig. 2. Operative endoscopy before a tracheotomy. The examiner, anesthetist, and room staff are able to visualize lesions obstructing the airway as a magnified, high-resolution image.

Table 2
Common causes of neonatal stridor by anatomic subsite

Anatomic Subsite	Pathologic Condition	Notes
Supraglottic larynx	Laryngomalacia	Most common cause of newborn stridor
		Mild cases are self-limited and do not require surgical consultation
	Vallecular cysts	
	Saccular cysts	
	Masses	Lymphatic malformations most common
Glottic larynx	Webs	Hoarseness and stridor
	Clefts	Stridor present only when associated with significant redundancy of mucosa
	Vocal fold immobility	May be associated with Chiari malformation
Subglottic larynx	Subglottic stenosis or cysts	Can be congenital or acquired (after prolonged intubation)
	Masses	Hemangiomas most commonly present at 3–4 mo of age
Trachea	Tracheomalacia Primary	Because of abnormal ratio of membranous to cartilaginous tracheal wall
	Secondary	Extrinsic compression from vascular anomalies (anomalous innominate, double aortic arch, pulmonary artery sling)
		Collapse due to presence of tracheoesophageal fistula
	Stenosis	Congenitally complete cartilaginous tracheal rings, or intubation injury

cuneiform cartilages into the airway. Other common findings include curling of the epiglottis upon itself and webbing of the aryepiglottic folds (**Fig. 3**). The severity of laryngomalacia is judged primarily by the degree of impairment of feeding and weight gain, and the presence of respiratory distress and/or apneic events. Symptoms usually resolve spontaneously by 12 to 24 months of age, but active management can reduce symptoms. Side positioning or semiprone positioning may be helpful in reducing sleep symptoms. Medical treatment of laryngopharyngeal reflux may also be considered, because there is an association between the 2 disorders. However, there has yet to be a randomized controlled trial examining the effect of acid-reducing medication on laryngomalacia symptoms, and there is no clear evidence that surgery for laryngomalacia reduces the frequency of reflux.[5,6] Providers may also consider instituting a high-calorie formula for patients with poor weight gain. In rare cases, supraglottoplasty is recommended to divide the aryepiglottic folds and reduce the cuneiform cartilages.[7] Patients with symptoms of aspiration and those being considered for supraglottoplasty should undergo a preoperative video swallow assessment, because aspiration may occur because of the pathologic condition or occasionally because of the surgical intervention.

Congenital cysts of the larynx are another supraglottic cause of neonatal stridor that can mimic laryngomalacia by causing prolapse of the epiglottis into the airway. Such lesions may originate in the vallecula (**Fig. 4**) or in the saccule of the laryngeal ventricle (**Fig. 5**). These cysts can easily be decompressed or marsupialized, but have a propensity to recur, and complete resection at the time of diagnosis is preferable. They are usually treated by excising the cyst and cauterizing the base deep to the vallecular mucosa.

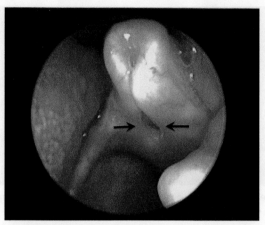

Fig. 3. Laryngomalacia. The epiglottis is seen curled upon itself. Arrows indicate webbing of aryepiglottic folds.

Glottic Obstruction

Glottic obstruction is usually due to a fixed lesion such as bilateral vocal fold immobility or laryngeal web. The associated stridor will usually be biphasic. Bilateral vocal fold paralysis is usually idiopathic, but may be due to an abnormality of the central nervous system, such as Chiari malformation, cerebral palsy, or hydrocephalus. In fact, stridor due to vocal fold paralysis can occasionally be the first presenting symptom of Chiari malformation.[8] In such cases, the stridor may improve with the correction of the central nervous system pathologic condition. Cases in which the paralysis is not reversible often require surgical intervention, which may include some combination of posterior laryngeal grafting, posterior vocal fold resection, or tracheotomy. In contrast, unilateral vocal fold paralysis results in stridor that, if present, is very mild and often improves in idiopathic cases. This disorder has been

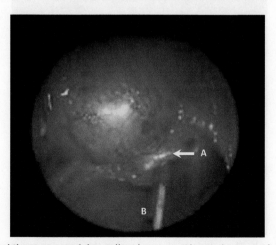

Fig. 4. Epiglottis (*A*) compressed by vallecular cyst. Airway is secured by endotracheal tube (*B*).

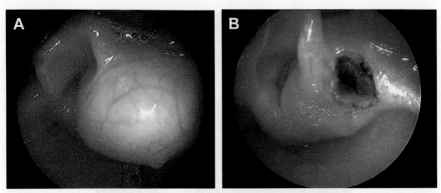

Fig. 5. (*A*) Laryngeal compression due to lateral saccular cyst. (*B*) Compression of larynx relieved following excision of cyst and laser cautery of its base.

reported to occur in more than 30% of patent ductus ligations examined postoperatively regardless of symptoms.[9] Laryngeal webs result from failure of the larynx to completely recanalize during embryogenesis (**Fig. 6**). In contrast to bilateral vocal fold paralysis, dysphonia is a prominent presenting symptom. This disorder may be associated with 22q11 deletion syndrome.[10] Management usually includes division of the web and stenting as well as laryngeal expansion with cartilage grafting.

Subglottic Obstruction

Subglottic obstruction will usually result in biphasic, predominantly inspiratory stridor. Subglottic stenosis may be congenital or acquired, even in the newborn period. In congenital cases, the cricoid cartilage is often elliptical (**Fig. 7**). Such cases can often

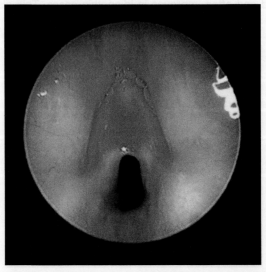

Fig. 6. Laryngeal web. These lesions always involve the anterior commissure, resulting in dysphonia. The more the lesion extends posteriorly, the greater the degree of stridor.

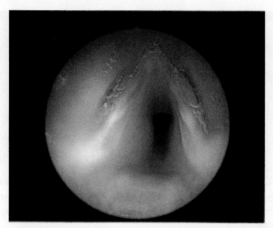

Fig. 7. Congenital subglottic stenosis. Patient has no history of endotracheal intubation. Note the elliptical shape of subglottic (cricoid cartilage).

be managed conservatively if the stridor is not severe, because the narrowed segment of the airway grows with the patient. Occasionally, division and grafting of the cricoid are necessary and may be performed using cartilage from the rib or thyroid cartilage. Acquired cases, most often due to prolonged endotracheal intubation in premature infants, have a less favorable prognosis and more often require some combination of serial balloon dilation, laryngotracheal cartilage grafting, and tracheotomy (**Fig. 8**).

Preterm infants who have been intubated may also develop progressive biphasic stridor due to subglottic cysts that slowly increase in size (**Fig. 9**). These lesions may be multiple, but usually respond quite well to laser or mechanical excision. The subglottis is also a site of predilection for infantile hemangiomas (**Fig. 10**). These lesions will rapidly increase in size during the first few weeks of age, with a presentation similar to that of the lesions above. Once diagnosed, subglottic hemangiomas usually respond well to medical therapy with propranolol, although refractory lesions may need to be addressed with steroid injection or surgical excision.[11]

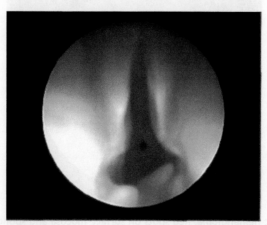

Fig. 8. Acquired subglottic stenosis in a patient with history of prematurity and endotracheal intubation.

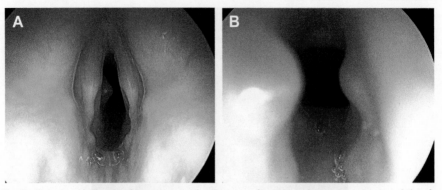

Fig. 9. Cysts in subglottis of a patient with a history of prematurity and intubation. (*A*) Left-sided cyst visible from above glottis. (*B*) Closeup view reveals second subglottic cyst slightly deeper on right side.

Tracheal Obstruction

Tracheal obstruction will usually result in a predominantly expiratory stridor as increased intrathoracic pressure predisposes the trachea to collapse during expiration. Tracheal obstruction may be due to primary tracheomalacia, secondary tracheomalacia (compression of trachea, usually vascular), and tracheal stenosis. Primary tracheomalacia results from a reduced ratio of cartilaginous to membranous trachea, resulting in flattening of the affected area due to lack of support. This finding is particularly common in cases of tracheoesophageal fistula (**Fig. 11**). Although it often improves over time, severe primary tracheomalacia occasionally must be managed with a tracheotomy to bypass the collapsing segment. Secondary tracheomalacia is most commonly due to vascular ring (double aortic arch, or right arch with left ligamentum arteriosum; **Fig. 12**), aberrant innominate artery, aberrant right subclavian artery, or pulmonary artery sling. Depending on the pathologic condition, the compression can be relieved either by suspension of the offending vessel or by surgical correction

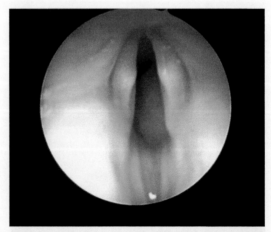

Fig. 10. Subglottic hemangioma. Red spots on surface mucosa and spongy texture are the key to diagnosis. Biopsy is rarely necessary, but intraoperative steroid injection is a good adjunct to medical therapy with propranolol.

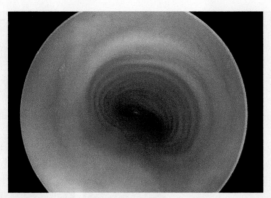

Fig. 11. Tracheomalacia in a patient with tracheoesophageal fistula. The trachea has a classic "fish-mouth" appearance.

of the vascular anomaly. It should be noted that the aberrant right subclavian artery may also cause significant esophageal compression, and that the association of pulmonary artery sling with tracheal stenosis has been reported to be as high as 50%.[12] Tracheal stenosis is usually due to a tracheal segment in which complete tracheal rings replace the usually membranous posterior wall (**Fig. 13**). Unless exceedingly mild, this condition must be surgically corrected by slide tracheoplasty. Tracheal sources of stridor often require multidisciplinary treatment from a variety of aerodigestive specialists, including pediatric otolaryngologists, pulmonologists, gastroenterologists, cardiothoracic surgeons, and speech and swallow therapists.

REPRESENTATIVE CASES
Case 1

A concerned mother brings her 4-week-old son to clinic with noisy breathing. He is the product of a full-term birth to a primipara mother, with no perinatal complications or concerning family history. He has had noisy breathing since birth, which is most noticeable when feeding or laying on his back. He does have relatively frequent spit ups, but is able to take 4 ounces of formula in under 10 minutes, and does not have coughing episodes while feeding. He has not had any cyanotic episodes and is gaining weight appropriately. He does have noisy breathing when sleeping in the supine

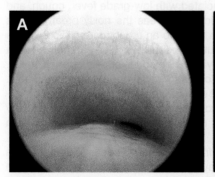
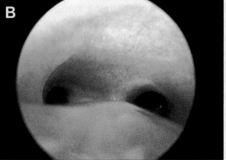

Fig. 12. (*A*) Posterior tracheal compression superior to carina due to double aortic arch. (*B*) Airway appears more patent immediately inferior to the area of vascular compression.

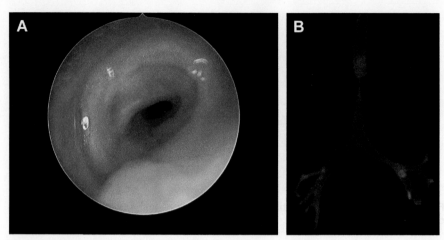

Fig. 13. Tracheal stenosis due to complete tracheal rings. (*A*) Endoscopic appearance. (*B*) Three-dimensional CT reconstruction.

position, but has not been noted to have pauses during sleep. On examination, he is of above-average body mass index and is well appearing, with no dysmorphic features, no skin lesions, no murmurs or rubs, clear lung fields, and a grossly normal neurologic examination. He does have intermittent high-pitched inspiratory stridor when supine or excited, in addition to mild stertor and mild subcostal retractions. His stridor and stertor do appear to diminish when he is placed on his side or held in the prone position.

This example is classic for mild laryngomalacia. The child's successful feeding and steady weight gain, as well as the absence of cyanotic episodes and sleep disturbance, are reassuring. If the diagnosis is in doubt, it may be confirmed in the otolaryngology office by FFL, and the patient can subsequently be followed in the outpatient primary care setting until the issue resolves with further growth and maturation. Conversely, poor weight gain and persistent airway distress should prompt further evaluation by the otolaryngologist.

Case 2

A 2-month-old girl is brought to clinic with 3 weeks of increasingly loud high-pitched breathing. This stridor had initially been associated with low-grade fever, cough, and rhinorrhea; however, these symptoms subsided, whereas the noisy breathing has continued to progress. She has already been taken to an urgent care clinic 2 weeks ago and treated with azithromycin and albuterol nebulizers. Her parents report a normal voice, snoring but no apnea, and no cyanotic episodes or respiratory distress. The remainder of her birth history, family history, and social history is unremarkable. Her physical examination reveals body weight at the 20th percentile, moderate generalized hypotonia, biphasic stridor that is more pronounced during the inspiratory phase, normal cry, and mild supraclavicular retractions. There are no notable skin lesions.

This case differs in several important ways from case 1. This patient's stridor is of a different character (constant, biphasic), is delayed in its onset, and is progressive. She also has the additional finding of hypotonia. Given this constellation of symptoms, a central nervous system abnormality, such as Chiari malformation, should be high in the differential. Management options for her would include semiurgent outpatient referral to an otolaryngologist to include FFL, or inpatient admission for further monitoring during which otolaryngology consultation may be obtained.

Case 3

A 6-week-old baby boy is brought to clinic by his parents for concerns of poor feeding and weight gain. His prenatal course had been complicated by premature rupture of membranes, with delivery at 32 weeks' gestation and subsequent 5-week stay in the neonatal intensive care unit. He had been intubated for 2 weeks after birth, before being extubated and weaned to room air. He was discharged without evidence of stridor, but has since had 2 episodes of croup that improved with courses of steroids. Even with treatment, however, his symptoms of noisy breathing and barky cough have never completely cleared. He has not gained any weight since leaving the hospital. Examination is significant for weight below the fifth percentile after adjusting for prematurity, mild subcostal retractions at rest, biphasic (predominantly inspiratory) stridor, and raised red lesions at the right mandibular angle and left parotid area.

Any newborn with a history of intubation and subsequent stridor, especially with barky cough, likely has fixed subglottic pathologic condition. The differential diagnosis in this case should include subglottic stenosis or subglottic cysts based on the history of prematurity and intubation, as well as subglottic hemangioma, given the prematurity and the skin lesions. All of these lesions present with a delay in onset, and none can be ruled out based on clinical presentation. In particular, the presence of hemangioma in the "beard" distribution increases the likelihood of such a lesion in the airway.[13] Regardless of the precise origin of his subglottic lesion, this child has a history and physical examination inconsistent with benign laryngomalacia and should be referred for expedient otolaryngologist assessment. The fact that the child also has failure to thrive suggests that he would benefit from admission to the hospital, with inpatient otolaryngologic consultation at that time.

Case 4

A 2-month-old girl is evaluated in clinic for chronic cough, intermittent fevers, spit ups, and noisy breathing. She was born full term without complication, has no history of intubations, and has no significant family history. On further questioning, her cough is most severe during and after feeding. Her noisy breathing is intermittent, "panting" in nature, and is exacerbated by supine positioning, by feeding, and during crying. She has had several cyanotic episodes during which she appears to struggle to breath for intervals of approximately 10 seconds, and she additionally has pauses in her breathing during sleep. She has had poor weight gain and is below the fifth percentile for weight. On examination, she appears underweight, has moderately increased work of breathing, and has a low-pitched, sputtering stridor during expiration, with copious secretions. The remainder of her examination is remarkable for a systolic murmur.

In this case, the presence of failure to thrive and cyanotic spells already mandates urgent otolaryngology referral and/or inpatient admission. These symptoms coupled with (low-pitched) expiratory stridor, should raise concern for tracheal pathologic condition, such as primary tracheomalacia or extrinsic compression of the trachea. An H-type tracheoesophageal fistula can be associated with chronic aspiration as well as tracheomalacia in the absence of esophageal atresia, and might account for her expiratory stridor as well as her chronic cough and cyanotic episodes. Another diagnostic possibility is a vascular ring compressing the trachea that could additionally contribute to her systolic murmur. Appropriate consultations with otolaryngology and pulmonology, operative endoscopy, and appropriate imaging should be ordered as an inpatient.

SUMMARY

Newborns with stridor who present to an outpatient pediatric office may be effectively evaluated, triaged, and diagnosed by applying history-taking principles, and a directed physical examination guided by a firm anatomic understanding of the origins of stridor. By recognizing the features that distinguish the various causes of stridor in the newborn, referrals for assessment may be appropriately triaged to either the emergency department or, less urgently, the office-based otolaryngologist.

REFERENCES

1. Bedwell J, Zalzal G. Laryngomalacia. Semin Pediatr Surg 2016;25:119–22.
2. Holinger LD. Diagnostic endoscopy of the pediatric airway. Laryngoscope 1989; 99:346–8.
3. Thompson DM. Abnormal sensorimotor integrative function of the larynx in congenital laryngomalacia: a new theory of etiology. Laryngoscope 2007; 117(6 Pt 2 Suppl 114):1–33.
4. Munson PD, Saad AG, El-Jamal SM, et al. Submucosal nerve hypertrophy in congenital laryngomalacia. Laryngoscope 2011;121:627–9.
5. Thompson DM. Laryngomalacia: factors that influence disease severity and outcomes of management. Curr Opin Otolaryngol Head Neck Surg 2010;18:564–70.
6. Hartl TT, Chadha NK. A systematic review of laryngomalacia and acid reflux. Otolaryngol Head Neck Surg 2012;147:619–26.
7. McCaffer C, Blackmore K, Flood LM. Laryngomalacia: is there an evidence base for management? J Laryngol Otol 2017;131:946–54.
8. Yousif S, Walsh M, Burns H. Bilateral vocal cord palsy causing stridor as the only symptom of syringomyelia and Chiari I malformation, a case report. Int J Surg Case Rep 2016;25:28–32.
9. Engeseth MS, Olsen NR, Maeland S, et al. Left vocal cord paralysis after patent ductus arteriosus ligation: a systematic review. Paediatr Respir Rev 2017;27: 74–85.
10. Sacca R, Zur KB, Crowley TB, et al. Association of airway abnormalities with 22q11.2 deletion syndrome. Int J Pediatr Otorhinolaryngol 2017;96:11–4.
11. Darrow DH. Management of infantile hemangiomas of the airway. Otolaryngol Clin North Am 2018;51:133–46.
12. Monnier P. Congenital tracheal anomalies. In: Monnier P, editor. Pediatric airway surgery. Berlin: Springer; 2011. p. 157–82.
13. Orlow S, Isakoff M, Blei F. Increased risk of symptomatic hemangiomas of the airway in association with cutaneous hemangiomas in a "beard" distribution. J Pediatr 1997;131:643–6.

Care of the Neonatal Intensive Care Unit Graduate after Discharge

Ricki F. Goldstein, MD[a],*, William F. Malcolm, MD[b]

KEYWORDS

- Infant, premature • Infant, newborn • Neonatal intensive care • Medical complexity
- Follow-up • Complex care • Pediatric care

KEY POINTS

- Premature and critically ill term infants are often discharged from the NICU with a variety of ongoing medical problems including: chronic lung disease; growth, nutrition, and feeding problems; and neurologic injury.
- At discharge, NICU graduates may be dependent on technology such as supplemental oxygen, tracheostomy, mechanical ventilation, surgically placed feeding tube and feeding pump, and various types of monitors.
- Primary care physicians must have special knowledge and understanding of the medical complications of NICU graduates to coordinate their post-discharge care and provide then with an effective medical home.

INTRODUCTION: POST-DISCHARGE CARE

Every primary care provider (PCP) who follows neonatal intensive care unit (NICU) graduates in their practice must be knowledgeable about the child's neonatal course and understand the various morbidities they have experienced. Providers should be familiar with the treatments for medical problems still present at discharge, be able to troubleshoot the technology that the infant is dependent on, and be able to co-ordinate the complicated care that they require. This Review will examine the most common post-discharge medical problems that may be present in former premature and critically ill term infants and inform the PCP about expected outcomes and possible new problems that may be encountered.

Disclosure Statement: The authors have no relationships with a commercial company that has a direct financial interest in the subject matter or materials discussed in this article.
[a] Pediatric Complex Care Program for Infants and Children, NICU Graduate Clinic, Department of Pediatrics/Neonatology, Kentucky Children's Hospital/University of Kentucky, 138 Leader Avenue, Lexington, KY 40508, USA; [b] Special Infant Care Follow-up Program, Department of Pediatrics/Neonatology, Duke University Medical Center, Box 2739, Durham, NC 27710, USA
* Corresponding author.
E-mail address: ricki.goldstein@uky.edu

Few outpatient clinics provide comprehensive medical follow-up for the myriad of medical problems still present at discharge in NICU graduates. Follow-up clinics for NICU graduates, in general, provide periodic developmental evaluations for high-risk infants and arrange intervention services when needed. A few will offer primary care and/or more specialized medical care (eg, weaning oxygen, adjusting or weaning off medications), Eligibility for NICU follow-up varies by center with respect to gestational age and/or birth weight and/or primary medical problems. However, many NICUs do not have their own follow-up clinic either for medical or developmental care. Instead, multiple subspecialty follow-up appointments are frequently scheduled at discharge (**Table 1**). It then becomes the responsibility of the PCP to integrate information from all subspecialists and coordinate care for the infant and family.[1,2]

Expectations of the PCP and Caregivers

Expectations of PCPs who care for medically complex NICU graduates are quite high. These include up-to-date knowledge and understanding of:

1. Neonatal technologies and therapies
2. Drug doses and indications
3. Laboratory tests that need to be followed
4. Indications for special formulas and recipes for adjusting calories
5. Various types of equipment (supplemental oxygen, nasogastric tube, gastrostomy tube [GT], ventriculoperitoneal [VP] shunt, ostomy, pulse oximeter, apnea monitor, tracheostomy, ventilator) and ability to recognize and troubleshoot problems

Parents are expected to understand the complex medical problems and needs of their NICU graduate, which include:

1. Multiple medications with fractional dosing and variable dosing intervals
2. Complicated feeding strategies and schedules, often throughout the day and night
3. Poor state regulation and sensitivity to sensory stimulation
4. Increased susceptibility to infection
5. Multiple subspecialty appointments
6. Multiple intervention services provided in and out of the home
7. Simultaneously, parents are expected to continue with their prior responsibilities (eg, care for siblings, return to work) despite having little or no respite time. They may also be struggling financially because of lost income

To provide optimal care for a medically complex infant, the PCP needs to have complete information about all medical problems and expectations at the time of discharge. PCPs should confirm that the parents are familiar with this content as well. A list of this content is included in **Table 2**. If information is missing from the discharge summary, the discharging physician should be contacted.

RESPIRATORY PROBLEMS AFTER NEONATAL INTENSIVE CARE UNIT DISCHARGE

Respiratory problems of NICU graduates may be congenital or acquired. Although the etiologies of problems in premature and term infants differ, treatments are similar. The most common respiratory problems are the sequelae of prolonged mechanical ventilation (bronchopulmonary dysplasia [BPD] or chronic lung disease) and congenital anomalies of the lungs and airways (congenital diaphragmatic hernia [CDH], tracheoesophageal fistula [TEF], pulmonary hypoplasia, tracheo- and/or bronchomalacia). Pulmonary hypertension may develop and persist in infants with

Table 1
Subspecialty clinic follow-up for medical problems in NICU graduates

Specialty Clinic	Medical Problems Followed
Pulmonary	Bronchopulmonary dysplasia Reactive airway disease Home ventilator management Interstitial disease
Cardiology	Patent ductus arteriosus Other congenital heart disease Pulmonary hypertension
Neurology	Seizures Spasticity Neuromuscular disease
Nephrology	Hypertension Renal failure Kidney anomaly
Endocrine	Hypothyroidism Adrenal insufficiency Hypopituitarism
Gastroenterology	Gastro-esophageal reflux Cholestatic jaundice Short gut syndrome Constipation
Infectious diseases	Cytomegalovirus infection Herpes simplex infection Other TORCH infections Perinatal human immunodeficiency virus exposure Perinatal hepatitis C exposure
Pediatric surgery	Congenital diaphragmatic hernia Surgical necrotizing enterocolitis Bowel atresia Nissen fundoplication Gastrostomy tube Hernias Ostomy
Urology	Hydronephrosis Vesico-ureteral reflux Meningomyelocele Other genital-urologic malformation
Otolaryngology	Tracheostomy Stridor Vocal cord dysfunction
Neurosurgery	Hydrocephalus Ventriculoperitoneal shunt Meningomyelocele
Orthopedic surgery	Hip dysplasia Vertebral anomalies Club foot Meningomyelocele Other skeletal dysplasia
Genetics	Suspected or documented chromosomal syndrome Metabolic disorder

(continued on next page)

Table 1
(continued)

Specialty Clinic	Medical Problems Followed
Ophthalmology	Retinopathy of prematurity
	Cortical visual impairment
	Cataract
	Glaucoma
Audiology	Failed hearing screen
	Risk of progressive hearing loss
Physical therapy	Abnormal muscle tone (decreased or increased)
	Torticollis/plagiocephaly
Occupational therapy	Brachial plexus injury
	Feeding (oral aversion)
	Other sensory integration problem
Speech/feeding	Feeding problem (dysphagia, swallowing problem)
	Vocal cord dysfunction
	Cleft lip and/or palate
Dietician (often in specialty clinic)	Special formulas and/or diets
	Advancement of gastrostomy tube feeds
	Failure to thrive

BPD, CDH, pulmonary hypoplasia or meconium aspiration syndrome. The most common reason for readmission in extremely low-birth-weight (ELBW) infants is respiratory problems.

Bronchopulmonary Dysplasia

1. Definition of bronchopulmonary dysplasia (BPD)[3]

Table 2
Necessary information for PCPs about NICU graduate

Category	Specifics
Prescribed medications	• Explanation of the "indication" for each medication and the problem it is treating
	• Whether the dose is calculated per kg of weight or is a standard dose
	• What to do if the infant misses a dose or vomits a dose
	• Where and when to refill the medication
	• Whether the medication needs to be adjusted for weight gain and, if so, how often
Feeding	• Indications for special formula
	• Mixing instructions for 2, 3, and 4 ounces of formula
	• Name of alternate formula (eg, Neocate/Elecare, Neosure/Enfacare, Alimentum/Nutramigen) to prevent substitution error
	• Local source for special formulas (pharmacy, grocery store)
	• How long special formula should be continued and what formula to transition to
Subspecialty clinic referrals	• Which clinic is for which problem?
	• What will be done at first visit (if repeat laboratory tests, can PCP order and send results to subspecialists)?
	• Which clinic to reschedule immediately if missed (eg, ophthalmology clinic for active ROP)

a. Old versus new BPD
  i. Old BPD refers to damage caused to lungs and airway by mechanical ventilation and/or oxygen resulting in inflammation and fibrosis. This type of BPD may occur in premature and term infants, and has been greatly reduced by the administration of surfactant and high frequency ventilation.
  ii. New BPD refers to abnormal or arrest in lung development (fewer and larger alveoli) and decreased microvascular development in ELBW infants.
b. Premature infants with severe respiratory distress syndrome, pulmonary interstitial emphysema, congenital pneumonia, or pulmonary hypoplasia are most likely to develop BPD.
c. Criteria for diagnosis in premature infants in the Vermont Oxford Network is the need for supplemental oxygen at 36 weeks post-menstrual age (PMA). Criteria for diagnosis in the NICHD Neonatal Research Network includes supplemental oxygen or any respiratory support at 36 weeks PMA.[4] Therefore, identification of an infant with BPD may vary from one NICU to another.
d. Diuretics and inhaled steroids are sometimes used to treat residual lung inflammation or fluid retention.
e. Full-term infants with meconium aspiration syndrome, CHD, or need for extracorporeal membrane oxygenation (ECMO) for another reason are the most likely to need treatment for BPD after discharge.
f. All infants with BPD are at increased risk of lower respiratory tract infections and need for rehospitalization during the first year of life.
g. Reactive airway disease (RAD)
  i. Infants with BPD have a high risk of developing RAD in infancy, and asthma in later childhood.
  ii. The most common symptoms are tachypnea either at rest or with exertion.
  iii. Occult RAD (ie, without wheezing) may be diagnosed based on response to a trial of bronchodilator treatment or results of pulmonary function testing.
h. Chronic home ventilation after discharge

Infants with severe BPD may require placement of a tracheostomy for prolonged mechanical ventilation at home. Timing of tracheostomy and age of discharge for infants receiving chronic mechanical ventilation varies among NICUs and often depends on the infant's clinical course, health care provider preferences, ability of the family to care for the infant at home, and medical resources (eg, home health nursing) in the community.

Congenital Anomalies of the Lungs and Airways

1. CDH/pulmonary hypoplasia
  a. CDH occurs when there is a defect in formation of one of the diaphragms, leading to herniation of the abdominal viscera into the pleural cavity on that side. This prevents normal growth and maturation of the lung parenchyma and pulmonary vasculature. This "hypoplasia" of the lungs results in pulmonary hypertension (PHTN) because of thickening of the muscular coat of arterioles, making these vessels more reactive to hypoxemia and acidosis. It is not a reason for premature birth (although it is often diagnosed in utero), so most infants are born at term or near term.
  b. Infants with CDH may recover completely after initial treatment in the NICU without residual lung problems, but most will develop some degree of chronic lung disease and have persistent PHTN requiring supplemental oxygen and other medications after discharge.

    c. Infants with premature and prolonged rupture of membranes often develop some degree of pulmonary hypoplasia due to oligohydramnios, which prevents normal growth of the lungs in utero. Premature infants born with pulmonary hypoplasia often require prolonged mechanical ventilation, develop significant BPD, and have associated PHTN. They are frequently discharged on supplemental oxygen and other medications.

2. Tracheoesophageal fistula
    a. TEF is a congenital malformation of the trachea and esophagus.
    b. There are three types of TEF, the most common being esophageal atresia with a fistula between the trachea and lower esophagus.
    c. Repair of this defect sometimes results in tracheal stenosis or an area of tracheomalacia (collapse) at the fistula site causing prolonged stridor.

3. Tracheo- and/or bronchomalacia
    Malacia or collapse of the proximal (trachea) or distal (bronchial) airways can result in stridor and increased work of breathing. This may be secondary to tracheal repair (as in TEF) or caused by an intrinsic weakness of the airway-supporting structures. Airway malacia almost always improves with growth of the child but may require prolonged ventilatory support (tracheostomy) during infancy and early childhood.

Pulmonary Hypertension

1. Some infants with severe BPD will develop secondary PHTN requiring increased oxygen and treatment with vasodilators (most commonly inhaled nitric oxide acutely followed by sildenafil chronically).
2. PHTN may develop before or after discharge from the NICU.
3. Infants with CDH or other etiology for pulmonary hypoplasia also often have significant PHTN requiring prolonged treatment after discharge.
4. Diagnosis of PHTN is made by evidence of increased pulmonary artery pressure (right ventricular hypertrophy, flattening of the intraventricular septum, tricuspid valve regurgitation) evident by echocardiography or cardiac catheterization.
5. This serious complication of BPD and other respiratory problems in term and preterm infants needs to be followed closely by a pediatric cardiologist and/or pulmonologist. Infants with PHTN will require periodic echocardiograms to determine if medications and oxygen should be weight adjusted or may be weaned.
6. Chronic aspiration (secondary to gastro-esophageal reflux disease [GERD] or swallowing problem) and infection should be prevented because they can exacerbate PHTN.

Follow-up of Infants with Bronchopulmonary Dysplasia

1. Infants with BPD with or without PHTN (ie, home on supplemental oxygen) should be followed in an NICU Graduate Clinic, and/or by a Pediatric Pulmonary Clinic, to determine when supplemental oxygen and medications should be adjusted or weaned.
    a. Good growth and medical stability should be established before decreasing the treatment.
    b. Oxygen is often weaned off first during the day and then at night.
    c. Infants who are unable to wean from oxygen as expected, should be evaluated for PHTN, if not already diagnosed.
2. Respiratory syncytial virus (RSV) prophylaxis with Synagis.[3]
    a. Eligibility for RSV prophylaxis changes each year. The most recent criteria are:

i. Infants born ≤28 weeks gestation who are less than 12 months old
ii. Infants less than 1 year old with hemodynamically significant congenital heart disease
iii. Children less than 2 years old with BPD who continue to require medical intervention (supplemental oxygen, chronic corticosteroid, or diuretic therapy)
iv. Children with pulmonary abnormality or neuromuscular disease that impairs the ability to clear secretions from the upper and lower airways in the first year of life
   b. Influenza vaccine—all infants with BPD greater than 6 months of age and their immediate family and other caretakers should receive a flu shot

FEEDING, GROWTH, AND NUTRITION IN THE NEONATAL INTENSIVE CARE UNIT GRADUATE

Feeding problems in the NICU are frequently a barrier for discharge.[5,6] These difficulties often persist, or even worsen, once the infant has transitioned to the home environment and are among the most common parental stressors post-discharge.[7] Whether these feeding problems are caused by physiologic immaturity in premature infants, comorbidities of prematurity, or a complication of an underlying diagnosis requiring NICU admission (eg, respiratory, cardiac, neurologic, genetic), they are also a primary reason for readmission.[8–10] It is important for the PCP to be aware of the different stages of feeding skills and factors that may interfere with their normal progression.

Common Feeding Problems by Age (Age Corrected for Prematurity in Premature Infants)

Birth to 3 months:
1. Oral feeding skills are driven by primitive reflexes. Rooting, sucking, and swallowing are the basic skills newborns possess to breast or bottle feed shortly after birth. Protective reflexes including gagging, coughing, and the laryngeal chemoreflex provide safety measures to allow for successful early feeding.
2. Any disturbance in the autonomic nervous system, as may be seen in extremely premature birth or neurologic injury, may interfere with this involuntary process.
3. Comorbidities such as BPD, necrotizing enterocolitis (NEC), or GERD that may interrupt normal breathing and feeding schedules (eg, nil per os, continuous feedings), may negatively impact the natural progression of early feeding.

3 to 6 months:
1. Feeding becomes a voluntary activity. Primitive reflexes integrate with brain development and the upper aerodigestive tract grows to resemble that of an adult by 5 months of age. With this, along with developing head control, a transition to solid foods is supported.
2. The infant must now coordinate the movement of food from the anterior oral cavity to the posterior pharynx to swallow, a much different eating pattern than sucking liquid from a nipple directly into the pharynx.
3. Oral exploration is abundant (hands, feet, clothing, toys to mouth) and works to desensitize the tongue to accept more textured foods.
4. Delays in head control or gross motor skills, as well as negative oral experiences (eg, orogastric and endotracheal tubes, suctioning, GERD), may disrupt this transition to voluntary feeding and may lead to oral aversion or difficulty in transition to textured foods.

6 to 9 months:

1. Infants begin eating thicker solids and finger foods, further increasing sensory stimulation with visual, auditory, tactile, taste, and smell contributing to the feeding process.
2. A more mature "munching" chewing pattern develops with vertical movement of the mandible and tongue protrusion coordinated with lip closure to retrieve food and keep it in the mouth.
3. Gross and fine motor skills begin to become more important as upright seating becomes the preferred feeding position, and reaching out and holding on to finger foods emerges.

9 to 12 months:

1. Infants begin eating mixed textures, including table foods. Infants also develop a more mature "rotary" chewing pattern required to shred more textured foods.
2. More advanced gross and fine motor skills are necessary for trunk stability, self-feeding, and initiating drinking from a cup.

Breastfeeding in Neonatal Intensive Care Unit Graduates

Problem:

1. Breastfeeding rates post-discharge from the NICU are low.
2. Only about one-fourth of very low-birth-weight infants are still receiving human milk at 6 months of age.
3. Less than one-fourth are actually feeding at the breast at the time of discharge.[11]

Barriers to maintaining breastfeeding in the home environment:

1. Common concerns of mothers and providers:
   a. Unknown volume of milk ingested when breastfeeding
      i. By using a breastfeeding scale to measure pre-/post-breastfeeding weights, mothers and providers can get a sense of how much breast milk the infant takes with each breastfeed, which will guide how much expressed breast milk or formula should be given by bottle or tube.[12]
      ii. Lactation specialists and skilled nurses should be available during discharge teaching, as well as post-discharge, to help support the mother and teach techniques to maximize efficiency at the breast.
      iii. Breastfeeding positions that help support the infant's head, neck, and shoulders will allow for more effective latch and transfer of milk. This will become less necessary as the infant shows increased gross motor strength and endurance.[13]
   b. Concern that the mother can keep up her milk supply once the infant is home
      i. A common misconception is that mothers of infants in the NICU only need to use a breast pump because they are separated from their infants, and, once their baby is discharged to home, they will feed their infant on demand and discontinue pumping.
      ii. Studies have shown that continuing pumping in the home environment actually helps maintain the mother's supply and allows for the transfer of milk despite a weaker suck in those first few months after going home from the NICU.[11]
   c. Whether human milk provides adequate nutrition for a growing premature or high-risk infant
      i. There is some controversy about whether or not exclusive human milk feedings provide adequate nutrition for premature and sick term infants post-discharge, if they are taking sufficient volumes.

ii. Because most very premature and high-risk infants sustain poor growth in the NICU and need to establish some catch-up growth post-discharge, breast milk alone usually has insufficient energy, protein, and minerals, such as calcium and phosphorous, to meet their nutritional needs after discharge (**Table 3**).

Growth in the Neonatal Intensive Care Unit Graduate

Poor growth is a common outcome of the NICU hospitalization, with postnatal growth failure the norm, and need for "catch-up growth" post-discharge the expectation.[14]

Reasons for growth failure:
1. Difficulty with feeding, food absorption, or tolerance.
2. Increased metabolic demands of conditions such as BPD, congestive heart failure, and hypertonia requiring increased caloric intake to establish a return to standardized growth curves.

Use of Growth Curves

1. Standardized World Health Organization (0–24 months) and Centers for Disease Control and Prevention (24–36 months) growth charts with weight, length, and head circumference plotted according to corrected age should be recorded at all follow-up visits of premature infants.
2. Weight should continue to be adjusted for degree of prematurity for 24 months, with length and head circumference adjusted closer to 36 months.[15]
3. Weight-to-length ratio is also an important growth parameter to monitor in premature infants, because body composition in very premature infants acquiring catch-up growth is a strong predictor for the development of the metabolic syndrome later in life.

Goals for Growth Post-discharge

1. The American Academy of Pediatrics recommends that the goal for growth of premature infants should match fetal growth rate and body composition.[15]
2. "Extra-uterine growth restriction" is a well-known entity in premature infants and is usually dealt with by altering calories of expressed breast milk or formula.
3. Post-discharge diet should also meet protein and mineral needs for linear growth, as rapid weight gain without an increase in length leads to increased adiposity and future risks for hypertension, cardiovascular disease, and type II diabetes.[16,17]

| Table 3 | | | | |
| Dietary intake requirements in infants based on 150 mL/kg/d | | | | |
	Energy	Protein	Calcium	Phosphorus
Recommended for premature infants after discharge	120–130 kcal/kg/d	2.5–3.1 g/kg/d	70–140 mg/kg/d	35–90 mg/kg/d
Human milk without fortification	100 kcal/kg	1.5 g/kg	44 mg/kg	14 mg/kg
Term infant formula	100 kcal/kg	2 g/kg	80 mg/kg	42 mg/kg
Post-discharge premature formula	110 kcal/kg	3.1 g/kg	117 mg/kg	69 mg/kg

4. Post-discharge diet should correct for deficiencies of micronutrients (essential fatty acids, iron), as well as calcium and phosphorous, protein and energy.
5. Conditions with increased metabolic demands and increase energy/protein needs include:
   a. Bronchopulmonary dysplasia
   b. Congenital heart disease, especially if uncorrected with pulmonary overflow
   c. Surgical NEC, especially if resulting in short bowel syndrome
   d. History of intrauterine growth restriction
6. Goals for growth
   a. Before term corrected age: weight increase of 18 g/kg/d and head circumference growth of 0.9 cm/wk.
   b. After term corrected age and over 2 kg: 25 to 30 g/d, length to match the weight velocity, and head circumference growth closer to 0.5 cm/wk.

Recommendations for Achieving Energy, Protein, and Mineral Needs

For premature infants receiving human milk:
1. Feed at the breast a couple of times daily and then supplement with either fortified expressed breastmilk by bottle or 2 to 4 feedings of a transitional preterm formula (Enfacare or Neosure concentrated to at least 24 cal/oz).
2. The growth chart and bone health indices (calcium, phosphorus, alkaline phosphatase) should be followed monthly until catch-up growth has been established. Simply fortifying the expressed breast milk with formula powder often does not meet the protein and mineral needs for these high-risk infants.
3. If an infant is not demonstrating appropriate linear growth to match weight gain or if bone health becomes a concern (phosphorus <4.2 mg/dL, alkaline phosphatase >400 IU/L), supplementing with 2 to 4 pure formula feedings daily for increased protein is recommended.

For infants receiving infant formula feedings:
1. Infant formulas have standard mixing instructions without regard to specific needs of the NICU graduate.
   a. Post-discharge premature infant formulas (Enfacare, Neosure) mixed to standard dilution are 22 cal/oz. Term infant standard and specialty formulas are 19 and 20 cal/oz. Specific formula recipes are available for increasing caloric density up to 30 cal/oz.
   b. The post-discharge premature formulas have increased protein and mineral content (especially calcium and phosphorous) intended for former premature infants; however, many NICU graduates are discharged home on special term infant formulas, regardless of gestational age at birth, because of comorbidities (eg, GERD, NEC, short gut) leading to poor linear growth and or osteopenia.
   c. As with the breastfed NICU graduate, all growth parameters need to be followed closely, and caloric density increased as tolerated to establish steady, symmetric catch-up growth.
   d. When increasing to 27 cal/oz or higher, the high osmolality can lead to intolerance with constipation (especially if on diuretics), malabsorption, or high serum calcium and phosphorous levels. These parameters should be closely monitored.

For infants >1-year adjusted age:
1. Many very premature or chronically sick term infants have not yet established appropriate catch-up growth in the first year of life. These children often have oral feeding difficulties as well.

2. Complete balanced milk-based toddler formulas, as well as specialty toddler formulas, can be used to supplement their age-appropriate diet or as a complete diet for tube-fed children.
   a. Toddler formulas are available as 30 cal/oz, and sometimes 45 cal/oz, to assist with the continuation of catch-up growth in the second year of life.
3. Older children may also benefit from blended diets of different food groups. A Pediatric Gastroenterology Clinic and/or dietician can help with appropriate food selection.

NEUROLOGIC PROBLEMS IN NEONATAL INTENSIVE CARE UNIT GRADUATES

Term and preterm infants may be born with a variety of malformations of the central nervous system or may develop ischemic damage or bleeding in the brain before birth or in the neonatal period due to prematurity, birth trauma, or severe illness.[18,19] All suspected or documented brain malformations or injury result in the infant being at increased risk for abnormal neurodevelopment in infancy and early childhood.

Malformations of the Central Nervous System

1. Hydrocephalus, congenital, or acquired
   a. Congenital hydrocephalus
      i. Aqueductal stenosis
         Obstruction of the aqueduct, which connects the third and fourth ventricle, is the most common cause of congenital hydrocephalus. Blockage of the aqueduct causes progressive enlargement of the lateral and third ventricles, which eventually requires either a VP shunt to be placed, or, later in infancy, a third ventriculostomy to be performed. A shunt may be placed in the neonatal period or after initial NICU discharge.
      ii. Dandy-Walker malformation
         Dandy-Walker malformation is a congenital defect affecting the cerebellum, which can potentially impact a child's movements, behavior, or cognitive ability. A Dandy-Walker malformation can cause obstruction of the normal drainage of cerebrospinal fluid (CSF) from the fourth ventricle, resulting in a build-up of CSF with resultant hydrocephalus.
   b. Acquired hydrocephalus
      i. Post-hemorrhagic hydrocephalus
         Infants with bleeding inside the ventricles (grade 3 or 4 intraventricular hemorrhage [IVH]) in premature infants, or a choroid plexus bleed in term infants, can lead to obstruction of the drainage of CSF out of the ventricles as a result of blockage of the ventricular lining secondary to inflammation (ie, ventriculitis) or from blood obstructing the aqueduct. This post-hemorrhagic hydrocephalus may self-resolve over time or require a VP shunt for permanent drainage of the CSF.

Infants with a diagnosis of hydrocephalus in the newborn period, with or without a shunt, must be followed closely for abnormal growth of the head and signs of increased intracranial pressure (lethargy, irritability, emesis, sun-setting of eyes). Parents must also be educated about these signs as well as the clinical presentation of shunt failure (ie, increased intracranial pressure or swelling around the shunt tubing or entrance site) or shunt infection (same as shunt failure plus fever).

2. Neural tube defect (with or without hydrocephalus)

A neural tube defect (or meningomyelocele) is failure of closure of a portion of the neural tube during development with resultant exposure of the spinal cord. This type of defect is typically repaired in the first days after birth. Infants may have an associated Dandy-Walker malformation. Problems following repair may be progressive hydrocephalus requiring a shunt, wound dehiscence or infection, neurogenic bladder, and urinary tract infection (UTI). Parents are often required to perform a straight catheterization of the bladder one or more times per day to prevent urine retention and UTI. Infants should be followed closely for acceleration of head growth, neurologic deficits, and signs of UTI (fever, blood in or discoloration of urine). Close follow-up with the PCP is integrated with follow-up with other subspecialties such as Pediatric Neurosurgery, Urology, and Orthopedics.

3. Microcephaly

Microcephaly (head circumference below the 3rd percentile) can be caused by intrauterine viral infections such as cytomegalovirus and Zika early in pregnancy, or by other environmental toxins (eg, alcohol). Infants with microcephaly must be watched closely for muscle tone abnormality and developmental delay. Depending on the cause, other problems should be screened for (eg, deafness, visual impairment, congenital heart defects).

Ischemic Brain Injury

Ischemic brain injury may be global or focal. The most common ischemic-type injuries include:

Hypoxic-ischemic encephalopathy

Hypoxic-ischemic encephalopathy (HIE) is a clinical diagnosis when an infant has suffered a period of decreased blood and oxygen to the brain, resulting in depression at birth and an abnormal neurologic exam. HIE is categorized as mild, moderate, or severe using the Sarnat scoring for encephalopathy. Treatment with therapeutic hypothermia (either whole body or head) in the NICU is now standard of care for infants ≥36 weeks gestation with moderate or severe HIE. Following cooling and rewarming, the infant will have a brain magnetic resonance imaging (MRI) to determine the presence and extent of brain injury. The history of a normal MRI after cooling carries a good prognosis for normal developmental outcomes. Patterns of brain injury after HIE may be focal or global. Injury in the basal ganglia and/or thalamus or global ischemic injury (diffuse cystic encephalomalacia being the most severe) is associated with a poor neurologic outcome including cerebral palsy (CP). Seizures in the first few days in infants with HIE are not predictive of a poor outcome; however, persistent seizures after rewarming are a poor prognostic sign.

Middle cerebral artery infarct/other focal stroke

Middle cerebral artery (MCA) stroke is the most common focal ischemic injury in full-term infants. It often presents with apnea and/or seizures in the first 24 hours of life. An electroencephalogram may be consistent with a focal lesion but definitive diagnosis will be by MRI. Moderate-to-severe MCA stroke is associated with hemiplegic CP on the opposite side. Small strokes may have no long-term neurologic sequelae. Close follow-up is warranted and physical therapy should be ordered when asymmetry of muscle tone or movement is detected.

Other focal strokes can result from arteriolar emboli. This is most frequently found in infants treated with ECMO, but may be diagnosed in other infants as well (eg, infants with congenital heart disease). These infarcts may not be clinically apparent before discharge unless detected on an MRI. Affected infants may present with asymmetry of tone and movement in later infancy.

Periventricular leukomalacia
Periventricular leukomalacia (PVL) is the most common ischemic brain injury in premature infants, but is also seen in some term infants after cardiac surgery and prolonged time on cardiac bypass. PVL can be cystic or non-cystic. Cystic PVL most commonly manifests as cysts in the temporoparietal periventricular white matter on postnatal ultrasonography. The cysts are usually bilateral and are associated with the development of CP (diplegia or quadriplegia). Non-cystic PVL may be suspected on head ultrasound by the appearance of mild ventriculomegaly without former IVH. Follow-up MRI will demonstrate thinning of the periventricular white matter, which is also associated with the development of CP. PVL can also be diagnosed in the frontal area and the long-term outcome of this injury is less certain.

Hemorrhagic Brain Injury

Hemorrhage or bleeding can occur in the ventricles or parenchyma of the brain. The most common types of hemorrhages include:

1. Intraventricular hemorrhage (IVH)
   a. An IVH arises from the germinal matrix in premature infants. The germinal matrix is a very vascular area of the brain during development that disappears by 36 weeks gestation. Hypoperfusion and reperfusion injury in this subependymal area causes rupture of tiny capillaries and bleeding to occur. A grading system (grades I–IV) had previously been used to describe the type of IVH; this has now been replaced with a preference of description of the finding. The mildest IVH is limited to the germinal matrix (formerly grade 1 IVH). A more severe type is blood that extends into the ventricle but does not cause ventricular dilatation (formerly grade II IVH). Infants can also have bleeding that extends into the ventricle resulting in ventricular dilatation (formerly grade III IVH); this can result in post-hemorrhagic hydrocephalus. The most significant IVH occurs when blood is noted in the parenchyma usually adjacent to the ventricle (formerly grade IV IVH), which can lead to post-hemorrhagic hydrocephalus and/or a porencephalic intraparenchymal cyst. This type of hemorrhage may be the result of bleeding into an area of infarction. The PCP needs to closely monitor the head circumference of infants with severe IVH; if a child has not yet received a shunt, head ultrasounds should be repeated until the ventricular dilation resolves (see post-hemorrhagic hydrocephalus section above).
   b. Choroid plexus bleed
      In term infants, a choroid plexus bleed may occur with severe illness or birth trauma resulting in an IVH. This may also result in post-hemorrhagic hydrocephalus. The infant's head circumference should be followed, and ultrasound should be repeated periodically until the blood and ventricular dilatation, if present, resolves.

Other Neurologic Problems

Other neurologic problems that are common in NICU graduates include:

Seizures

a. Both term and preterm infants can develop seizures secondary to brain injury or infection. Efforts to wean off seizure medication may be unsuccessful before discharge, so many infants will be discharged on continuing seizure medications.

b. Follow-up with a pediatric neurologist should be scheduled to determine when the medication needs to be weight adjusted or weaned off. Seizure medication should not be stopped abruptly.

c. Parents should be educated in detecting signs of seizure activity, such as jerking of arms or legs (which is not stopped with restraint), eye deviation, or stiffening of the body. A seizure may be followed by a period of somnolence (post-ictal period).

d. Infants with brain injury are at risk of developing seizures after discharge, and parents should be aware of the signs and symptoms.

e. Fever in an infant can lower the seizure threshold so parents should be instructed on proper temperature control during times of illness and after immunizations.

Muscle tone abnormalities

Abnormalities of muscle tone (increased or decreased) are common in premature and sick term infants and may be transient in nature or persist and result in a diagnosis of CP. Some NICU follow-up clinics have physical therapists who will teach home exercise programs. If this is not available, infants with abnormal muscle tone should be referred for physical therapy after hospital discharge.

a. Hypotonia
1. The most common abnormality of muscle tone following discharge in an NICU graduate is hypotonia (low muscle tone), either central (just in the trunk) or generalized (in the trunk and extremities). Sometimes this is secondary to muscle wasting from poor nutrition and other times from weakness secondary to illness.
2. Truncal hypotonia is manifested early on by poor head control and poor prone skills and later by delay in reaching motor milestones (rolling, sitting, and walking). However, low muscle tone usually improves over time as the underlying chronic illness improves. This is particularly true for infants with BPD.
3. Significant generalized hypotonia can also be seen with severe brain injury (eg, HIE, severe IVH, particularly in the early months), cerebellar injury, and various genetic syndromes (eg, Prader-Willi, Trisomy 21).

b. Hypertonia
1. Transiently increased muscle tone, particularly in the lower extremities, is common in premature infants. These infants often have an imbalance in flexion and extension of various muscle groups from lack of movement and exercise. Mild-to-moderate hypertonia may improve over time with exercise and physical therapy.
2. Significant hypertonia in the extremities, particularly when coupled with decreased truncal tone and exaggerated primitive reflexes, may represent early precursors of CP.

Cerebral Palsy (CP)

a. Definition: NICU graduates who have experienced severe IVH, HIE, or other ischemic brain injury causing damage to the motor cortex or pathways may have persistent abnormalities of muscle tone and motor function known as cerebral palsy. Patterns of increased muscle tone can affect the upper and lower extremity on the same side (hemiplegia), both lower extremities (diplegia) or all 4 extremities (quadriplegia). CP is characterized as mild, moderate, or severe based on degree of functional impairment by the Gross Motor Function Score. Hypotonic CP is associated with ataxia.

b. Diagnosis and intervention: it is important for infants who have sustained significant brain injury to be followed closely for early signs of CP. This is best accomplished in an NICU follow-up clinic or by a pediatric neurologist. Appropriate early intervention with physical and occupational therapy will help to prevent contractures and maximize functional outcomes.

Sensory impairment

a. Vision problems

Retinopathy of prematurity (ROP)

- Characterized by abnormal growth of the retinal vessels with tortuosity and clumping.
- Occurs in premature infants to varying degrees depending on gestational age and severity of early illness.
- Severe stages of ROP, if not detected and treated, can result in retinal detachment and blindness. Less severe stages of ROP can result in either myopia or hyperopia requiring refraction.
- Because growth of the retinal vessels is not complete until approximately 44 weeks gestation, follow-up visits will often be scheduled for premature infants soon after discharge from the NICU.
- The PCP should be aware of the infant's ROP status and make sure that follow-up with an ophthalmologist is scheduled and attended.

Cortical visual impairment

- Results from injury to the occipital lobe of the brain or generalized ischemic damage to the cerebral cortex.
- Most commonly seen in term infants with HIE, infants born with microcephaly secondary to intrauterine infection or in utero ischemic damage, and kernicterus.
- Cortical visual impairment is not corrected by refraction (ie, glasses). However, visual therapy is usually available from early intervention programs to help infants accommodate to this disability.

b. Hearing problems

- Hearing loss in premature and term infants may be sensorineural, conductive, or mixed.
- Sensorineural hearing loss involves injury to the auditory nerve and can be genetic in origin or secondary to various medications or illnesses (TORCH infections, kernicterus).
- Conductive hearing loss is caused by a problem in conduction of sound through bone and inner ear. Premature infants, in particular, have an increased incidence of Eustachian tube dysfunction resulting in conductive hearing loss. Improvement in hearing can be achieved by inserting myringotomy tubes to drain fluid from the middle and inner ear. Premature infants with repeated otitis should be evaluated by a pediatric otolaryngologist to determine if tubes are indicated.
- Hearing loss in both premature and term infants may improve with hearing aids or cochlear implants. Close follow-up with a pediatric otolaryngologist is essential to maximize hearing before 1 year of age to maximize potential for language development.

Developmental delay

Risk for developmental problems in NICU graduates can be identified at the time of discharge. Infants with conditions associated with moderate to high risk of neurodevelopmental delay should be followed in an NICU follow-up clinic if available. These include:

1. Prematurity (please see article "Neurodevelopmental Follow-up of Preterm Infants: What is new?" by Elisabeth McGowan and Betty R. Vohr, in this issue.)
   a. Extremely low birth weight (<1000 g)
   b. Extreme prematurity (≤26 weeks gestation)
2. Serious neonatal illness/morbidity
   a. Bronchopulmonary dysplasia
   b. PHTN treated with nitric oxide
   c. Respiratory failure treated with ECMO
   d. Surgical NEC
3. Suspected or documented brain injury
   a. Severe IVH (grade 3 or 4)
   b. PVL/other stroke (eg, MCA)
   c. HIE
   d. Neonatal seizures
   e. Hydrocephalus (congenital or acquired)
   f. Central nervous system malformation
   g. Meningitis, encephalitis
4. Poor intrauterine environment
   a. Intrauterine growth restriction
   b. Neonatal abstinence syndrome
   c. Intrauterine viral infections

TECHNOLOGY DEPENDENCE IN THE NEONATAL INTENSIVE CARE UNIT GRADUATE

NICU graduates with medical complexity are often discharged with dependence on one or more forms of technology.[20] It is important for PCPs to understand why they are being used and know how to troubleshoot common problems.

Oxygen

1. As many as 60% of infants with moderate-severe BPD will be discharged home on oxygen therapy, most being weaned off in the first year of life.
2. Oxygen therapy is a first-line treatment for infants with PHTN.
3. Infants requiring supplemental oxygen should be sent home with an oximeter to measure peripheral oxygen saturations (SpO_2) with a goal of greater than 90% in infants with BPD and greater than 94% with concerns of PHTN. The oximeter is also a valuable tool to be used during room air trials when weaning off oxygen.
4. Administration of supplemental oxygen.
   a. Supplemental oxygen is provided by nasal cannula in infants without an artificial airway.
   b. Infants with a tracheostomy who require oxygen: use a trach collar or oxygen is entrained into a home ventilator.
   c. Most infants will be discharged on ≤0.5 L/min. Oxygen gauges are either in decimal (0.1 increments) or fractions of a liter. Oxygen can be delivered from as little as 1/16 L/min (0.03 L/min) to several liters/minute. Patients have small portable oxygen tanks (typically for travel, lasting ~ 4 hr) and a larger tank with a concentrator for home use.
5. Important points:
   • Infants discharged home on oxygen therapy should also have a portable oximeter.

- Humidification should be placed on all condensers for delivery of supplemental oxygen greater than 1.0 L O_2.
- Higher oxygen requirement in the home environment can be due to the length of oxygen tubing going to the condenser.
- If a child is suddenly desaturating at home, caregivers should check for mechanical errors first and attempt to increase oxygen delivery to solve the problem (eg, unplugged tubing or power source, empty oxygen tank)
- Oxygen is generally weaned in step-wise fashion over a period of time (weeks to months) with no consensus statement on standardized protocol.
    - Weaning oxygen therapy first versus diuretics or bronchodilators is clinician dependent, but often oxygen is weaned off first.
    - Daytime oxygen is usually discontinued first, allowing freedom for travel, therapies and developmental playtime, while maintaining oxygen use at night.
    - Continuous overnight pulse oximetry to evaluate nocturnal saturations is generally used to evaluate ability to discontinue overnight oxygen.

Apnea Monitor

Indications

1. Monitoring of infants at increased risk of life-threatening episodes of apnea, bradycardia, and hypoxemia.
    a. Persistent apnea of prematurity treated with caffeine
    b. Persistent central or obstructive apnea secondary to neurologic, metabolic, or other disorders
    c. Severe GERD
    d. Frequent seizures
    e. History of apparent life-threatening event post-discharge from NICU
    f. History of sibling dying from sudden infant death syndrome
2. Important points
    - Discharge settings: low heart rate alarm at 80 bpm (70 bpm if >44 weeks PMA), high heart rate alarm at 220 bpm, and apnea alarm at 20 seconds.
    - Frequent alarms and artifact may occur if electrodes are placed incorrectly or if the chest strap is too loose. Use of stick-on electrodes, as used in the hospital setting, may alleviate the problem.
    - As the infant grows older, low heart rate alarm will need to be decreased from 80 bpm to 70 or 60 bpm to prevent false alarms during deep sleep periods.
    - Apnea monitors should have memory-recording ability; these are generally downloaded by durable medical equipment companies and information outsourced. Apnea monitor use and event occurrences are reported to the PCP in a print out.
    - Parents and other caretakers should be taught infant cardiopulmonary resuscitation before discharge and have an emergency plan for frequent or prolonged alarming or equipment failure.

Tracheostomy and Home Ventilator

1. Indications for tracheostomy:
    a. Prolonged respiratory failure
    b. Subglottic stenosis
    c. Severe tracheo- and/or bronchomalacia

    d. Vocal cord paralysis or dysfunction
    e. Congenital airway malformations
    f. Tumors
    g. Craniofacial anomalies
    h. Neuromuscular disorders
2. Description:
    a. Made of either polyvinyl chloride (Shiley) or silicone (Bivona).
3. Important points:
- Decimal point and the number zero (no. 4.0) are used to designate a neonatal or pediatric tracheostomy tube. Tracheostomy tubes are identified as either no. 3.5 NEO Shiley or no. 3.5 PED Shiley on the neck plates of the tracheostomy tube.
- Pre-measured suctioning depth not longer than the trach cannula is essential to prevent epithelial tissue damage.
- Tracheostomy care should be performed twice daily and more frequently, as needed, to prevent skin breakdown.
- Clean technique should be used for tracheostomy changes in the home environment. Sterile technique does not decrease infections.
- Parents and/or caregivers should demonstrate proficiency in tracheostomy tube change, suctioning, and trouble-shooting before discharge. Caregivers should be taught assessment skills and be aware of and know how to implement emergency measures.
- All patients with a tracheostomy tube should have an emergency supply bag containing a replacement tracheostomy of the same size and one tracheostomy tube one size smaller, flexible suction catheter and suction machine, scissors, spare tracheostomy ties, gloves, water-based lubricant, Ambu bag, and oral endotracheal tube.
- Ventilated patients and those with thick secretions should always use humidification. Use of the motto "When in doubt, change it out" may be applied to most situations where tracheostomy tubes require action due to the inability to diagnose the problem during patient emergency.

Home Ventilator; Laptop Ventilator

1. Indications: Provide ventilation for infants with chronic respiratory failure due to various disease processes such as BPD, bronchomalacia, congenital and acquired central hypoventilation syndrome, and neuromuscular disease in the home setting.
2. Description: Small, laptop-sized, portable ventilator for home use.
3. Important points:
- Patients with a home ventilator should always have an Ambu bag readily available in case of ventilator failure.
- Condensation in ventilator tubing can cause ventilator to auto-cycle and trigger additional ventilator breaths. Troubleshoot by emptying ventilator limbs to remove water.
- Local emergency services and power company should be notified of the dependent infant's address in case of future emergency or power outage.

Feeding Tube

1. Indications: for children with dysphagia, aspiration, oral aversion, and/or those who have failure to thrive for other reasons.
2. Description:

a. The gastrostomy tube (GT) is generally placed in the left upper quadrant to deliver liquid feedings at prescribed volume ("dose") and rate.

b. The feeding tubes can be placed directly in the stomach, jejunum, or passed from the stomach into the jejunum (trans-gastric jejunal or "GJ" tube).

3. Important points:

- Bolus feedings should only be attempted with GT feedings.
- Continuous feedings only are permitted through a jejunal tube secondary to risk for dumping syndrome, diarrhea, or intestinal injury.
- Patients who cannot tolerate large daytime bolus feedings may benefit from continuous nighttime feedings at a lower rate for 8 to 10 hours per night with smaller daytime bolus feedings. This is also a strategy for transitioning to oral feedings if unable to take enough by mouth during awake periods.
- The skin around the tube should be cleansed twice daily with soap and water, and should be assessed daily for leakage, irritation, infection, or granulation tissue.
- The GT should be rotated a quarter of a turn with every diaper change to prevent skin breakdown, and the water volume (generally 3–7 mL) in the balloon should be assessed weekly (if Mic-Key or AMT Mini ONE)
- The GT button should be replaced every 3 months and the parents should be comfortable in doing this after the first change, as it is not uncommon for a GT with an established tract to become dislodged.
- Skin irritation due to leakage or infection may occur. Typically, over-the-counter skin barriers assist with local irritation from gastric leakage. True skin infections around the GT are relatively uncommon but intense redness, tenderness, or systemic signs of fever or malaise may occur. Mild local infections may be treated with topical antibiotics, whereas true cellulitis requires oral or intravenous antibiotics covering typical skin organisms. Rashes may also occur and are typically yeast and may be treated topically.
- Granulation tissue is excessive reactive tissue around the GT. It is often moist with mucous discharge and bleeds easily. It can lead to leakage around and, sometimes, dislodgement of the GT. It is usually treated by chemically cauterizing with silver nitrate, and, if chronic, may be treated at home with topical steroid ointment.
- Infants discharged home with gastrostomy, jejunostomy, or nasogastric feeding tubes should be provided with a feeding pump so that feedings can be given at a consistent rate.

Home Nursing Services for Technology-Dependent Infants

- Caring for an NICU graduate with medical complexity, particular one who is technology dependent, can be very expensive financially, and emotionally draining, for parents and siblings.
- Availability of home nursing services varies by location and type of insurance coverage.
- The PCP should investigate what might be available for their patient and family through their established insurance coverage or additional Medicaid waiver services for which they may be eligible.

REFERENCES

1. The role of the primary care pediatrician in the management of high-risk newborn infants. American Academy of Pediatrics. Committee on Practice

and Ambulatory Medicine and Committee on Fetus and Newborn. Pediatrics 1996;98:786.

2. Hospital discharge of the high-risk neonate. American Academy of Pediatrics Committee on Fetus and Newborn. Pediatrics 2008;122(5):1119–26.
3. Chronic respiratory conditions of the preterm infant. In: Malcolm WF, editor. Beyond the NICU: comprehensive care of the high-risk infant. 1st edition. New York: McGraw-Hill; 2014. p. P42–56.
4. Ehrenkranz RA, Walsh MC, Vohr BR, et al. Validation of the National Institutes of Health consensus definition of bronchopulmonary dysplasia. Pediatrics 2005; 116(6):1353.
5. Jadcherla SR, Khot T, Moore R, et al. Feeding methods at discharge predict long-term feeding and neurodevelopmental outcomes in preterm infants referred for gastrostomy evaluation. J Pediatr 2017;181:125–30.e1.
6. Walsh MC, Bell EF, Kandefer S, et al. Neonatal outcomes of moderately preterm infants compared to extremely preterm infants. Pediatr Res 2017;82(2):297–304.
7. Pridham K, Saxe R, Limbo R. Feeding issues for mothers of very low birth weight, premature infants through the first year. J Perinat Neonat Nurs 2004;18:161–9.
8. Jadcherla SR, Wang M, Vijayapal AS, et al. Impact of prematurity and co-morbidities on feeding milestones in neonates: a retrospective study. J Perinatol 2010;30(3):201–8.
9. DeMauro SB, Patel PR, Medoff-Cooper B, et al. Postdischarge feeding patterns in early- and late-preterm infants. Clin Pediatr (Phila) 2011;50(10):957–62.
10. Feeding issues in the NICU graduate. In: Malcolm WF, editor. Beyond the NICU: comprehensive care of the high-risk infant. 1st edition. New York: McGraw-Hill; 2014. p. P812–34.
11. Meier PP, Engstrom JL, Patel AL, et al. Improving the use of human milk during and after the NICU stay. Clin Perinatol 2010;37(1):217–45.
12. Meier PP, Engstrom JL. Test weighing for term and premature infants is an accurate procedure. Arch Dis Child Fetal Neonatal Ed 2007;92(2):F155–6.
13. Breastfeeding. In: Malcolm WF, editor. Beyond the NICU: beyond the NICU: comprehensive care of the high-risk infant. 1st edition. New York: McGraw-Hill; 2014. p. P121–32.
14. Ehrenkranz RA, Younes N, Lemons J, et al. Longitudinal growth of hospitalized very-low birth-weight infants. Pediatrics 1999;104:280–9.
15. Adamkin DH. Nutritional management of the very low birthweight infant, optimizing enteral nutrition and postdischarge nutrition. NeoReviews 2006;e608(7):12.
16. Adamkin DH. Nutritional strategies for the very low birthweight infant. New York: Cambridge University Press; 2009. p. 141–2.
17. Euser AM, Finken MJ, Keijzer-Veen MG, et al. Associations between prenatal and infancy weight gain and BMI, fat mass, and fat distribution in young adulthood: a prospective cohort study in males and females born very preterm. Am J Clin Nutr 2005;81(2):480–7.
18. Volpe JJ. Neurology of the newborn. 5th edition. Oxford (United Kingdom): Elsevier Limited; 2008.
19. IVH, PVL and hydrocephalus. In: Malcolm WF, editor. Beyond the NICU: comprehensive care of the high-risk infant. 1st edition. New York: McGraw-Hill; 2014. p. 320–46.
20. Home equipment. In: Malcolm WF, editor. Beyond the NICU: comprehensive care of the high-risk infant. 1st edition. New York: McGraw-Hill; 2014. p. 910–23.

Neurodevelopmental Follow-up of Preterm Infants
What Is New?

Elisabeth C. McGowan, MD[a,b], Betty R. Vohr, MD[a,b,*]

KEYWORDS

- Neurodevelopment • Cerebral palsy • Premature infants
- Developmental coordination disorder • Language • Socioeconomic status

KEY POINTS

- Although the rate of severe cerebral palsy (CP) has decreased among preterm infants, the rate of mild CP and the identification of developmental coordination disorder (DCD) have increased in this population.
- DCD has been shown to have effects persisting throughout school age and adolescence.
- There is increasing recognition of the importance of early interactive language exposure on the language development of infants.
- Although maternal education level continues to be the most frequently reported socioeconomic status indicator, there is increasing evidence of the impact of psycho-socioeconomic adversities on preterm neurodevelopmental and behavioral outcomes.
- Identification of adverse maternal mental health in the neonatal ICU and postdischarge provides an opportunity for intervention in former preterm infants and their mothers.

There is increasing evidence of ongoing changes occurring in short-term and long-term motor and language outcomes in the preterm population. In addition, there is increased awareness of the negative impact of family psycho-socioeconomic adversities on preterm outcomes. This review provides updates on 3 areas of reported change in neurodevelopmental follow-up and outcomes in preterm infants: motor impairments, language delays and disorders, and the impact of family psycho-socioeconomic adversities on outcomes.

MOTOR IMPAIRMENTS AMONG PRETERM INFANTS—A CHANGING PICTURE

Modern neonatal intensive care has contributed to increased survival of infants at the limits of prematurity,[1–4] and changes in the rates of neonatal morbidities[5] and

The authors have nothing to disclose.
[a] Department of Pediatrics, Alpert Medical School of Brown University, Women & Infants Hospital of Rhode Island, 101 Dudley Street, Providence, RI 02905-2499, USA; [b] Department of Pediatrics, Alpert Medical School of Brown University, Neonatal-Follow-up Clinic, Women & Infants Hospital of Rhode Island, 101 Dudley Street, Providence, RI 02905-2499, USA
* Corresponding author. 101 Dudley Street, Providence, RI 02905-2499.
E-mail address: bvohr@wihri.org

Pediatr Clin N Am 66 (2019) 509–523
https://doi.org/10.1016/j.pcl.2018.12.015
0031-3955/19/© 2018 Elsevier Inc. All rights reserved.

neurodevelopmental impairments.[1,3] A key component of neurodevelopmental impairment is cerebral palsy (CP).[6] During the early years of neonatology, a primary focus of follow-up studies was on identification of rates of CP.[7-9] CP is often associated with other long-term sequelae, including cognitive, sensory, and language impairments; seizure disorders; and growth abnormalities. Confirmation of this diagnosis is difficult to achieve before 18 months to 24 months of age, especially if the manifestation is mild. Categorization of degree of CP severity based on the Gross Motor Function Classification System[10] into mild (level 1), moderate (levels 2 and 3), and severe to profound (levels 4 and 5) is well accepted.

Recent studies suggest changes in both the rates of CP and the degree of severity.[5,11-14] The Neonatal Research Network study of extreme preterm infants less than or equal to 27 weeks' gestation born from 2011 to 2014 and evaluated at 18 months to 26 months of age showed that the rate of CP decreased during this time period from 16% to 12%.[5] In addition, whereas the rate of severe CP decreased by 43%, the rate of mild CP increased by 13% during the study period. An additional 19% of children had a suspect neurologic examination. This indicates that improvement of motor outcomes is occurring in conjunction with the increased survival of the most preterm neonates. This finding supports that just as there is a spectrum of white matter abnormalities among preterm infants, there is a spectrum or continuum of motor findings ranging from mild to profound.[15,16]

Former preterm infants are at risk of a range of motor abnormalities, including delayed motor milestones, balance abnormalities, challenges with manual dexterity, and generalized coordination abnormalities now codified as developmental coordination disorder (DCD) with the Movement Assessment Battery for Children (MABC)–Second Edition (MABC-2).[17-19] The American Psychiatric Association in 2013 defined DCD as impairment in coordinated motor skills that significantly interfere with performance in everyday activities. Abilities assessed include manual dexterity, aiming, and catching and balance. Scores above the 15th percentile are considered normal, scores in the 6th to 15th percentiles are at risk, and scores in less than or equal to the 5th percentile are consistent with significant motor difficulty. Although motor delays are evident in early childhood, the diagnosis of DCD is often not made until school age.[20] A series of studies reporting DCD at ages 3 years to 24 years is shown in **Table 1**.

Kwok and colleagues[21] examined the predictive value of the MABC-2 at 3 years to predict DCD at 4.5 years among very preterm (VPT) children, defined by the investigators as 24 weeks' to 32 weeks' gestation, and reported a sensitivity of 90% and specificity of 69%, indicating many false-positive results. The investigators concluded that at this early age, the MABC is highly sensitive but with limited specificity in identifying VPT children who are at risk of DCD. The Griffiths and colleagues' study[22] reported that 25% of infants born at less than 30 weeks' gestation had scores consistent with significant motor difficulty ($\leq$5%) at both 4 years of age and 8 years of age, and the MABC-2 at 4 years had high sensitivity (79%) and specificity (93%) for predicting motor impairment at 8 years. Bolk and collegues[23] examined a large cohort of apparently healthy extreme preterm infants (defined as 22–26 weeks' gestation) compared with term controls at 6.5 years of age and reported the highest rate of DCD of 37.1% in preterm infants versus 5.5% in term infants. Three studies from the Victorian Infant Collaborative Study Group[24] of infants born at 22 weeks' to 27 weeks' gestation identified consistently low but increasing rates of DCD during 3 time periods between 1991 and 2005, with increasing rates of 2%, 8%, and 7%. The findings are similar to those of Setanen and colleagues[25] in a Finish cohort at 11 years of age. Finally, a study[26] from Norway reported rates of DCD of 29% in a

Table 1
Developmental coordination disorder

Authors, Year Published	Gestational Age	Date of Birth or Visits	Sample Size	Age of Assessment	Movement Assessment Battery for Children Coordination Disorder	
Kwok et al,[21] 2018 Canada	24–32 wk	Visits 2010–2015	165	3 y 4.5 y	Prediction Sensitivity 90% Specificity 69%	
Griffiths et al,[22] 2017 Australia	<30 wk	2005–2007	96	4 y 8 y	<5th% 25th% 25th%	
Bolk et al,[23] 2018 Sweden	22–26 wk	Birth 2004–2007	229 preterm 244 term	6.5 y	<5th% Preterm Term	37.1% 5.5%
Davis et al,[28] 2007 Australia; Victorian Infant Collaborative Study Group	22–27 wk	Birth 1991–1992	163	8 y	<15th% <5th%	10% 2%
Roberts,[27] 2011 Australia; Victorian Infant Collaborative Study Group	22–27 wk	1997	132 154 term	8 y	EP <15th% EP <5th % T <5th%	23% 16% 5%
Spittle et al,[24] 2018 Australia: Victorian Infant Collaborative Study Group	22–27 wk	1991–2005	Study Year 1991–1992 226 1997 172 2005 189	8 y	<5th% <5th% <5th%	2% 8% 7%
Setanen et al,[25] 2016 PIPARI Study Group Finland	23–35 wk	2001–2004	82	11 y	<5th%	8%
Husby et al,[26] 2013 Norway	VLBW <1500 g	1986–88	36 VLBW 37 term	14 y 23 y	<5th% <5th%	29% 29%

small cohort of former very-low-birthweight (VLBW) infants, less than 1500 g, born from 1986 to 1988 at both ages 14 years and 23 years. At 23 years, the VLBW subjects had poorer total motor scores and subscores for manual dexterity and balance compared with the term comparison group. After exclusion of the 4 VLBW subjects with CP, however, the difference in total MABC-2 score between study groups was no longer significant.[26] This study has a small sample size and the results need to be replicated in larger studies. The percentage identified in reports are impacted if children with CP are excluded.[27] The findings overall suggest that early motor coordination challenges among former preterm infants have lasting effects.

Risk factors of DCD include preterm birth, male gender,[28] and decreased brain volume at term age.[25] Setanen and colleagues[25] propose that volumetric brain MRI at term age may provide a tool to identify infants at risk for later neuromotor impairment. Relative to longer-term outcomes, CP is fairly consistently associated with a spectrum of more severe neurosensory morbidities, including seizure disorders, blindness, and hearing impairment.[29] In addition to coordination deficits, including difficulties writing and balancing, DCD can be associated with academic challenges, behavior problems, and decreased participation in sports.[30] At school age, DCD is associated with lower cognitive and academic test scores and greater behavior problems.[28]

Prenatal medical interventions, including antenatal steroids[31] and magnesium sulfate,[32,33] and neonatal interventions, including indomethacin[34] and caffeine,[35,36] have been shown associated with at least partial reduction in rates of CP and DCD. Several motor and education-based interventions have shown some efficacy in reducing the manifestations coordination disorder.[37–39] Steps can be taken in the neonatal ICU (NICU) to identify infants potentially at risk of CP or DCD, provide physical therapy/occupational therapy support during the NICU stay, facilitate referrals to neurology for follow-up as needed, provide anticipatory guidance for parents, and refer all high-risk infants to early intervention programs at the time of discharge.[40,41]

PRETERM LANGUAGE IMPAIRMENTS: CAN MORE BE DONE TO IMPROVE OUTCOMES?

Early development of language is critically important because it is the building block for basic communication, cognitive processes, literacy, and social interactions. Preterm infants are at increased risk of speech and language morbidities, including mild to moderate delays/deficiencies in vocabulary development,[42] phonological processing,[43] language comprehension,[44] verbal short-term memory,[45,46] and grammatical development.[43] In addition to brain injury, environmental factors, including both nonwhite race and Hispanic ethnicity, have been associated with early speech and language delays among VPT infants with less than 1000-g birthweight. Black and Hispanic toddlers had lower language scores than whites at 18 months to 22 months, even after adjustment for confounders.[47] A Neonatal Research Network study reported that children born at less than 28 weeks' gestation whose primary language was Spanish had lower Bayley Scales of Infant and Toddler Development (BSID) language scores but similar cognitive scores compared with children whose primary language was English.[48] The investigators suggested the findings may, in part, be secondary to use of English language–based testing tools that introduce bias. In addition, low socioeconomic status (SES) is well known to be associated with alterations in the language environment, decreased early language exposure, and subsequent language delay.[49,50]

Responses to the language environment begin in fetal life. The cochlea of the inner ear completes development between 24 weeks' and 26 weeks' gestation, and auditory reception starts during this time period. Blink-startle responses to vibroacoustic stimuli are first elicited in the fetus at 24 weeks' to 26 weeks' gestation, with consistent responses by 27 weeks' to 28 weeks' gestation.[51] At 27 weeks' to 29 weeks' gestation, the hearing threshold in utero is approximately 40 dB. The fetus differentiates the maternal voice from a stranger's voice at approximately 32 weeks' to 37 weeks' gestation by changes in heart rate, suggesting a preattention reaction.[52] Fetuses have the ability to differentiate a maternal voice from a paternal voice.[53] Term infants prefer human voice to other acoustic stimuli and prefer a maternal voice to other female voices and to a paternal voice.[54–57]

The extreme preterm infant, however, leaves the protective sound environment of the uterus as early as 22 weeks' to 23 weeks' gestation and enters the noisy and stressful NICU nonoptimal language environment for extended periods of up to 2 months to 6 months. The first 3 years of age represent a sensitive period of brain plasticity, with the sensory environment impacting brain growth, structures, connectivity, and function.[58] Exposure of the preterm brain to the NICU environment alters neuronal differentiation, which may alter subsequent development.[59,60] The term infant, however, goes home in 1 day to 3 days and is exposed to the touch, talk, sounds, and social interactions within a typical family unit.

Despite the nonoptimal environment, the early preterm infant begins to respond to auditory stimuli by 24 weeks' gestation, with consistent responses by 28 weeks and distinct preferences shown for maternal voice.[61] Preterm infants have also been shown to respond to recordings of maternal sounds and voice by lowering their heart rate, which has been interpreted as increased infant relaxation.[62]

Should language intervention be provided in the NICU? It has been shown that increased exposure to early language experience for term children in the form of conversations and talk with family members is associated with improved child vocabulary size and IQ.[49,50] The authors' team investigated preterm vocalizations and the language environment of the NICU with 16-hour audio recordings of adult speech, child vocalizations, conversation turns (CTs), silence, and noise. The 2-oz recording device can be placed into a small vest the infant wears or can be placed immediately adjacent to the infant. Language Environment Analysis (LENA) speech-identification algorithms have been determined to be reliable, with 82% accuracy for adults and 76% accuracy for infants and children.[63] Output of a typical recording, which is used to provide feedback to the parent, is shown in **Fig. 1**. It is divided into 4 domains, including the audio environment, child vocalizations, CTs, and number of adult words spoken each hour. The printout is reviewed with the parents, awake times with high and low interactions are identified, and goals can be set for timing and intensity of child-directed conversations.

Study findings revealed that extremely-low-birthweight (ELBW) infants vocalize as early as 8 weeks before their due date, that parent talk is a significant predictor of both infant vocalizations and CTs at 32 weeks' and 36 weeks' gestation, and that ELBW infants are exposed to significantly more words from their parents than from NICU caretakers.[64] In addition, every increase in 100 adult word count (AWC)/h in the NICU at 32 weeks' gestation was associated with a 2-point increase in the BSID, Third Edition, language composite score ($P = .04$) at 18 months. Every increase in 100 AWC/h at 36 weeks' gestation was associated with a 1.2-point increase in BSID, Third Edition, cognitive composite score ($P = .004$) and a 0.3-point increase in expressive communication at 18 months ($P = .07$). This is highly suggestive that parent talk in the NICU 4 weeks and 8 weeks prior to an infant's due date has a powerful impact on subsequent infant language and cognitive development.[65]

A recent study[66] of term 3-year-old to 6-year-old children using LENA recordings and functional MRI identified that increased CTs were associated with higher parent education, higher income, higher child composite verbal scores, and bilateral MRI superior temporal lobe activation. Correlations between activation during language processing and CTs remained significant after adjustment for parent education, test scores, AWC, and child vocalizations. In a mediation model, the effect of CTs on language scores was mediated by activation of the left inferior frontal gyrus. The investigators concluded that this is the first evidence that neural activation patterns underlay

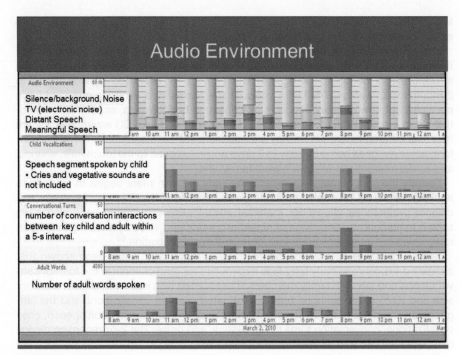

Fig. 1. Recording output.

the relationship between interactive language exposure reflected by CTs and child language abilities.[66]

These findings strongly support the concept of implementing family-integrated care[67] in the NICU and suggest that preterm infants benefit from enhanced parent presence and interaction, including caretaking, kangaroo care, cuddling, talking, singing, and reading. Open visiting and the single-room NICUs[68-70] with enhanced maternal involvement and developmental care are beneficial. Policies that remove barriers and encourage parent presence and participation in the NICU are encouraged.

SOCIOECONOMIC RISKS, MATERNAL EDUCATION LEVEL, AND BEYOND

Childhood health is closely linked to social advantage, and, typically, improvement in SES is associated with more optimal outcomes.[71-73] Measurement of social advantage or disadvantage is often difficult to capture but may include a variety of indicators, such as education status, income level, occupation, and insurance status. In the preterm population, there is evidence that both low SES and specific biologic variables are risk factors for poor developmental outcomes.[74-78] As the long-term influence of these risks is beginning to be explored, particularly in the post-surfactant era, complex interactions among these factors are becoming evident.

Current studies examining the effects of SES continue to highlight the important influence of educational status on neurodevelopmental outcomes. Linsell and colleagues,[79] in a systematic review, showed that low parental education and nonwhite race/ethnicity were predictors of pre-school (before school age, specifically 1.5 – 2.5 years of age) global impairments in VPT infants. Asztalos and colleagues,[80] of the Canadian Neonatal Follow-Up Network, reported positive association of 18-month to 21-month developmental outcomes with maternal education level. For infants born at less than 29 weeks' gestation, cognitive and language scores improved as caregiver education increased, and scores approached mean values of 100 only for infants of mothers with the highest levels of education.

The impact of parent education level seems to persist into early school years, particularly on cognitive and behavior outcomes. In a cohort of preterm infants less than 28 weeks' gestation without morbidities, such as CP, blindness, or deafness, child IQ was positively associated with higher maternal education.[81] In the EPIPAGE cohort, Beaino and colleagues[74] defined SES as both maternal and paternal education status. Low parental education was the main predictor for mild cognitive delay (adjusted odds ratio [OR] 3.43; 95% CI, 2.01–5.83) and a significant predictor for severe cognitive delay (OR 2.6; 95% CI, 1.29–5.24) at 5 years of age, along with small-for-gestational-age status and cystic periventricular leukomalacia.[74] Potharst and colleagues[82] reported on 5-year outcomes for infants less than 30 weeks' gestation, and, compared with term controls, the preterm-term mean IQ difference was 5 points, if parent education was high, and increased to 15 points, if parent education was low. Similar patterns were seen for behavior. Maternal IQ, income, occupation, and single-parent household as either independent or composite variables show similar associations with cognitive and behavior outcomes.[83–86]

As more preterm cohorts are followed longitudinally, investigators are now able to evaluate the longer-term contribution of social influences. Joseph and colleagues[87] reported that children of mothers in the lowest education stratum in the ELGAN cohort were more likely to score greater than or equal to 2 SDs below the mean on a battery of neurocognitive tests at 10 years of age. The risks of unfavorable SES, particularly in association with brain injury, have also been explored. In a European cohort of 200 ELBW infants born between 1993 and 1998, low maternal education was the most significant risk factor for decreased IQ; however, grade III/IV intraventricular hemorrhage or periventricular leukomalacia continued to have a negative impact at 13 years of age.[88] For this study, the developmental trajectories for children of mothers with higher versus lower education were different irrespective of brain injury. Children of mothers with the highest education had increases in composite IQ scores between 6 years and 13 years of age, whereas those with lower maternal education remained essentially unchanged. An Australian cohort from the same study era, comprising both early preterm/ELBW infants and normal birthweight controls,[89] reported a strong and persistent influence of intraventricular hemorrhage on cognition and academic performance at 2 years, 5 years, 8 years, and 18 years of age. Maternal education and social class, however, did not reach statistical significance until years 8 and beyond.

The interpretation of the effects of socioeconomic variables on long-term outcomes is challenging. Many adverse social situations are inter-related, tend to cluster, and have dose-response relationships with poor health.[90,91] Positive mental health is shaped by various socioeconomic and physical environments and is an integral component of enriched relationships, particularly for the mother-infant dyad. Maternal depression, anxiety, and stress have been associated with low maternal self-efficacy, defined as a mother's belief in her ability to parent.[92,93] At NICU discharge, mothers with a history of mental health disorders report decreased self-confidence compared with mothers without a history of mental health disorders.[94] Hawes and colleagues[95] report that decreased NICU discharge readiness is associated with postdischarge depressive symptoms. Importantly, within the first year of age, maternal depression and anxiety have been linked to infant dysregulation, difficult temperament, and sleep disturbances as well as compromised parent-infant interactions and inadequate parental caregiving practices.[96–99]

Less has been published on the long-term effects of maternal depression and anxiety on preterm infant outcomes; results are often conflicting and portray different patterns of symptoms.[100–102] A prospective cohort of VLBW infants born in Finland was followed from infancy to school age, and, after adjustment for maternal education level, significant associations of parental depression and stress symptoms with child cognitive, behavior, and socioemotional problems were reported between 2 years to 5 years of age.[103–105] It has been suggested that over time, parents of vulnerable infants experience increasing levels of stress. Singer and colleagues[106] reported that mothers of high-risk VLBW infants perceived increased stress extending from early childhood through adolescence compared with mothers of term or low-risk VLBW children.

It is important to recognize these long-term studies cannot determine causal pathways, because associations between parent psychological wellness and infant health/development are multifactorial and bidirectional. Mediators of maternal stress, depression, and anxiety, however, include low birthweight, low maternal education, infant and child behavior difficulties, lack of family social supports, and poor child health, all of which are more prevalent in the preterm population.[100,106–109] Additionally, the emerging field of epigenetics is beginning to uncover the effects of early adverse advents on the developing infant. One mechanism in particular, DNA methylation of genes encoding for stress regulators of the hypothalamus-pituitary-adrenal axis, shows promise.[110] In the preterm population, links between maternal anxiety and depression and alteration of infant stress-related genes have been reported, highlighting yet another pathway influencing developmental outcomes.[111–113]

In conclusion, investigations targeting psycho-socioeconomic risks provide opportunities for improving outcomes of the vulnerable preterm infant. Evidence suggests that early interventions, in particular those that focus on strengthening parent-infant relationships, have a positive influence on motor, cognitive, and behavior outcomes and may decrease parental symptoms of depression and anxiety.[38,114–116] The importance of supporting parental mental health is now widely recognized, and guidelines encourage starting this in the NICU.[117] Continued exploration of the complex interactions of psychological, social, and medical contributions is needed as efforts are made to identify effective strategies that optimize long-term outcomes for preterm infants and their families.

REFERENCES

1. Rysavy MA, Li L, Bell EF, et al. Between-hospital variation in treatment and outcomes in extremely preterm infants. N Engl J Med 2015;372(19):1801–11.
2. Stoll BJ, Hansen NI, Bell EF, et al. Trends in care practices, morbidity, and mortality of extremely preterm neonates, 1993-2012. JAMA 2015;314(10):1039–51.
3. Younge N, Goldstein RF, Bann CM, et al. Survival and neurodevelopmental outcomes among periviable infants. N Engl J Med 2017;376(7):617–28.
4. Bashir RA, Thomas JP, MacKay M, et al. Survival, short-term, and long-term morbidities of neonates with birth weight < 500 g. Am J Perinatol 2017;34(13):1333–9.
5. Stoll BJ, Hansen NI, Bell EF, et al. Neonatal outcomes of extremely preterm infants from the NICHD Neonatal Research Network. Pediatrics 2010;126(3):443–56.
6. Graham HK, Rosenbaum P, Paneth N, et al. Cerebral palsy. Nat Rev Dis Primers 2016;2:15082.

7. Palisano R, Rosenbaum P, Walter S, et al. Development and reliability of a system to classify gross motor function in children with cerebral palsy. Dev Med Child Neurol 1997;39(4):214–23.
8. O'Shea TM, Dammann O. Antecedents of cerebral palsy in very low-birth weight infants. Clin Perinatol 2000;27(2):285–302.
9. Robertson CM, Watt MJ, Yasui Y. Changes in the prevalence of cerebral palsy for children born very prematurely within a population-based program over 30 years. JAMA 2007;297(24):2733–40.
10. Palisano RJ, Hanna SE, Rosenbaum PL, et al. Validation of a model of gross motor function for children with cerebral palsy. Phys Ther 2000;80(10):974–85.
11. Vohr BR, Stephens BE, Higgins RD, et al. Are outcomes of extremely preterm infants improving? Impact of bayley assessment on outcomes. J Pediatr 2012; 161(2):222–8.e3.
12. Wilson-Costello D. Is there evidence that long-term outcomes have improved with intensive care? Semin Fetal Neonatal Med 2007;12(5):344–54.
13. Hintz SR, Kendrick DE, Vohr BR, et al. Changes in neurodevelopmental outcomes at 18 to 22 months' corrected age among infants of less than 25 weeks' gestational age born in 1993-1999. Pediatrics 2005;115(6):1645–51.
14. Hack M, Costello DW. Trends in the rates of cerebral palsy associated with neonatal intensive care of preterm children. Clin Obstet Gynecol 2008;51(4): 763–74.
15. de Kieviet JF, Piek JP, Aarnoudse-Moens CS, et al. Motor development in very preterm and very low-birth-weight children from birth to adolescence: a meta-analysis. JAMA 2009;302(20):2235–42.
16. Bracewell M, Marlow N. Patterns of motor disability in very preterm children. Ment Retard Dev Disabil Res Rev 2002;8(4):241–8.
17. Barnett A, Henderson S, Sugden D. The movement assessment battery for children-2. London: Pearson Assessment; 2007.
18. Spittle AJ, Orton J. Cerebral palsy and developmental coordination disorder in children born preterm. Semin Fetal Neonatal Med 2014;19(2):84–9.
19. Vohr BR, Msall ME, Wilson D, et al. Spectrum of gross motor function in extremely low birth weight children with cerebral palsy at 18 months of age. Pediatrics 2005;116(1):123–9.
20. Missiuna C, Moll S, King S, et al. A trajectory of troubles: parents' impressions of the impact of developmental coordination disorder. Phys Occup Ther Pediatr 2007;27(1):81–101.
21. Kwok C, Mackay M, Agnew JA, et al. Does the movement assessment battery for children-2 at 3 years of age predict developmental coordination disorder at 4.5 years of age in children born very preterm? Res Dev Disabil 2018. https://doi.org/10.1016/j.ridd.2018.04.003.
22. Griffiths A, Morgan P, Anderson PJ, et al. Predictive value of the movement assessment battery for children - second edition at 4 years, for motor impairment at 8 years in children born preterm. Dev Med Child Neurol 2017;59(5): 490–6.
23. Bolk J, Farooqi A, Hafstrom M, et al. Developmental coordination disorder and its association with developmental comorbidities at 6.5 years in apparently healthy children born extremely preterm. JAMA Pediatr 2018;172(8):765–74.
24. Spittle AJ, Cameron K, Doyle LW, et al, Victorian Infant Collaborative Study Group. Motor impairment trends in extremely preterm children: 1991-2005. Pediatrics 2018;141(4) [pii:e20173410].

25. Setanen S, Lehtonen L, Parkkola R, et al. The motor profile of preterm infants at 11 y of age. Pediatr Res 2016;80(3):389–94.
26. Husby IM, Skranes J, Olsen A, et al. Motor skills at 23 years of age in young adults born preterm with very low birth weight. Early Hum Dev 2013;89(9): 747–54.
27. Roberts G, Anderson PJ, Davis N, et al. Developmental coordination disorder in geographic cohorts of 8-year-old children born extremely preterm or extremely low birthweight in the 1990s. Dev Med Child Neurol 2011;53(1):55–60.
28. Davis NM, Ford GW, Anderson PJ, et al, Victorian Infant Collaborative Study Group. Developmental coordination disorder at 8 years of age in a regional cohort of extremely-low-birthweight or very preterm infants. Dev Med Child Neurol 2007;49(5):325–30.
29. Himmelmann K, Beckung E, Hagberg G, et al. Gross and fine motor function and accompanying impairments in cerebral palsy. Dev Med Child Neurol 2006;48(6):417–23.
30. Edwards J, Berube M, Erlandson K, et al. Developmental coordination disorder in school-aged children born very preterm and/or at very low birth weight: a systematic review. J Dev Behav Pediatr 2011;32(9):678–87.
31. Linsell L, Malouf R, Morris J, et al. Prognostic factors for cerebral palsy and motor impairment in children born very preterm or very low birthweight: a systematic review. Dev Med Child Neurol 2016;58(6):554–69.
32. Nelson KB, Chang T. Is cerebral palsy preventable? Curr Opin Neurol 2008; 21(2):129–35.
33. Hirtz DG, Weiner SJ, Bulas D, et al. Antenatal magnesium and cerebral palsy in preterm infants. J Pediatr 2015;167(4):834–9.e3.
34. Allan WC, Vohr B, Makuch RW, et al. Antecedents of cerebral palsy in a multicenter trial of indomethacin for intraventricular hemorrhage. Arch Pediatr Adolesc Med 1997;151(6):580–5.
35. Doyle LW, Schmidt B, Anderson PJ, et al. Reduction in developmental coordination disorder with neonatal caffeine therapy. J Pediatr 2014;165(2):356–9.e3.
36. Schmidt B, Roberts RS, Anderson PJ, et al. Academic performance, motor function, and behavior 11 years after neonatal caffeine citrate therapy for apnea of prematurity: an 11-Year follow-up of the CAP randomized clinical trial. JAMA Pediatr 2017;171(6):564–72.
37. Spittle A, Orton J, Anderson P, et al. Early developmental intervention programmes post-hospital discharge to prevent motor and cognitive impairments in preterm infants. Cochrane Database Syst Rev 2012;(12):CD005495.
38. Spittle A, Orton J, Anderson PJ, et al. Early developmental intervention programmes provided post hospital discharge to prevent motor and cognitive impairment in preterm infants. Cochrane Database Syst Rev 2015;(11):CD005495.
39. Smits-Engelsman B, Vincon S, Blank R, et al. Evaluating the evidence for motor-based interventions in developmental coordination disorder: a systematic review and meta-analysis. Res Dev Disabil 2018;74:72–102.
40. Blank R, Smits-Engelsman B, Polatajko H, et al, European Academy for Childhood Disability. European Academy for Childhood Disability (EACD): recommendations on the definition, diagnosis and intervention of developmental coordination disorder (long version). Dev Med Child Neurol 2012;54(1):54–93.
41. Camden C, Foley V, Anaby D, et al. Using an evidence-based online module to improve parents' ability to support their child with developmental coordination disorder. Disabil Health J 2016;9(3):406–15.

42. Foster-Cohen SH, Friesen MD, Champion PR, et al. High prevalence/low severity language delay in preschool children born very preterm. J Dev Behav Pediatr 2010;31(8):658–67.

43. Sansavini A, Guarini A, Alessandroni R, et al. Are early grammatical and phonological working memory abilities affected by preterm birth? J Commun Disord 2007;40(3):239–56.

44. Jansson-Verkasalo E, Korpilahti P, Jantti V, et al. Neurophysiologic correlates of deficient phonological representations and object naming in prematurely born children. Clin Neurophysiol 2004;115(1):179–87.

45. Omizzolo C, Scratch SE, Stargatt R, et al. Neonatal brain abnormalities and memory and learning outcomes at 7 years in children born very preterm. Memory 2014;22(6):605–15.

46. Grunewaldt KH, Skranes J, Brubakk AM, et al. Computerized working memory training has positive long-term effect in very low birthweight preschool children. Dev Med Child Neurol 2016;58(2):195–201.

47. Freeman Duncan A, Watterberg KL, Nolen TL, et al. Effect of ethnicity and race on cognitive and language testing at age 18-22 months in extremely preterm infants. J Pediatr 2012;160(6):966–71.e2.

48. Lowe JR, Nolen TL, Vohr B, et al. Effect of primary language on developmental testing in children born extremely preterm. Acta Paediatr 2013;102(9):896–900.

49. Hart B, Risley TR. Meaningful differences in the everyday experience of young American children. Baltimore (MD): P.H. Brookes; 1995.

50. Suskind DL, Leffel KR, Graf E, et al. A parent-directed language intervention for children of low socioeconomic status: a randomized controlled pilot study. J Child Lang 2015;43(2):1–41.

51. Birnholz JC, Benacerraf BR. The development of human fetal hearing. Science 1983;222(4623):516–8.

52. Kisilevsky BS, Hains SM, Brown CA, et al. Fetal sensitivity to properties of maternal speech and language. Infant Behav Dev 2009;32(1):59–71.

53. Lee GY, Kisilevsky BS. Fetuses respond to father's voice but prefer mother's voice after birth. Dev Psychobiol 2014;56(1):1–11.

54. DeCasper AJ, Fifer WP. Of human bonding: newborns prefer their mothers' voices. Science 1980;208(4448):1174–6.

55. DeCasper AJ, Prescott PA. Human newborns' perception of male voices: preference, discrimination, and reinforcing value. Dev Psychobiol 1984;17(5):481–91.

56. DeCasper AJ, Prescott P. Lateralized processes constrain auditory reinforcement in human newborns. Hear Res 2009;255(1–2):135–41.

57. Granier-Deferre C, Bassereau S, Ribeiro A, et al. A melodic contour repeatedly experienced by human near-term fetuses elicits a profound cardiac reaction one month after birth. PLoS One 2011;6(2):e17304.

58. Bennet L, Van Den Heuij L, Dean JM, et al. Neural plasticity and the Kennard principle: does it work for the preterm brain? Clin Exp Pharmacol Physiol 2013;40(11):774–84.

59. Huppi PS, Schuknecht B, Boesch C, et al. Structural and neurobehavioral delay in postnatal brain development of preterm infants. Pediatr Res 1996;39(5):895–901.

60. Webb AR, Heller HT, Benson CB, et al. Mother's voice and heartbeat sounds elicit auditory plasticity in the human brain before full gestation. Proc Natl Acad Sci U S A 2015;112(10):3152–7.

61. Krueger C. Exposure to maternal voice in preterm infants: a review. Adv Neonatal Care 2010;10(1):13–8 [quiz: 19–20].

62. Rand K, Lahav A. Maternal sounds elicit lower heart rate in preterm newborns in the first month of life. Early Hum Dev 2014;90(10):679–83.

63. Gilkerson J, Richards JA, Warren SF, et al. Mapping the early language environment using all-day recordings and automated analysis. Am J Speech Lang Pathol 2017;26(2):248–65.

64. Caskey M, Stephens B, Tucker R, et al. Importance of parent talk on the development of preterm infant vocalizations. Pediatrics 2011;128(5):910–6.

65. Caskey M, Stephens B, Tucker R, et al. Adult talk in the nicu with preterm infants and developmental outcomes. Pediatrics 2014;133(3):1–7.

66. Romeo RR, Leonard JA, Robinson ST, et al. Beyond the 30-million-word gap: children's conversational exposure is associated with language-related brain function. Psychol Sci 2018;29(5):700–10.

67. Bracht M, O'Leary L, Lee SK, et al. Implementing family-integrated care in the NICU: a parent education and support program. Adv Neonatal Care 2013; 13(2):115–26.

68. Lester BM, Hawes K, Abar B, et al. Single-family room care and neurobehavioral and medical outcomes in preterm infants. Pediatrics 2014;134(4):754–60.

69. Lester BM, Salisbury AL, Hawes K, et al. 18-month follow-up of infants cared for in a single-family room neonatal intensive care unit. J Pediatr 2016;177:84–9.

70. Vohr B, McGowan E, McKinley L, et al. Differential effects of the single-family room neonatal intensive care unit on 18- to 24-month Bayley scores of preterm infants. J Pediatr 2017;185:42–8.

71. Wolke D, Meyer R. Cognitive status, language attainment, and prereading skills of 6-year-old very preterm children and their peers: the Bavarian Longitudinal Study. Dev Med Child Neurol 1999;41(2):94–109.

72. Tong S, Baghurst P, Vimpani G, et al. Socioeconomic position, maternal IQ, home environment, and cognitive development. J Pediatr 2007;151(3):284–8, 288.e1.

73. Moore TG, McDonald M, Carlon L, et al. Early childhood development and the social determinants of health inequities. Health Promot Int 2015;30(Suppl 2): ii102–15.

74. Beaino G, Khoshnood B, Kaminski M, et al. Predictors of the risk of cognitive deficiency in very preterm infants: the EPIPAGE prospective cohort. Acta Paediatr 2011;100(3):370–8.

75. Vohr BR, Wright LL, Dusick AM, et al. Neurodevelopmental and functional outcomes of extremely low birth weight infants in the National Institute of Child Health and Human Development Neonatal Research Network, 1993-1994. Pediatrics 2000;105(6):1216–26.

76. Wood NS, Costeloe K, Gibson AT, et al. The EPICure study: associations and antecedents of neurological and developmental disability at 30 months of age following extremely preterm birth. Arch Dis Child Fetal Neonatal Ed 2005; 90(2):F134–40.

77. Wang LW, Wang ST, Huang CC. Preterm infants of educated mothers have better outcome. Acta Paediatr 2008;97(5):568–73.

78. Hack M, Wilson-Costello D, Friedman H, et al. Neurodevelopment and predictors of outcomes of children with birth weights of less than 1000 g: 1992-1995. Arch Pediatr Adolesc Med 2000;154(7):725–31.

79. Linsell L, Malouf R, Morris J, et al. Prognostic factors for poor cognitive develop-ment in children born very preterm or with very low birth weight: a systematic review. JAMA Pediatr 2015;169(12):1162–72.

80. Asztalos EV, Church PT, Riley P, et al. Association between Primary caregiver education and cognitive and language development of preterm neonates. Am J Perinatol 2017;34(4):364–71.

81. Leversen KT, Sommerfelt K, Ronnestad A, et al. Prediction of neurodevelopmen-tal and sensory outcome at 5 years in Norwegian children born extremely pre-term. Pediatrics 2011;127(3):e630–8.

82. Potharst ES, van Wassenaer AG, Houtzager BA, et al. High incidence of multi-domain disabilities in very preterm children at five years of age. J Pediatr 2011; 159(1):79–85.

83. Lean RE, Paul RA, Smyser CD, et al. Maternal intelligence quotient (IQ) predicts IQ and language in very preterm children at age 5 years. J Child Psychol Psy-chiatry 2018;59(2):150–9.

84. Potijk MR, Kerstjens JM, Bos AF, et al. Developmental delay in moderately preterm-born children with low socioeconomic status: risks multiply. J Pediatr 2013;163(5):1289–95.

85. Potijk MR, de Winter AF, Bos AF, et al. Behavioural and emotional problems in moderately preterm children with low socioeconomic status: a population-based study. Eur Child Adolesc Psychiatry 2015;24(7):787–95.

86. Manley BJ, Roberts RS, Doyle LW, et al. Social variables predict gains in cogni-tive scores across the preschool years in children with birth weights 500 to 1250 grams. J Pediatr 2015;166(4):870–6.e1-2.

87. Joseph RM, O'Shea TM, Allred EN, et al. Maternal educational status at birth, maternal educational advancement, and neurocognitive outcomes at age 10 years among children born extremely preterm. Pediatr Res 2018;83(4):767–77.

88. Voss W, Jungmann T, Wachtendorf M, et al. Long-term cognitive outcomes of extremely low-birth-weight infants: the influence of the maternal educational background. Acta Paediatr 2012;101(6):569–73.

89. Doyle LW, Cheong JL, Burnett A, et al. Biological and social influences on out-comes of extreme-preterm/low-birth weight adolescents. Pediatrics 2015; 136(6):e1513–20.

90. Jimenez ME, Wade R Jr, Lin Y, et al. Adverse experiences in early childhood and kindergarten outcomes. Pediatrics 2016;137(2):e20151839.

91. Folger AT, Eismann EA, Stephenson NB, et al. Parental adverse childhood expe-riences and offspring development at 2 years of age. Pediatrics 2018;141(4) [pii:e20172826].

92. Leahy-Warren P, McCarthy G. Maternal parental self-efficacy in the postpartum period. Midwifery 2011;27(6):802–10.

93. Porter CL, Hsu HC. First-time mothers' perceptions of efficacy during the transi-tion to motherhood: links to infant temperament. J Fam Psychol 2003;17(1): 54–64.

94. McGowan EC, Du N, Hawes K, et al. Maternal mental health and neonatal inten-sive care unit discharge readiness in mothers of preterm infants. J Pediatr 2017; 184:68–74.

95. Hawes K, McGowan E, O'Donnell M, et al. Social emotional factors increase risk of postpartum depression in mothers of preterm infants. J Pediatr 2016;179: 61–7.

96. Treyvaud K, Anderson VA, Lee KJ, et al. Parental mental health and early social-emotional development of children born very preterm. J Pediatr Psychol 2010; 35(7):768–77.

97. Field T. Postpartum depression effects on early interactions, parenting, and safety practices: a review. Infant Behav Dev 2010;33(1):1–6.

98. Minkovitz CS, Strobino D, Scharfstein D, et al. Maternal depressive symptoms and children's receipt of health care in the first 3 years of life. Pediatrics 2005; 115(2):306–14.

99. Field T. Postnatal anxiety prevalence, predictors and effects on development: a narrative review. Infant Behav Dev 2018;51:24–32.

100. Schappin R, Wijnroks L, Uniken Venema MM, et al. Rethinking stress in parents of preterm infants: a meta-analysis. PLoS One 2013;8(2):e54992.

101. Miceli PJ, Goeke-Morey MC, Whitman TL, et al. Brief report: birth status, medical complications, and social environment: individual differences in development of preterm, very low birth weight infants. J Pediatr Psychol 2000;25(5):353–8.

102. Piteo AM, Yelland LN, Makrides M. Does maternal depression predict developmental outcome in 18 month old infants? Early Hum Dev 2012;88(8):651–5.

103. Huhtala M, Korja R, Lehtonen L, et al. Parental psychological well-being and cognitive development of very low birth weight infants at 2 years. Acta Paediatr 2011;100(12):1555–60.

104. Huhtala M, Korja R, Lehtonen L, et al. Parental psychological well-being and behavioral outcome of very low birth weight infants at 3 years. Pediatrics 2012;129(4):e937–44.

105. Huhtala M, Korja R, Lehtonen L, et al. Associations between parental psychological well-being and socio-emotional development in 5-year-old preterm children. Early Hum Dev 2014;90(3):119–24.

106. Singer LT, Fulton S, Kirchner HL, et al. Longitudinal predictors of maternal stress and coping after very low-birth-weight birth. Arch Pediatr Adolesc Med 2010; 164(6):518–24.

107. Taylor HG, Klein N, Schatschneider C, et al. Predictors of early school age outcomes in very low birth weight children. J Dev Behav Pediatr 1998;19(4): 235–43.

108. Halpern LF, Brand KL, Malone AF. Parenting stress in mothers of very-low-birth-weight (VLBW) and full-term infants: a function of infant behavioral characteristics and child-rearing attitudes. J Pediatr Psychol 2001;26(2):93–104.

109. Ong LC, Chandran V, Boo NY. Comparison of parenting stress between Malaysian mothers of four-year-old very low birthweight and normal birthweight children. Acta Paediatr 2001;90(12):1464–9.

110. Provenzi L, Guida E, Montirosso R. Preterm behavioral epigenetics: a systematic review. Neurosci Biobehav Rev 2018;84:262–71.

111. Oberlander TF, Weinberg J, Papsdorf M, et al. Prenatal exposure to maternal depression, neonatal methylation of human glucocorticoid receptor gene (NR3C1) and infant cortisol stress responses. Epigenetics 2008;3(2):97–106.

112. Essex MJ, Boyce WT, Hertzman C, et al. Epigenetic vestiges of early developmental adversity: childhood stress exposure and DNA methylation in adolescence. Child Dev 2013;84(1):58–75.

113. Murgatroyd C, Quinn JP, Sharp HM, et al. Effects of prenatal and postnatal depression, and maternal stroking, at the glucocorticoid receptor gene. Transl Psychiatry 2015;5:e560.

114. Spencer-Smith MM, Spittle AJ, Doyle LW, et al. Long-term benefits of home-based preventive care for preterm infants: a randomized trial. Pediatrics 2012;130(6):1094–101.
115. Spittle AJ, Barton S, Treyvaud K, et al. School-age outcomes of early intervention for preterm infants and their parents: a randomized trial. Pediatrics 2016; 138(6) [pii:e20161363].
116. van Wassenaer-Leemhuis AG, Jeukens-Visser M, van Hus JW, et al. Rethinking preventive post-discharge intervention programmes for very preterm infants and their parents. Dev Med Child Neurol 2016;58(Suppl 4):67–73.
117. Hynan MT, Steinberg Z, Baker L, et al. Recommendations for mental health professionals in the NICU. J Perinatol 2015;35(Suppl 1):S14–8.

Moving?

Make sure your subscription moves with you!

To notify us of your new address, find your **Clinics Account Number** (located on your mailing label above your name), and contact customer service at:

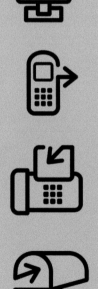

Email: journalscustomerservice-usa@elsevier.com

800-654-2452 (subscribers in the U.S. & Canada)
314-447-8871 (subscribers outside of the U.S. & Canada)

Fax number: 314-447-8029

Elsevier Health Sciences Division
Subscription Customer Service
3251 Riverport Lane
Maryland Heights, MO 63043

*To ensure uninterrupted delivery of your subscription, please notify us at least 4 weeks in advance of move.